Trypanosomiasis
and Leishmaniasis

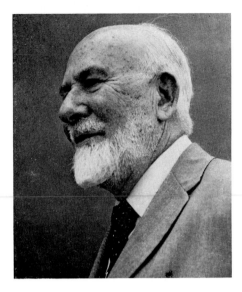

Dr E. Tejera

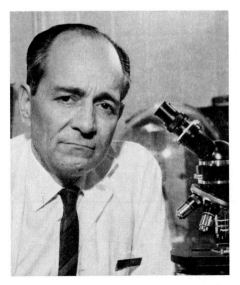

Professor F. Pifano

Guests of honour at the symposium

*The Ciba Foundation for the promotion of international cooperation in
medical and chemical research is a scientific and educational charity established by
CIBA Limited – now CIBA-GEIGY Limited – of Basle. The Foundation operates
independently in London under English trust law.*

*Ciba Foundation Symposia are published in collaboration with
Associated Scientific Publishers (Elsevier Scientific Publishing Company, Excerpta Medica,
North-Holland Publishing Company) in Amsterdam.*

Associated Scientific Publishers, P.O. Box 211, Amsterdam

Trypanosomiasis and Leishmaniasis with special reference to Chagas' disease

Ciba Foundation Symposium 20 (new series)

Held jointly with the Venezuelan Academy of
Sciences and 'La Trinidad' Medical Center, Caracas

1974

Elsevier · Excerpta Medica · North-Holland

Associated Scientific Publishers · Amsterdam · London · New York

ISBN Excerpta Medica 90 219 4021 3
ISBN American Elsevier 0 444-15017-x

Library of Congress Catalog Card Number 73-88892

Published in 1974 by Associated Scientific Publishers, P.O. Box 211, Amsterdam, and American Elsevier, 52 Vanderbilt Avenue, New York, N.Y. 10017.

Suggested series entry for library catalogues: Ciba Foundation Symposia.

Suggested publishers' entry for library catalogues: Associated Scientific Publishers

Ciba Foundation Symposium 20 (new series)

Printed in The Netherlands by Van Gorcum, Assen

Contents

Participants

Symposium on Trypanosomiasis and Leishmaniasis, with special reference to Chagas' disease, held jointly with the Venezuelan Academy of Sciences and 'La Trinidad' Medical Center at the Tamanaco Hotel, Caracas on 13-15 February 1973

B. A. NEWTON (*Chairman*) MRC Unit for Biochemical Parasitology, Molteno Institute, University of Cambridge, Downing Street, Cambridge CB2 3EE

A. ANSELMI Universidad Central de Venezuela, Instituto de Medicina Tropical, Ciudad Universitaria, Apartado 59019, Caracas, Venezuela

J. R. BAKER MRC Unit for Biochemical Parasitology, Molteno Institute, University of Cambridge, Downing Street, Cambridge CB2 3EE

I. B. R. BOWMAN Department of Biochemistry, University of Edinburgh Medical School, Teviot Place, Edinburgh EH8 9AG

R. S. BRAY *Wellcome Parasitology Unit No. 2, Haile Sellassie I University, PO Box 1176, Addis Ababa, Ethiopia

J. CONVIT Instituto Nacional de Dermatología, Apartado de Correos 4043, Caracas 101, Venezuela

P. DE RAADT Parasitic Disease Unit, World Health Organization, Avenue Appia, 1211 Geneva 27, Switzerland

F. C. GOBLE Department of Infectious Diseases, Cooper Laboratories Inc., Research and Development Division, 110 E. Hanover Avenue, Cedar Knolls, NJ 07927, USA

L. G. GOODWIN Nuffield Institute of Comparative Medicine, The Zoological Society of London, Regent's Park, London NW1 4RY

---

* *Present address:* MRC Laboratories, Fajara, nr Bathurst, The Gambia.

F. KERDEL-VEGAS I. de N. de la Academia de Medicina, Apartado 60391, Caracas, Venezuela

F. KÖBERLE Department of Pathology, Faculty of Medicine, University of São Paulo, Ribeirão Preto, Brazil

W. H. R. LUMSDEN Department of Protozoology, London School of Hygiene and Tropical Medicine, Keppel Street, Gower Street, London WC1E 7HT

G. A. MAEKELT Universidad Central de Venezuela, Instituto de Medicina Tropical, Ciudad Universitaria, Apartado 8250, Caracas, Venezuela

R. MARTINEZ-SILVA Zone Office 1, PAHO/WHO, Apartado 6722 (Carmelitas), Caracas, Venezuela

A. R. NJOGU East African Trypanosomiasis Research Organization, PO Box 96, Tororo, Uganda

J. A. O'DALY Instituto Venezolano de Investigaciones Cientificas (IVIC), Apartado 1872, Caracas, Venezuela

W. PETERS Department of Parasitology, Liverpool School of Tropical Medicine, Pembroke Place, Liverpool L3 5QA

F. PIFANO Instituto de Medicina Tropical, Universidad Central de Venezuela, Ciudad Universitaria, Apartado 8250, Caracas, Venezuela

P. PULIDO Centro Medico Docente 'La Trinidad', 50 Piso Oficina 502, Avenida Andres Bello, Apartado 50676, Caracas, Venezuela

A. SANABRIA Instituto Venezolano de Investigaciones Cientificas (IVIC), Apartado 1872, Caracas, Venezuela

R. J. TONN WHO Chagas' Disease Vector Research Unit, Apartado 11, Acarigua, Venezuela

W. TRAGER Parasitology Department, The Rockefeller University, New York, NY 10021, USA

K. VICKERMAN Department of Zoology, University of Glasgow, Glasgow G12 8QQ

R. ZELEDÓN Department of Parasitology, Universidad de Costa Rica, Ciudad Universitaria, 'Rodrigo Facio', Costa Rica, Central America

Editors: KATHERINE ELLIOTT, MAEVE O'CONNOR and G. E. W. WOLSTENHOLME

Observers

IMELDA CAMPO AASEN Instituto de Dermatologia, Hospital J. M. Vargas, Caracas, Venezuela

H. GARCIA BARRIOS Division de Enfermedades Cardiovasculares, Ministerio de Sanidad y Asistencia Social, Torre Sur Centro Simón Bolívar, Caracas, Venezuela

FLORENCE DELAFOSSE-GUIRAMAND Departmento de Dermatología, Universidad Central de Venezuela, Caracas, Venezuela

OLINDA DELGADO Instituto de Medicina Tropical, Universidad Central de Venezuela, Ciudad Universitaria, Apartado 8250, Caracas, Venezuela

N. ERCOLI Instituto de Biologica Tropical, Universidad Central de Venezuela, Caracas, Venezuela

YVONNE GÓMEZ Facultad de Farmacia Cátedra de Parasitología, Universidad Central de Venezuela, Caracas, Venezuela

J. C. GÓMEZ-NÚÑEZ División de Endemias Rurales Dirección de Malariología Saneam Ambiental, Ministerio de S.A.S. Maracay, Edo. Aragua, Venezuela

OLINDA GONZALEZ Sección de Patología Celular, Instituto de Medicina Tropical, Universidad Central de Venezuela, Caracas, Venezuela

L. E. ITURRIZA Instituto Nacional de Dermatología, Apartado de Correos 4043, Caracas 101, Venezuela

LYLE LANSDELL Department of Dermatology, University of Miami, 1600 N.W. 10 Avenue, Miami, Florida, USA

J. J. PUIGBO   Cátedra de Cardiología, Facultad de Medicina, Universidad Central de Venezuela, Hospital Universitario, Caracas, Venezuela

J. ROMERO   Instituto de Medicina Tropical, Universidad Central de Venezuela, Ciudad Universitaria, Apartado 8250, Caracas, Venezuela

V. RUESTA   Sección de Cardiología Experimental, Instituto de Medicina Tropical, Universidad Central de Venezuela, Caracas, Venezuela

CECILIA DE SCORZA   Facultad de Ciencias, Universidad de Los Andes, Mérida, Edo. Mérida, Venezuela

J. V. SCORZA   Facultad de Ciencias, Universidad de Los Andes, Mérida, Edo. Mérida, Venezuela

H. SERRANO   Facultad de Medicina, Universidad de Zulia, Maracaibo, Edo. Zulia, Venezuela

D. TAPLIN   Department of Dermatology, University of Miami, 1600 N.W. 10 Avenue, Miami, Florida, USA

W. TORREALBA   Departmento de Patología Tropical, Facultad de Medicina, Universidad de Carabobo, Valencia, Venezuela

MARIAN ULRICH   Instituto de Dermatología, Hospital J. M. Vargas, Caracas, Venezuela

Introduction

B. A. NEWTON

MRC Unit for Biochemical Parasitology, Molteno Institute, University of Cambridge

The South American and African forms of trypanosomiasis, together with the cutaneous and visceral forms of leishmaniasis, affect in diverse ways many millions of people in tropical and subtropical areas of the world. Over the years since the causative organisms were identified, we have learned a great deal about these diseases and about the parasites, but in spite of this progress methods for prevention and control are still far from adequate.

The parasites differ in many ways but as we learn more about them we are coming to appreciate that they also have some important features in common. I believe there is much to be gained by workers concerned with these three diseases coming together now to exchange information and to discuss common problems in an attempt to define the most important lines for future research.

This is the aim of our symposium—and to that end the programme is necessarily a broad one but it has a logical structure. We start with a general comparison of the parasites from a taxonomic point of view and go on to discuss epidemiology, pathogenicity and problems of immunity. Then we take a closer look at the parasites, their ultrastructure, nutrition and metabolism, and finally consider problems of chemotherapy and drug resistance.

However, the very breadth of this programme and the fact that the people here represent many different disciplines creates a hazard we must try to avoid if the symposium is to be a success, namely the danger of specialists using the jargon of their subject. I therefore appeal to the speakers to present their material in a form which can be readily understood by us all and not just by a specialist group.

Leishmaniasis and trypanosomiasis: the causative organisms compared and contrasted

W. H. R. LUMSDEN

Department of Medical Protozoology, London School of Hygiene and Tropical Medicine

Abstract The order Kinetoplastida comprises those protozoa which exhibit extranuclear DNA in the form of a kinetoplast—a self-replicating organelle associated with the mitochondrion; practically all its members are parasitic. Of the 18 or so genera into which the order is divided, most are of minor importance, being mainly parasites of insects; the main mass of the huge literature on the order relates to *Leishmania* and *Trypanosoma* because these genera include organisms seriously pathogenic to man and to his domestic animals.

Despite the close taxonomic affinity between these two genera, studies of the diseases which they respectively cause have remained rather separate. Nevertheless, there are clearly many aspects of these diseases where comparison between the two would be likely to be rewarding. Common to both is the manifest ability of organisms of identical morphology to be associated with different pathological outcomes or with different patterns of transmission in nature. How far such differences are determined by differences in the potential of the infecting organisms and how far by differences in the reactions of the hosts is at present largely unknown. Before the host component of the association can be properly appreciated, much more precise characterization of organisms is essential. Morphological criteria are clearly inadequate and other criteria for the recognition of populations of organisms of particular biological potential need to be found, such as those based on immunological or biochemical experiment. Studies for this purpose should be concentrated on populations of organisms of known homogeneity (clones), stabilated as close as possible to their natural origins.

A peculiarity of tropical medicine has been a tendency for its various sections to develop rather in isolation from one another, even when they might have been expected to be related scientifically. Many factors have contributed to this 'situation—the discontinuous geographical distribution of many tropical diseases, the geographical separation of the areas where the diseases occurred from integrative centres of medical science, the partition of the tropics into spheres of influence of extra-tropical states, the complexity of the epidemiology of many of the diseases which led necessarily to specialization by workers on individual diseases, and so on. However, in recent years many influences have been at work to dissolve these divisions and to promote the exchange of ideas and methods between sections. In this context it is impossible not to mention the influence of Dr N. Ansari, Chief, Parasitic Diseases, World Health Organization, who has greatly contributed to the integration of work on African trypanosomiasis in eastern and western Africa, and more recently to the integration of this field with that of South American trypanosomiasis.

The present symposium is another welcome influence in this respect and leads to a situation which would have been impossible a few years ago—that of a worker primarily experienced in arbovirus epidemiology, and then in trypanosomiasis in East Africa, attempting to contribute to the comparison of two fields in which he has had no direct practical involvement, leishmaniasis and Chagas' disease. I hope that from this somewhat detached position I shall be able to make some useful contribution.

MORPHOLOGICAL TAXONOMY

The essentials of the taxonomic position of the organisms under discussion, extracted from the classification of Honigberg *et al.* (1964) and relying mainly on Kudo (1966) for the placing of genera, are as follows:

Phylum Protozoa

Subphylum I Sarcomastigophora (of four Subphyla). Flagella, pseudopodia, or both types of locomotory organelles; single type of nucleus except ... Foraminiferida; typically no spore formation; sexuality, when present, essentially syngamy.

Superclass I Mastigophora (of three Superclasses). One or more flagella typically present in trophozoites; solitary or colonial; asexual reproduction basically by symmetrogenic binary fission; sexual reproduction unknown in many groups, nutrition phototrophic, heterotrophic, or both.

Class 2 Zoomastigophorea (of two Classes). Chromatophores absent; one to many flagella; additional organelles may be present in mastigonts; amoeboid forms with or without flagella, in some groups; sexuality known in a few groups; species predominantly parasitic.

Order 4 Kinetoplastida (of nine Orders). One to four flagella; kinetoplast argentophilic and Feulgen-positive, present as self-replicating organelle with mitochondrial affinities; most species parasitic.

Suborder 1 Bodonina (of two Suborders). Typically two unequal flagella, one directed anteriorly, one posteriorly; no undulating membrane; kinetoplast absent secondarily in some species; free-living or parasitic.

Genera: Bodo, Pleuromonas, Rhynchomonas, Proteromonas, Phyllomitus, Colponema, Cercomonas, Cryptobia.

Suborder 2 Trypanosomatina. One flagellum, either free, or attached to the body by means of an undulating membrane; all species parasitic.

Genera: Proleptomonas, Leptomonas, Phytomonas, Crithidia, Blastocrithidia, Herpetomonas, Rhynchoidomonas, Leishmania, Trypanosoma, Endotrypanum.

We may, at this stage, neglect the Bodonina and concentrate on the Trypanosomatina. These latter flagellates may exist in a variety of morphological forms distinguished primarily by the site of origin of the single flagellum; a convenient nomenclature for these morphological forms is that proposed by Hoare & Wallace (1966) (Fig. 1). This nomenclature is simple and straightforward and has rapidly come into general use. There are, however, some difficulties with regard to forms whose cell body is round or nearly so.

The round form in the Hoare & Wallace (1966) system is without a flagellum—an amastigote. For certain flagellated round forms of *Trypanosoma* (*Schizotrypanum*) *cruzi* seen in the gut of *Rhodnius prolixus*, Brack (1968) introduced the term 'sphaeromastigote'. This term seems to me to be unfortunate in that it departs from what Garnham (1971) described as the 'uniform Greek etymology' of the terms proposed by Hoare & Wallace (1966), which relate specifically to the condition of the flagellum, whether or not it exists and, where it does, to its position of origin. The sphaeromastigote term refers not to this, but to the shape of the body. It is further unfortunate that the term is being applied without distinction to rounded forms with a short uncomplicated flagellum (Fig. 1g), to rounded forms with a long flagellum and a circumferential undulating membrane (Fig. 1i), and to organisms whose flagellar development is intermediate between these extremes (Fig. 1h). These different forms, all at present designated as 'sphaeromastigotes', may well be stages in significantly different lines of development, as indeed was suggested by Brack herself. It would seem preferable, so as not to distort the excellent Hoare and Wallace system, and yet give a full description of the round forms occurring, to separate the descriptions of body form and those of flagellar position. By and large, these flagellated round (so-called 'sphaeromastigote') forms appear to run through the same gamut of flagellar modification as do the more elongate forms and they could be classified, respectively, as promastigote,

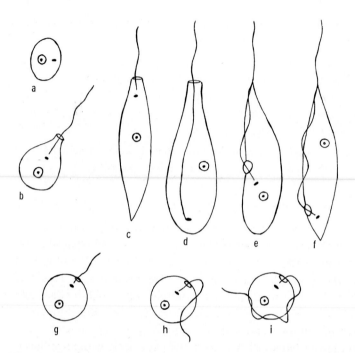

FIG. 1. The forms adopted by the Trypanosomatina (after Hoare & Wallace 1966).
(*a*) Amastigote, (*b*) choanomastigote, (*c*) promastigote, (*d*) opisthomastigote, (*e*) epimastigote,
(*f*) trypomastigote (Hoare & Wallace, 1966); (*g*)–(*i*) sphaeromastigotes (Brack 1968).

epimastigote or trypomastigote, depending on whether the flagellum arises immediately from the kinetoplast, or runs round the organism about 90°, or about 180°, before becoming free. Thus, Fig. 1g would be a round promastigote, Fig. 1h a round epimastigote, and Fig. 1i a round trypomastigote.

These round forms which occur in the cycles of development of vertebrate-infecting organisms are not apparently associated with any attribute of resistance to adverse circumstance. They are located in the interior of the cell, in vessels or in the insect gut. There are, however, other types of amastigote to which are accredited faculties of resistance and which occur in the midgut of insects infected with *Leptomonas* (McGhee 1968). Two kinds of true cysts are described for insect trypanosomatids (Wallace 1966): 'strap-hanger' cysts which arise from unequal division of the parent organism, the small daughter cell adhering to the flagellum of the larger, moving distally and encysting; and the secretion of a jelly-like coat around the flexed organism within which it continues to be motile. Wallace (1966) quotes, also, a number of cases in which flagellates survived 'drying' for long periods, suggesting that such cysts may be important stages in the life history of the organism. In fact he states later that transmission of insect flagellates is generally through contamination, in which such stages would seem likely to be of great importance. Little attention has been paid to the possibility of resistant stages occurring in the trypanosomatids parasitic in vertebrates, and so the relevance of these observations on insect trypanosomatids is at present uncertain.

Individually, all these named forms are of little use taxonomically, as any given form may occur, and be morphologically indistinguishable, in the course of the developmental cycle of two or more organisms which are clearly differentiable on other grounds. McGhee (1968) provocatively states the problem by pointing out that: '...one may not state with certainty, for example, whether the trypanosomatid [? promastigote form] seen in the rectum of a phytophagous hemipteron, *Oncopeltus fasciatus*, is of the genus *Phytomonas*, *Leptomonas*, *Crithidia*, *Blastocrithidia*, *Rhynchoidomonas*, *Trypanosoma*, *Leishmania*, *Herpetomonas*, or even possibly *Proleptomonas*, much less to allocate it to a 'species'.'

Within the Trypanosomatina, present classification depends on the summation of a number of characteristics ranging from morphological to clinical and epidemiological. Levine (1972) provides a useful table of these characteristics: positions of kinetoplast and reservoir, state of development of the undulating membrane, the number of forms occurring in the life cycle, host relationships and number and provenance of the species described. This is a very useful summary of the group but it must be remembered that the numbers of species described in groups are largely products of the amount of attention devoted to the groups and of the propensities of the workers concerned, whether they were 'lumpers' or 'splitters'. Thus the validity of a 'species' inevitably varies widely from genus to genus.

TAXONOMY OF LEISHMANIA

Leishmania is primarily characterized by existing in two forms—amastigote in the cells of its vertebrate host and promastigote in the gut of its insect vector. Because of the virtual morphological identity of the organisms throughout the genus, they are here classified mainly according to the clinical conditions which they produce in man. Lainson & Shaw (1972) say, in discussing the classification of New World *Leishmania* on the basis of vernacular terms applied to the clinical condition:

'...while a given *Leishmania* may produce an over-all similar clinical picture in man, individuals may react differently to the same parasite and the appearance of the disease may vary greatly at different stages of the infection'.

Reacting, thus, from the confusion likely to be engendered by too great reliance on clinical appearance alone as a basis of classification, Lainson & Shaw (1972) proposed a more widely based classification based on a variety of characters—rate of growth in culture or in experimental animals, geographical distribution, epidemiological patterns, as well as clinical characters. Briefly, this classification, extended on the same principles to include the other *Leishmania* spp. summarized by Garnham (1971) and Belding (1965), is as follows:

Leishmania donovani complex

Organisms tending to 'visceralize' in man (i.e. with a predilection for infecting cells in the viscera, particularly in the spleen); main vectors *Phlebotomus* of the 'major' group.

L. d. donovani: Asia, mainly India and China; infects adults; no known extra-human vertebrate host.

L. d. infantum: Mediterranean countries; infects mainly children; extra-human vertebrate hosts, dogs.

L. d. chagasi: South America; infects adults and children; extra-human hosts, wild dogs.

Leishmania tropica complex

Organisms confined to cutaneous locations, not tending to visceralize; main vectors *Phlebotomus papatasi* and *P. sergenti.*

L. t. tropica (= minor): Asia; aetological agent of 'dry' sore; no known extra-human hosts.

L. t. major: Asia; aetiological agent of 'moist' sore; extra-human vertebrate hosts, *Rhombomys* (gerbil), *Meriones* (jird), etc.

Leishmania mexicana complex

'Fast-growing' organisms in culture and in hamsters. In hamsters cell response is poor and lesions are packed with amastigotes; there is metastatic spread. Lesions in man are mild, cutaneous, with no nasopharyngeal involvement. Lesions in wild animal hosts (rodents, *Didelphis*) inconspicuous, mainly on tail. Vectors *Lutzomyia intermedia* group, mainly *L. olmeca* and *L. flaviscutellata*; promastigotes not developing in the hindgut triangle.

L. m. mexicana: Mexico, Guatemala, British Honduras. Causes mild infection, a single cutaneous lesion which is self-healing, or persistent chronic ear lesions; but no nasopharyngeal involvement. Chiclero's ear, Bay sore; one recorded case of 'anergid' diffuse cutaneous leishmaniasis (DCL).

L. m. amazonensis: Amazon basin to Mato Grosso State, Brazil; Trinidad; perhaps elsewhere. Rarely infects man, causing mild, single or limited, cutaneous lesions; no predilection for ear tissue or for nasopharynx. Occasional DCL cases.

L. m. pifanoi: Venezuela. Only known from DCL cases.

Leishmania enriettii

Brazil. An anomalous species discovered in laboratory *Cavia porcellus* (guinea pig); not infective for *C. aperea* (Brazilian wild guinea pig).

Leishmania braziliensis complex

'Slow-growing' organisms in culture and in hamsters. In hamsters cell response is marked and lesions have moderate or scanty amastigotes; there is no metastatic spread. Lesions in man, single or multiple, often extensive and disfiguring; nasopharyngeal involvement in one species. Lesions in wild animal hosts (rodents, procyonids, marmosets), limited discrete inconspicuous skin lesions, or inevident. Vectors *Lutzomyia intermedia* and *Psychodopygus* groups; parasites developing in the hindgut triangle.

L. b. braziliensis: Brazil, and forest areas east of Andes in other states. Causes destructive cutaneous leishmaniasis, lesions frequently large, persistent and disfiguring, with frequent nasopharyngeal metastases. Espundia.

L. b. guyanensis: Guyanas, Surinam, Brazil, Venezuela. Causes single lesion or spreads to many crateriform ulcers over body, metastasizes along lymphatics; probably not metastasizing to nasopharynx. Pian bois.

L. b. panamensis: Panama, possibly extending to north and south. Causes single, or few, shallow crateriform ulcers, metastasizing as nodules along lymphatics; probably not metastasizing to nasopharynx.

L. peruviana

Peru, western slopes of Andes to 3000 m; the only form not associated with forest areas. Causes single or limited number of self-healing lesions; no naso-pharyngeal involvement. Uta.

TAXONOMY OF TRYPANOSOMA

Trypanosoma is primarily characterized by manifesting, in at least some stage of the life history, trypomastigote forms; amastigote and epimastigote forms may also occur. There may be, also, a variety of flagellate round forms of as yet uncertain significance (Ormerod & Venkatesan 1971*a*, *b*).

A classification of the genus has been proposed by Hoare (1966, 1972) but this deals only with the species infecting mammals. It is, in summary, as follows:

(A) *Stercoraria*

Free flagellum present; kinetoplast large, not terminal; posterior end of body pointed; multiplication in mammal discontinuous, typically in epimastigote or amastigote forms; typically non-pathogenic; development in vector in posterior station, transmission contaminative.

Subgenus *Megatrypanum:* Large species; kinetoplast typically near nucleus, far from posterior end of body; includes *T. (M.) theileri, tragelaphi, ingens, melophagium* and others.

Subgenus *Herpetosoma:* Medium-sized species; kinetoplast subterminal; includes *T. (H.) lewisi, duttoni, nabiasi,* and others.

Subgenus *Schizotrypanum:* Small species, trypomastigotes typically curved; kinetoplast voluminous, close to posterior end of body; includes *T. (S.) cruzi, vespertilionis, pipistrelli* and others.

(B) *Salivaria*

Free flagellum present or absent; kinetoplast terminal or subterminal; posterior end of body usually blunt; multiplication in mammal continuous in trypomastigote stage; typically pathogenic; development in vector (*Glossina*

—tsetse-fly) in anterior station and transmission inoculative; includes also some atypical species transmitted non-cyclically by arthropod vectors, or by coitus.

Subgenus *Duttonella:* Monomorphic species; posterior end of body rounded; kinetoplast large, terminal; free flagellum present; development in *Glossina* in proboscis only; includes *T. (D.) vivax, uniforme.*

Subgenus *Nannomonas:* Small species; monomorphic or polymorphic; kinetoplast of medium size, typically marginal; free flagellum usually absent; development in *Glossina* in midgut and proboscis; includes *T. (N.) congolense, dimorphon, simiae.*

Subgenus *Pycnomonas:* Short, stout species; monomorphic; kinetoplast small, subterminal; free flagellum short; development in *Glossina* in midgut and salivary glands; includes *T. (P.) suis.*

Subgenus *Trypanozoon:* Typically pleomorphic species with small subterminal kinetoplast; development in *Glossina* in midgut and salivary glands; includes some aberrant species transmitted non-cyclically or by coitus; includes *T. (T.) brucei, gambiense, rhodesiense, evansi, equinum, equiperdum.*

Levine (1972), discussing Hoare's (1966, 1970) classification of the *Trypanosoma* spp. of mammals, observes: (*a*) that, as the classification of the genus does not include its type species—*Trypanosoma rotatorium* (Mayer, 1843)—it will be necessary to erect one subgenus additional to the seven proposed by Hoare (see also Hoare 1972), and (*b*) that all members of the 'group' (= genus) are so similar morphologically that splitting them into several subgenera is not justified.

The first proposal is unexceptionable, but not the second. In fact a main criticism of Hoare's classification could be based on the morphological heterogeneity of the trypanosomes of mammals, in particular the occurrence of amastigote intracellular forms in some of the subgenera but not in others, e.g. in *Herpetosoma* in the insect host and in *Schizotrypanum* in the mammal host. Although amastigote forms may not be confined to these subgenera—Ormerod & Venkatesan (1971*a*, *b*) advance the occurrence of a similar phase in *(T.T.) brucei,* though not as an intracellular organism—this seems to be an important distinction, as recognized in Baker's (1965) phylogenetic chart by the grouping of *T. (S.) cruzi* with *Leishmania* rather than with the other species of *Trypanosoma* (see below).

TAXONOMY OF ENDOTRYPANUM

Brief mention should be made here of this genus, included by Hoare (1966) as a subgenus in the Stercoraria but deserving generic status. Epimastigote and trypomastigote forms occur within the erythrocytes of the host (*Choloepus* and *Bradypus*; sloths). The genus includes only two species, *E. schaudinni* and *E. monterogeii* (Shaw 1969).

Insufficient is known of the genus to make it very profitable to discuss it. However, it has a similarity to *Leishmania* and to *T. (S.) cruzi* in that it shows an intracellular form in its vertebrate hosts. However, this is only a slender connection in that the invaded cells are erythrocytes and the cell-invading form is not especially adapted to intracellular existence—it is an epimastigote or trypomastigote, not an amastigote.

PHYLOGENY OF THE TRYPANOSOMATINA

Conjectures as to the phylogeny of the Trypanosomatina are based mainly on the variety and upon the order of the morphological forms through which the organisms pass in the course of their development. Wallace (1966) distinguishes between a 'life cycle' (in which a more or less constant and obligate sequence of stages is followed by an individual organism) and a 'population cycle' (in which a sequence of changes is superimposed on an indeterminate number of individual generations). By these definitions the developmental processes of the Trypanosomatina are probably population cycles. Considerable confusion exists in described life histories because the infections studied were frequently mixed; Wallace (1966) emphasizes the need to study clone populations.

Wallace (1966) suggests that the kinetoplast originated as an adaptation in organisms subject to sudden changes in the oxygen (or nutrient) content of their surroundings. He points out that the *Bodo*-like flagellates are subject to such changes and selects them, therefore, as the group in which the kinetoplast may well have originated. Such flagellates, later established in the intestine of a vertebrate host, found themselves ready equipped to invade the tissues and become transmitted by haematophagous arthropods. From this point (Fig. 2) Wallace derives the two 'parasitic' lines *Leishmania* and *Trypanosoma*, differentiated by the position of the reservoir (equivalent to kinetoplast), these leading, respectively, to arthropod parasites of similar morphology. He does not explain the loss of one of the two flagella.

Baker (1965) proposes a line of evolution almost diametrically the opposite

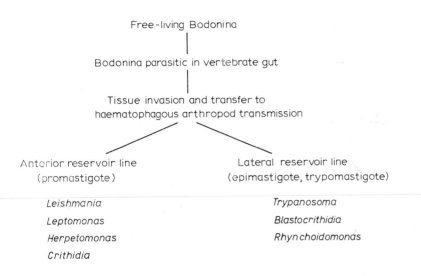

FIG. 2. Phylogenetic history of the genera of the Trypanosomatina, according to Wallace (1966).

of this (Fig. 3), starting from primitive (free-living) *Leptomonas* by a progressive elaboration through forms parasitic in insects to those parasitic in vertebrates, though again, as with Wallace's theory, in two lines, one promastigote, one epimastigote.

One may not place too much reliance on such conjectural evolutionary plans but it is interesting to note that: (*a*) both theories regard *Leishmania* as a homogeneous genus; (*b*) one theory (Wallace's) does the same for *Trypanosoma*, but the other (Baker's) splits *Trypanosoma* into three widely separated groups: the generality of the insect-transmitted *Trypanosoma* grouped with the flagellates of insects; the annelid-transmitted and *Glossina*-transmitted trypanosomes; *Trypanosoma cruzi* grouped with *Endotrypanum*.

One wonders why such weight is given to the promastigote–epimastigote difference, with so much less to other of the form differences and to even more fundamental differences such as habitat in the vertebrate body. One of the most striking of the last is whether or not the organisms show an essential stage of their life cycle within cells of the vertebrate host.

This happens in three groups—*Leishmania* spp., *Trypanosoma (Schizotrypanum) cruzi* and *Endotrypanum* spp. We may disregard *Endotrypanum* as a probably highly aberrant genus and consider the other two vertebrate-infecting genera.

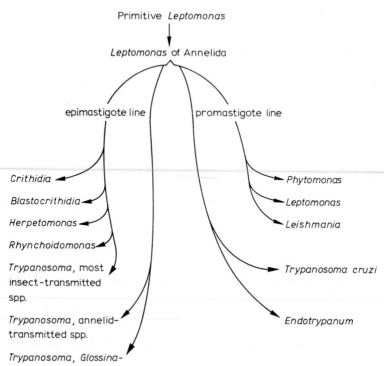

FIG. 3. Phylogenetic history of the genera of the Trypanosomatina; modified from Baker (1965).

COMPARISON OF LEISHMANIA AND TRYPANOSOMA

Morphology and transmission

Leishmania. These occur, as far as the vertebrate host is concerned, in reptiles and in mammals.

The *Leishmania* spp. occurring in reptiles may be rather separate. They exist in the vertebrate host mainly in the promastigote form (Garnham 1971). According to Garnham (1971), there is a consistent difference between reptile-infecting and mammal-infecting *Leishmania* in the interval between the sub-pellicular microtubules, which is 58–67 nm in the reptile-infecting and 35–42 nm in the mammal-infecting species. Considering the antiquity of the reptiles phylogenetically, it is remarkable that the reptile-infecting *Leishmania* are (? completely) confined to the Old World; this might indicate that the leishmanial colonization of the reptile was a rather recent event. The absence of reports of leishmanial infection in birds, also, is arresting.

The *Leishmania* spp. infecting mammals seem to be a very homogeneous group. Only two morphological forms are exhibited, amastigotes related to intracellular existence in the vertebrate host and promastigotes related to extracellular life in the gut of the insect host. All species are transmitted by phlebotomine (Diptera) flies. The range of mammalian hosts which they infect is comparatively restricted—only rodents, canids and primates.

Trypanosoma. This seems to be a much less homogeneous collection of organisms than is *Leishmania.* Organisms may exhibit themselves as amastigotes, epimastigotes and trypomastigotes. The variety of form exhibited within the trypomastigotes is extremely wide, varying from nearly spherical forms to extremely long, slender, ribbon-like forms. *Trypanosoma* spp. are transmitted by a wealth of vectors, mainly annelids (leeches) and a wide range of insects, including Siphonaptera, Hemiptera, Diptera. The range of vertebrate hosts infected is also very wide, including fish, reptiles, amphibia, birds and mammals.

Considering this heterogeneity in relation to Hoare's (1966, 1972) classification of the *Trypanosoma* spp. infecting mammals, it may be seen that the heterogeneity lies mainly in the Stercoraria. The Salivaria are a homogeneous group comprising species transmitted by the highly aberrant muscid fly genus —*Glossina*—in cycles which involve only artiodactyls, perissodactyls and primates, together with species likely to be derived directly from that transmission pattern.

The Stercoraria, on the other hand, include organisms transmitted by Hemiptera, Siphonaptera and Diptera (Tabanidae) and cover an extremely wide range of mammal host species—rodents, marsupials, canids, felids, artiodactyls, primates, cheiroptera, etc. Most of this diversity of mammal host species is, however, contributed by the one subgenus, *Schizotrypanum*, which includes *T. (S.) cruzi.* This subgenus is also aberrant among the Stercoraria in showing intracellular amastigote forms in the vertebrate host.

In summary, then, it appears that *Leishmania* is a very homogeneous genus while *Trypanosoma* is not. Further, the subgenus *Schizotrypanum* is the most aberrant one in the genus *Trypanosoma* and shares with *Leishmania* the ability to invade the cells of the host vertebrate and multiply within them. There seems, therefore, possibly to be some phylogenetic affinity between *Leishmania* and *T. (S.) cruzi* to justify further consideration of their relationship. Baker (1969) regarded *Trypanosoma (S.) cruzi* as at the end of the *Trypanosoma* spectrum most closely related to *Leishmania*.

Distribution in the vertebrate host

The distribution of these two groups of organisms in the body of the vertebrate host is as follows:

Leishmania appear to invade exclusively cells of the mononuclear phagocyte system (van Furth *et al.* 1972).

Trypanosoma (S.) cruzi. Andrade & Andrade (1971) accept that the earliest cells invaded are cells of the mononuclear phagocyte system but very soon a wide variety of other cells are involved. In fact *T. (S.) cruzi* is vastly catholic in the cells which it invades—cells of the mononuclear phagocyte system, glial cells, muscle cells, vascular endothelial cells, neurons, fat cells, etc. (Köberle 1968; Weinman 1968). However, muscle cells of all types—cardiac, intestinal, skeletal—are those especially affected.

The contrast between the types of cells selected by these two different groups of organisms is paralleled by the amount of attention which seems to have been devoted to consideration of the mechanisms of transfer of infection from cell to cell within the host in the two groups. No discussion of this matter with relation to *Leishmania* has been noticed; it does not seem to be known whether this is accomplished by phagocytosis of organisms in whole or disrupted infected cells, or by conversion of the amastigotes to promastigotes and reinvasion, or whether the dissemination of infection simply accompanies multiplication of the cells. In this latter respect it is interesting to recall the studies of Hulliger *et al.* (1964, 1966), who found that *Theileria* multiplied at about the same rate as their host cells. The organisms were associated with the spindle fibres of the host cells and were pulled apart and distributed to the daughter cells. Van den Ende & Edlinger (1971), from studies of the multiplication of *Theileria annulata* in mixed male and female lymphoid cell cultures (separable on the basis of their chromosome patterns), concluded that cell-to-cell infection *in vitro* did not take place. Cells containing parasites were induced to multiply more actively than unparasitized cells. One may conjecture that something of the same sort occurs with *Leishmania*-infected macrophages.

On the other hand, this matter of cell-to-cell infection seems to have been the focus of considerable interest in *T. (S.) cruzi*, as discussed by Köberle (1968). Transformation of amastigotes to trypomastigotes takes place within the pseudocyst and on rupture the transformed organisms distribute themselves and infect other cells. Amastigotes not transformed at the time of pseudocyst rupture are believed to be non-viable and it is to their degeneration in the vicinity of the pseudocyst that lesions of nearby ganglion cells are ascribed (Köberle 1968).

Thus, although *Leishmania* and *T. (S.) cruzi* share the characteristic of invading the cells of their vertebrate hosts, there appears to be a clear distinction between them as regards the types of cell invaded and perhaps also in the routes of cell-to-cell distribution of the organisms.

Systems of classification

We have seen above that, in default of usable morphological or other criteria that can be applied directly to the causative organisms, a system of classification has been built up for the genus *Leishmania* which includes such characteristics as clinical outcome and epidemiological transmission pattern.

With Chagas' disease, if an equivalent approach were to be adopted, we might, as very rough 'cockshies' arrive at something like the following:

T. (S.) cruzi cardiodamnum: Venezuela. Acute infections in children frequently recognized (Romaña's sign occurs in 80% of cases); main long-term pathological effect, cardiopathy—myocardial fibrosis and conduction defects. Vertebrate reservoirs: wild hosts little involved, main transmission intra-human although domestic animals may be important. Vectors: mainly *Rhodnius prolixus.*

T. (S.) cruzi viscerodilatans: South Brazil. Acute attacks in children rarely recognized; long-term pathological effects mainly damage to gut function leading to both megaoesophagus and megacolon, though cardiopathy also commonly occurs; these effects determined by ganglion cell destruction. Vertebrate reservoirs: mainly *Dasypus* (armadillo), *Didelphis* (opossum). Vectors: mainly *Triatoma infestans.*

T. (S.) cruzi innoxia: Southern parts of North America. Rarely infects man and then only causes very mild clinical signs, mild fever with no notable long-term pathological effect. Vertebrate reservoirs: *Neotoma* (wood-rat), *Didelphis* (opossum), *Procyon* (raccoon). Vectors: *Triatoma protracta, T. gerstaeckeri, T. heidemanni.*

And so on.

That such a system of classification has not been built up for Chagas' disease is perhaps simply because the clinical outcomes are not so easily classified as are the more obvious end-results of cutaneous leishmaniasis and because the background epidemiological pattern is more difficult to work out.

METHODS OF CHARACTERIZATION OF ORGANISMS

Classification of leishmaniases, and perhaps also of Chagas' disease, on this very wide range of characters is valuable in assisting the codification of the characters of the several disease situations and in directing attention towards informative comparisons. But such systems beg the question of how much the differences between disease situations are due to actual biological differences between the organismal populations concerned and how much to differences in host susceptibility and reaction or to other environmental factors. Examples of different clinical outcomes occurring with identical organismal populations are the reduction of virulence of *T. (T.) brucei* strains to mice by exposing the host to a high environmental temperature (Otieno 1972), and the lesser virulence of *Plasmodium falciparum* to individuals with S than to those with A haemo-globin. Further, organismal populations existing in particular localities may be adapted to other local components of the epidemiology. Collaborative studies between the Republic of Panama and Argentina indicate that there are affinities between the *T. (S.) cruzi* strains being transmitted in these two countries with the respective triatomine vectors concerned. *Rhodnius pallescens* and *Triatoma dimidiata*, the principal vectors in Panama, did not become in-fected when fed on Argentinian cases of Chagas' disease although *T. infestans*, the vector in Argentina, did. Conversely, the Panama vectors became 'better infected' when fed on Panamanian cases than did the Argentinian vector (Gorgas Memorial Laboratory 1972).

Basically it seems to me that, so long as both main components contributing to the ultimate outcome—the organism and the host—are unfixed, progress in our understanding will be limited. If we were able, however, to recognize particular organismal populations we would be able to fix one component of the picture and so we would be the more confident in our interpretation of the effect of other factors. It is appropriate, therefore, in conclusion, to quote briefly some examples of lines of research which might afford methods for the characterization of organismal populations. In the first place it will be im-portant to work with populations which are close to their wild origin. Any differences existing are likely to be lost if the organisms are maintained for long periods in uniform laboratory conditions and so convergently selected. Thus cryopreservation at a low passage level will be an essential component of any study. Secondly, populations studied must be known to be homogeneous and this can only be ensured by cloning. I have discussed elsewhere the basic considerations operative in such studies (Lumsden 1972).

Examples of recent attempts to develop methods for characterizing protozoal populations are as follows:

(a) Recent work on *Plasmodium* has shown that different populations of the same species may be separated on the basis of enzyme variants. Carter (1970) showed this with the rodent-infecting *Plasmodium berghei*. Carter & Voller (1973) have now shown the same kind of distinction between *Plasmodium falciparum* materials derived from south-east Asia, and East and West Africa, by means of horizontal starch-gel electrophoresis. A fast-moving form of glucose phosphate isomerase occurred in the south-east Asian and East African materials, but only a slow-moving form in the West African material. So far such studies refer to only a very few examples of *P. falciparum* from the various regions concerned and to strains passaged for long periods in laboratory animals (*Aotus*), and it is not yet known how characteristic such differences are of the *P. falciparum* strains circulating in particular geographical areas.

(b) Enzyme ratios have been computed, the activity of one enzyme being expressed relative to the activity of a second enzyme. Since the rates of enzyme synthesis in an organism are dependent on its genetic constitution, it may be expected that different 'types' of trypanosome will show different ratios (Parr & Godfrey 1973; Godfrey & Kilgour 1973).

(c) Burnett (1973) characterized the kinetoplast DNA of '*Trypanosoma brucei*'. Newton *et al.* (1973) drew attention to the differences in buoyant density of kinetoplast and nuclear DNA and suggested that these differences were related to dissimilarities in DNA base composition. They synthesized tritium-labelled complementary RNA on purified kinetoplast DNA, using RNA polymerase from *Escherichia coli*, and found that the RNA-binding was 'species-specific'.

(d) Organismal populations may sometimes be distinguished by differences in their physiology (Guttman & Wallace 1964). A recent experimental study in this area has been the blood-incubation–infectivity test—an attempt to differentiate man-infecting from non-man-infecting strains of *Trypanosoma* (*Trypanozoon*) *brucei* by comparing their ability to retain their infectivity to small mammal hosts after incubation with human serum (Rickman & Robson 1970; Targett & Wilson 1973).

(e) Immunological identification of organismal populations has been attempted. Trypanosome populations may perhaps be distinguished on the basis of the 'spectrum' of antigenic types which they produce (McNeillage *et al.* 1969) or on the patterns of precipitation which they yield in Ouchterlony gel systems (González Cappa & Kagan 1969). Schnur *et al.* (1972) have found that metabolic factors excreted *in vitro* by promastigotes of *Leishmania* precipitate with antisera raised against homologous, but not with antisera raised against heterologous, promastigotes.

In the foregoing rather discursive review of the subject, I have attempted to select some points of interest rather than to be systematic. I hope that this will provoke some useful discussion and comment.

References

ANDRADE, Z. A. & ANDRADE, S. G. (1971) Chagas' disease (American trypanosomiasis), in *Pathology of Protozoal and Helminthic Diseases* (Marcial-Rojas, R. A., ed.), Williams & Wilkins, Baltimore

BAKER, J. R. (1965) The evolution of parasitic Protozoa, in *Evolution of Parasites* (Taylor, A. E. R., ed.), Blackwell Scientific Publications, Oxford

BAKER, J. R. (1969) *Parasitic Protozoa*, Hutchinson, London

BELDING, D. L. (1965) *Textbook of Parasitology*, 3rd edn, Appleton-Century-Crofts, New York

BRACK, C. (1968) Elektronmikroskopische Untersuchungen zum Lebenszyklus von *Trypanosoma cruzi*. *Acta Trop.* **25**, 289-356

BURNETT, J. K. (1973) Further characterization of kinetoplast DNA from *Trypanosoma brucei*. *Trans. R. Soc. Trop. Med. Hyg.* **67**, 254-255

CARTER, R. (1970) Enzyme variation in *Plasmodium berghei*. *Trans. R. Soc. Trop. Med. Hyg.* **64**, 401-406

CARTER, R. & VOLLER, A. (1973) Enzyme typing of malaria parasites. *Br. Med. J.* **1**, 149-150

GARNHAM, P. C. C. (1971) The genus *Leishmania*. *Bull. W.H.O.* **44**, 477-489

GODFREY, D. G. & KILGOUR, V. (1973) The relative activities of alanine and aspartate aminotransferases in bloodstream trypanosomes. *Trans. R. Soc. Trop. Med. Hyg.* **67**, 260

GONZÁLEZ CAPPA, S. M. & KAGAN, I. G. (1969) Agar gel and immunoelectrophoretic analysis of several strains of *Trypanosoma cruzi*. *Exp. Parasitol.* **25**, 50-57

GORGAS Memorial Laboratory (1972) Forty-third annual report, U.S. Government Printing Office, Washington, D.C.

GUTTMAN, H. N. & WALLACE, F. G. (1964) Nutrition and physiology of the trypanosomatidae, in *Biochemistry and Physiology of the Protozoa* (Hutner, S. H., ed.), vol. 3, pp. 459-494, Academic Press, New York

HOARE, C. A. (1966) The classification of mammalian trypanosomes. *Ergeb. Mikrobiol. Immunitätsforsch Exp. Ther.* **39**, 43-57

HOARE, C. A. (1970) The mammalian trypanosomes of Africa, in *The African Trypanosomiases* (Mulligan, H. W., ed.), Allen & Unwin, London

HOARE, C. A. (1972) *The Trypanosomes of Mammals*, Blackwell Scientific Publications, Oxford

HOARE, C. A. & WALLACE, F. G. (1966) Developmental stages of trypanosomatid flagellates: a new terminology. *Nature (Lond.)* **212**, 1385-1386

HONIGBERG, B. M., BALAMUTH, W., BOVEE, E. C., CORLISS, J. O., GOJDICS, M., HALL, R. P., KUDO, R. R., LEVINE, N. D., LOEBLICH, A. R., WEISER, J. & WENRICH, D. H. (1964) A revised classification of the phylum Protozoa. *J. Protozool.* **11**, 7-20

HULLIGER, L., WILDE, J. K. H., BROWN, C. G. D. & TURNER, L. (1964) Mode of multiplication of *Theileria* in cultures of bovine lymphocytic cells. *Nature (Lond.)* **203**, 728-730

HULLIGER, L., BROWN, C. G. D. & WILDE, J. K. H. (1966) Transition of developmental stages of *Theileria parva in vitro* at high temperature. *Nature (Lond.)* **211**, 328-329

KÖBERLE, F. (1968) Chagas' disease and Chagas' syndromes: the pathology of American trypanosomiasis. *Adv. Parasitol.* **6**, 63-116

KUDO, R. R. (1966) *Protozoology*, Thomas, Springfield, Ill.

LAINSON, R. & SHAW, J. J. (1972) Leishmaniasis in the New World: taxonomic problems. *Br. Med. Bull.* **28**, 44-48

LEVINE, N. D. (1972) Relationship between certain protozoa and other animals, in *Research in Protozoology* (Chen, T.-T., ed.), Pergamon, Oxford

LUMSDEN, W. H. R. (1972) Principles of viable preservation of parasitic Protozoa. *Int. J. Parasitol.* **2**, 327-332

McGHEE, R. B. (1968) Development and reproduction (vertebrate and arthropod host), in *Infectious Blood Diseases of Man and Animals* (Weinman, D. & Ristic, M., eds.), Academic Press, New York

McNEILLAGE, G. J. C., HERBERT, W. J. & LUMSDEN, W. H. R. (1969) Antigenic type of first relapse variants arising from a strain of *Trypanosoma (Trypanozoon) brucei. Exp. Parasitol.* **25**, 1-7

NEWTON, B. A., STEINERT, M. & BORST, P. (1973) Differentiation of haemoflagellate species by hybridization of complementary RNA with kinetoplast DNA. *Trans. R. Soc. Trop. Med. Hyg.* **67**, 259-260

ORMEROD, W. E. & VENKATESAN, S. (1971a) The occult visceral phase of mammalian trypanosomes with special reference to the life cycle of *Trypanosoma (Trypanozoon) brucei. Trans. R. Soc. Trop. Med. Hyg.* **65**, 722-735

ORMEROD, W. E. & VENKATESAN, S. (1971b) An amastigote phase of the sleeping sickness trypanosome. *Trans. R. Soc. Trop. Med. Hyg.* **65**, 736-741

OTIENO, L. H. (1972) Studies on the effect of variations in ambient temperature on pathogenicity and on host immune response in trypanosome infections; with special reference to *Trypanosoma (Trypanozoon) brucei* infections in mice. Ph.D. Thesis, University of London

PARR, C. W. & GODFREY, D. G. (1973) The measurement of enzyme ratios as a means of differentiating trypanosomes. *Trans. R. Soc. Trop. Med. Hyg.* **67**, 260

RICKMAN, L. R. & ROBSON, J. (1970) The blood incubation infectivity test. A simple test which may serve to distinguish *Trypanosoma brucei* from *T. rhodesiense. Bull. W.H.O.* **42**, 650-651

SCHNUR, L. F., ZUCKERMAN, A. & GREENBLATT, C. L. (1972) *Leishmania* serotypes distinguished by the gel diffusion of factors excreted *in vitro* and *in vivo. Isr. J. Med. Sci.* **8**, 932-942

SHAW, J. J. (1969) *The Haemoflagellates of Sloths* (London School of Hygiene and Tropical Medicine, Memoir No. 13), Lewis, London

TARGETT, G. A. T. & WILSON, V. C. L. C. (1973) The blood incubation infectivity test as a means of distinguishing between *Trypanosoma brucei brucei* and *T. brucei rhodesiense. Int. J. Parasitol.* **3**, 5-11

VAN DEN ENDE, M. & EDLINGER, E. (1971) Culture de lignées lymphocytaires bovines infectées par *Theileria annulata. Arch. Inst. Pasteur Tunis* **48**, 45-54

VAN FURTH, R., COHN, Z. A., HIRSCH, J. G., HUMPHREY, J. H., SPECTOR, W. H. & LANGEVOORT, H. L. (1972) The mononuclear phagocyte system: a new classification of macrophages, monocytes, and their precursor cells. *Bull. W.H.O.* **46**, 845-852

WALLACE, F. G. (1966) The trypanosomatid parasites of insects and arachnids. *Exp. Parasitol.* **18**, 124-193

WEINMAN, D. (1968) The human trypanosomiases, in *Infectious Blood Diseases of Man and Animals* (Weinman, D. & Ristic, M., eds.), Academic Press, New York

Discussion

Baker: You rightly said that there needs to be a nominate subgenus of *Trypanosoma* to contain the type species, Professor Lumsden, but this has been proposed by Hoare (1964).

Secondly, in the evolutionary scheme of the trypanosomes that I drew up and that you showed (in Fig. 3), the line deriving the Salivaria from the annelid-transmitted forms was put in very tentatively. I now prefer Woo's (1970) suggestion that the Salivaria instead developed quite recently from trypanosomes of reptiles in Africa.

You also wondered why both Wallace (1966) and I (1963) stressed the difference between the promastigote and epimastigote lines, rather than between intracellular or extracellular habitats. I regard the fundamental morphological difference between these two lines (i.e. the posterior migration of the kinetoplast and basal body) as more important than a mere difference in habitat. It is like the difference between a vertebrate or an invertebrate rather than that between an animal living in the sea or on the land.

Lumsden: But is there not an equally fundamental morphological difference between the flagellate and the aflagellate forms? I agree that they are associated with a different habitat but there exists also a fundamental difference in morphological form between the flagellate forms, whether epimastigote or promastigote, and the non-flagellate amastigote form.

Baker: I would have thought probably not, since the amastigote has the potentiality of producing a flagellum; it has a basal body. But these things are obviously very subjective.

Zeledón: Dr Lumsden said that Brack's term sphaeromastigote is perhaps unfortunate. I do not quite agree with this, particularly now that we know that sphaeromastigotes play an important role in the *T. cruzi* cycle in the vector. As Brack (1968) herself mentioned, and as indicated by Brener (1972) more recently, a promastigote type, as defined by Hoare & Wallace (1966), is not really present in the *T. cruzi* cycle in the insect. The term sphaeromastigote probably would be a good one if we kept it for a round form with a small free flagellum.

Lumsden: You are suggesting that 'sphaeromastigote' should be limited to what I was calling a round promastigote. The trouble is that it is being applied to the whole range of the development of the flagellum in the round form.

Sanabria: Creemers & Jadin (1967) suggested that a more suitable name for the amastigote is micromastigote because this form has a very short flagellum visible in the electron microscope.

Bray: One way round that is simply to say that the amount of flagellum seen in an amastigote is called an axoneme and not a flagellum at all. It is then still aflagellate; it just happens to have an axoneme.

Trager: Could we just retain the term promastigote and talk about round promastigotes, especially as even the so-called amastigote has a bit of a flagellum when viewed by electron microscopy? The flagellum may stick out a little bit or it may stick out a little more, and we may be trying to make too fine a distinction.

Newton: I agree. The terminology is extremely complicated and confusing already and the introduction of yet more terms just confuses me further. I believe we ought to consider the developmental stages in the life cycle of trypanosomes as forming a continuum and not as a number of discrete morphological forms which can be specifically identified and named.

Lumsden: I quite agree.

de Raadt: McNeillage *et al.* (1969) in your laboratory, Professor Lumsden, using clone populations in mice, showed that the first relapse variant was antigenically not homogeneous and also that there was a difference in virulence, at least for mice amongst the different variants in such populations (McNeillage & Herbert 1968). Would there be much point in cloning, as the clone population itself seems to be already a mixture?

Lumsden: The cloning there was to try to see whether a given population (the first relapse variant: see McNeillage *et al.* 1969) was antigenically homogeneous. The individual organisms were separated and then grown in mice at passage intervals of less than three days, so that they could be presumed to stay antigenically the same as the individual organisms which were isolated to begin with (Lourie & O'Connor 1937). The antigenic type of the population which develops at the end is therefore likely to be representative of the antigenic type of the original organism. That work showed that the population of organisms existing in the mouse at a given moment was not homogeneous as far as the antigenic type was concerned.

de Raadt: Yes, I agree that McNeillage's experiments were started with a mixture, but I thought that from the clones taken from that experiment, she saw again more than one variant occurring among the first relapse population.

Lumsden: This may well happen but at least one knows that the genetic constitution of the population one started with is the same as that of the population ensuing, although, as Dr Vickerman (1971) has suggested, that population of organisms may be able to manifest different antigenic types from the same genetic basis. What often seems confusing is that in any wild situation, genetically different populations may well be transmitted at the same time. One must work with populations known to be homogeneous if one is to disentangle the effect of different populations from the variations occurring within one population. This is comparable to trying to work out the fermentative capabilities, of, say, *Salmonella*, by working always with a whole *Salmonella* population instead of cloning the organisms first to separate them into different fermentative types.

de Raadt: But one may also discover that the fermentative characteristics will change again, depending on the circumstances under which they are cultivated.

Lumsden: That is so, but at least you know that you have started with something homogeneous.

Peters: Obviously clones have to be produced if pure lines of these parasites are to be identified, but how many clones should one try to set up? Any wild population is genetically mixed. If, for example, one of these lines is present in the proportion of one in 100, we may have to set up at least 100 clones to produce that one. If perhaps half a dozen clones all turn out to be the same, and we assume that these are really representative of the population, we may be misleading ourselves.

O'Daly: How many biochemical markers can be defined in the clone?

Lumsden: That question can't be answered yet. All that I am suggesting is that we should work with populations that we know are homogeneous and then use whatever methods of classification are available, whether biochemical or immunological, to classify these organisms at a sub-morphological level.

Newton: What evidence is there that no antigenic variation takes place during the three-day intervals between passage of trypanosomes from one animal to another?

Lumsden: Lourie & O'Connor (1937) tested this in about 5000 different infections and only got changes in about two out of this 5000. In this short interval, which is before the first antigenic type starts to be selected out by the antibody response of the host, one can reasonably assume that the population usually stays undeviant.

Newton: But what is the sensitivity of a method like that? What percentage of the total population would be detected if they were antigenically different?

Lumsden: Some organisms could well change in antigenic type but they are not going to extend their representation in the population unless there is selection of some sort. If one avoids the selection by transmitting at three-day intervals then the population stays stable in antigenic type, as far as anyone's experience goes.

Zeledón: I think the species or subspecies *L.m.pifanoi* in Lainson & Shaw's (1972) classification of leishmania should be considered now as a *species inquerenda.*

In relation to the terms *T. (S.) cruzi cardiodamnum* and *T. (S.) cruzi viscerodilatans,* I believe you said, Professor Lumsden, that these subspecies or strains, or whatever they are, are somehow related to certain species of bugs and that some southern South American strains have a preference for the cardiac fibres. I think that some of the most cardiotropic strains are those here in Venezuela, transmitted by *Rhodnius prolixus.* I don't think that what you call *T. (S.) cruzi viscerodilatans* is related to *Triatoma brasiliensis*, for instance. If it is especially related to some insect, it would be to *T. infestans*.

Lumsden: My rough classification was simply an attempt to stimulate thought. You have risen to the bait and started to produce such a classification, Dr Zeledón. Those names are just rough examples and are not based on precise knowledge of the particular systems.

Bray: I entirely agree about *L.m.pifanoi*. We are in no doubt at all that in Ethiopia exactly the same parasite produces diffuse cutaneous leishmaniasis and normal cutaneous leishmaniasis. We are looking at an immunological defect, not a change in the organism.

Peters: We have had a look at the organism associated with diffuse leishmaniasis from the Amazon region and the same thing applies there: this is the local *L. mexicana amazonensis*. I am hoping to obtain some of these strains from Dr Convit to see how they come out in our biochemical classification.

Bray: A lot of work has been done on *Theileria parva* and on its dissemination in the host through parallel division with and inside its host cell. We have been interested in this too, with Dr D. J. Bradley in Oxford. The evidence at present seems to be that *Leishmania* does not disseminate in that way. As far as one can see, the mature macrophage does not divide after it has been infected, but blood monocytes are recruited into the area and are invaded and become new host cells.

Trager: What do you consider are good methods for cloning, Professor Lumsden? For example, if one were going to clone *T. cruzi*, would one begin with blood forms from an infected mouse or would one get it in culture first and try to clone these forms? Or would it be best to clone from the blood first and then, having got that in culture, clone from that?

Lumsden: I would have thought that one would have to relate the material as closely as possible to the original epidemiological situation. Our material from Salvador comes to the UK in bugs infected from whatever the wild epidemiological situation is, whether it is an animal or a human patient or an infected bug gathered in the field. Probably the best methods for cloning are with metacyclic or first passage bloodstream forms inoculated into immunodepressed mice.

Martinez-Silva: I think the best method for cloning *T. cruzi* is provided by tissue culture, since most cells are infected by a single parasite. Once it is infected the cell can be isolated, with the result that the entire parasite population comes from a single parasite. However, it is difficult to affirm that this cloned population is homogeneous in all its characteristics. Using tissue-cultured cells in a perfusion chamber, we were able to follow the course of infection of single cells with a single parasite. Usually the course of intracellular multiplication follows a regular pattern in which all the amastigotes undergo division with a generation time characteristic for a given strain. However, we observed on one occasion that the penetrating parasite, after the usual lag period, divided into two daughter amastigotes, from which only one pursued multiplication, while the other remained non-dividing until the cell was disrupted by the trypomastigotes originating from the active dividing amastigote. If we consider a clone as the population originating from a single ancestor, it is obvious that we had a clone with members showing very different properties. If we look for more subtle criteria, such as the synthesis by the parasites of a specific protein, we would assume the existence of a homogeneous population; this, however, would not be the case. Therefore, I agree with Dr de Raadt and others that the question of cloning is not going to solve many of the problems, since the descendants will have genetic information, but the rate of mutation will be expressed in a certain proportion of them.

Baker: One snag about trying to clone from cultures, particularly cultures *in vitro* rather than tissue cultures, is that this has to be done aseptically. Several of my assistants in Cambridge have gone completely mad trying to do this.*

Martinez-Silva: It is pretty easy to work under aseptic conditions by using antibiotics. One does not need a micromanipulator, but simply to put small drops of saline solution in a petri dish. The parasite suspension can be diluted with a fine pasteur pipette and observed with an inverted microscope. Work is easy if the whole is in a hood with a laminar flow system, which provides an aseptic environment. In tissue culture one can manipulate the single infected cells by the standard methods and so obtain a parasite population derived from a single ancestor.

Newton: Although many antibiotics are not trypanocidal or leishmanicidal we should remember that they may modify these parasites in ways we don't yet know about. Wherever possible we should avoid the use of antibiotics in culturing protozoa.

References

BAKER, J. R. (1963) Speculations on the evolution of the family Trypanosomatidae Doflein, 1901. *Exp. Parasitol.* **13**, 219-233

BRACK, C. (1968) Elektronmikroskopische Untersuchungen zum Lebenszyklus von *Trypanosoma cruzi. Acta Trop.* **25**, 289-356

---

* *Note added in proof:* One (Mrs S. M. Green) managed to clone from culture, in May, 1973. J. R. B.

BRENER, Z. (1972) A new aspect of *Trypanosoma cruzi* life-cycle in the invertebrate host. *J. Protozool.* **19**, 23-27

CREEMERS, J. & JADIN, J. M. (1967) Etude de l'ultrastructure et de la biologie de *Leishmania mexicana* Biagi 1953. I: Les modifications qui surviennent lors de la transformation leishmania-leptomonas. *Bull. Soc. Pathol. Exot.* **60**, 53-58

HOARE, C. A. (1964) Morphological and taxonomic studies on mammalian trypanosomes. X: Revision of the systematics. *J. Protozool.* **11**, 200-207

HOARE, C. A. & WALLACE, F. G. (1966) Developmental stages of trypanosomatid flagellates: a new terminology. *Nature (Lond.)* **212**, 1385-1386

LAINSON, R. & SHAW, J. J. (1972) Leishmaniasis of the New World: taxonomic problems. *Br. Med. Bull.* **28**, 44-48

LOURIE, E. M. & O'CONNOR, R. J. (1937) A study of *Trypanosoma rhodesiense* relapse strains *in vitro*. *Ann. Trop. Med. Parasitol.* **31**, 319-340

MCNEILLAGE, G. J. C. & HERBERT, W. J. (1968) Infectivity and virulence of *Trypanosoma (Trypanozoon) brucei* for mice. *J. Comp. Pathol.* **78**, 345-349

MCNEILLAGE, G. J. C., HERBERT, W. J. & LUMSDEN, W. H. R. (1969) Antigenic type of first relapse variants arising from a strain of *Trypanosoma ((Trypanozoon) brucei*. *Exp. Parasitol.* **25**, 1-7

VICKERMAN, K. (1971) Morphological and physiological considerations of extracellular blood protozoa, in *Ecology and Physiology of Parasites* (Fallis, A. M., ed.), University of Toronto Press, Toronto

WALLACE, F. G. (1966) The trypanosomatid parasites of insects and arachnids. *Exp. Parasitol.* **18**, 124-193

WOO, P. T. K. (1970) The origin of mammalian trypanosomes which develop in the anterior station of blood-sucking arthropods. *Nature (Lond.)* **228**, 1059-1062

Epidemiology of African sleeping sickness

J. R. BAKER

MRC Unit for Biochemical Parasitology, Molteno Institute, University of Cambridge

Abstract   The two forms of Africanum han trypanosomiasis differ markedly in their epidemiology, largely because of differences in their virulence to mammalian hosts. *Trypanosoma brucei gambiense* is unable to maintain parasitaemias adequate to infect *Glossina* in most of the mammals which are regularly fed upon by these flies, and which could therefore serve as reservoirs of infection, with the exception of man. Thus this parasite depends essentially on a man–fly–man cycle. *Trypanosoma brucei rhodesiense*, on the other hand, is more virulent and maintains higher (though fluctuating) parasitaemias in a variety of mammals, including man, that are favoured hosts of *Glossina*. Its virulence to man may be so great that the chance of transmission to *Glossina* is reduced, as the patient feels too ill to leave his home and all too soon dies (if untreated); thus his contact with *Glossina* is reduced or prevented. Hence, *T. b. rhodesiense* depends for survival on an ungulate–fly–ungulate cycle, and man is usually only adventitiously infected when he impinges on this cycle and converts it into a 'triple-contact' relationship.

It is suggested that *T. b. gambiense* and *T. b. rhodesiense* evolved independently from a common ancestral species resembling *T. b. brucei*. *T. b. rhodesiense* may have evolved extremely recently (even within the last 100 years), probably in south-east Africa, whence it is spreading north.

The parasites and their vectors

African human trypanosomiasis (sleeping sickness) is caused by parasitic protozoa of the genus *Trypanosoma* (subgenus *Trypanozoon*). Classically the causative organisms were regarded as two distinct species—*T. gambiense* and *T. rhodesiense*. Lately the view is prevailing that these two organisms are less distinct than specific separation would imply, and they are now often treated as either subspecies or even nosodemes ('clinical races') of their presumed ancestral species, *T. brucei* (which, by definition, does not infect man). The argument has been summarized by Hoare (1972); without entering into it, I shall here adopt the subspecific terminology as a convenient compromise. The parasites are transmitted cyclically by various species of *Glossina* (tsetse flies) and perhaps, during epidemics, sometimes non-cyclically by these and other blood-sucking Diptera also. The life cycle of the parasites in *Glossina* is complex. It consists essentially of three stages: initial establishment and multiplication within the endoperitrophic cavity of the midgut; colonization of the ectoperitrophic space and then the proventriculus; and finally invasion of the salivary glands. Only the so-called metacyclic trypomastigotes which develop in this last situation are infective to mammals. Perhaps partly because of the complexity of this cycle, *Glossina* spp. are in general surprisingly resistant to infection with *T. brucei rhodesiense* or *T. b. gambiense*; even under the best obtainable experimental conditions, fewer than 10% of flies which are known to have ingested infective trypanosomes eventually have metacyclic trypomastigotes within their salivary glands. Natural populations of *Glossina* rarely have infection rates greater than one-hundredth of this figure and this fact is important epidemiologically (see below). An exceptionally high natural infection rate (4.8%) has however been reported recently for *G. fuscipes* (Rogers *et al.* 1972). Further information on the trypanosomes and their vectors can be found in monographs by Hoare (1972) and Buxton (1955) respectively.

The diseases

Human trypanosomiasis in Africa is restricted to the region between the two tropics (Fig. 1), roughly to the area where the annual rainfall exceeds 500 mm (Fig. 2). This restriction is due to the effect of the climate on *Glossina*, the pupa of which is particularly vulnerable to desiccation. Within this area, there are two main types of human disease produced by trypanosomes. One is chronic, lasting (if untreated) a matter of years before the patient finally succumbs. This, the 'Gambian' form caused by *T. b. gambiense*, is found mainly in the western half of tropical Africa, though it also occurs—or used to occur—on the eastern side of the continent around the north of Lake Victoria and up into the Sudan. Its range includes most of the areas of evergreen forest in Africa as well as some of the surrounding savannah (Fig. 1). The other, 'Rhodesian', disease is caused by *T. b. rhodesiense* and is restricted to the eastern third or so of tropical Africa, from the northern boundary of South Africa up into Ethiopia. This form of disease is much more acute, and usually kills untreated persons in a matter of weeks or months. The distinction between the two forms is not always as clear-cut as this, however, and intermediate types of infection

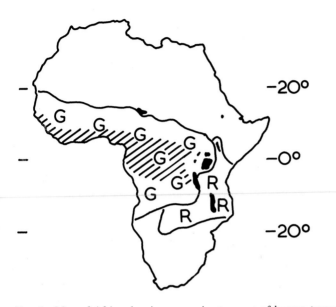

FIG. 1. Map of Africa showing approximate range of human trypanosomiasis due to *T. b. gambiense* (G) and *T. b. rhodesiense* (R). Hatched area denotes main extent of evergreen hygrophytic forest. (Based on *World Health Organization Chronicle*, 1963, **17**, 444 and the Oxford Atlas, Oxford University Press, 1966.)

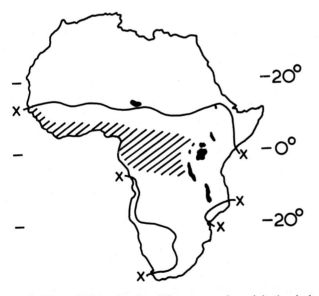

FIG. 2. Map of Africa showing 500 mm annual precipitation isohyets (×——×) and evergreen hygrophytic forest (hatched). (Based on the Oxford Atlas, Oxford University Press, 1966.)

exist, though they are probably rare. A recent compendium of knowledge on African trypanosomiasis has been edited by Mulligan & Potts (1970).

EPIDEMIOLOGY

In this paper I propose to treat epidemiology as the relationship between the disease and the total environment—the interaction of parasite, its arthropod and mammalian hosts (including man) and the geophysical nature of the areas in which they coexist. In other words, I shall deal with the ecological relationships of the parasites, viewed anthropocentrically with the emphasis on the human disease part of the situation. These relationships are not fully understood, but I shall try to outline what seem to me the more important features of what is known about them, treating the chronic and acute (that is, Gambian and Rhodesian) forms of the disease separately but comparatively and drawing extensively on the ideas of Ashcroft (1959, 1963). Fuller treatments of the subjects have been made recently by Scott (1970) for the Gambian, and Apted (1970) for the Rhodesian, diseases and by Ford (1971).

The Gambian disease

The chronicity of this infection is the key to its epidemiology. In mammals —and experimentally it can infect quite a large range of species from laboratory rodents through herbivores to primates—the parasite is rare in the circulating blood, being found more commonly in lymph and other tissue fluids. The number of organisms in the blood and elsewhere, though fluctuating throughout the infection, never becomes very high and the parasites may often be subpatent, that is, too scanty to be detected by microscopic examination. It has never been demonstrated conclusively whether this is due to an inherently reduced multiplication rate of the parasite, or to the fact that it is highly antigenic and thus the host is able to produce enough antibodies, and produce them quickly enough, to keep the parasite population under control. Perhaps it is a combination of both these mechanisms. At any rate, the effect of the low parasitaemia is to reduce the probability that a parasite will be ingested by a feeding *Glossina*. As already stated, never more than 10% (usually considerably less) of *Glossina* which ingest trypanosomes develop salivary gland infections and so become capable of transmitting the parasite. So if the number of parasites in the blood is so low that only, say, one in ten flies ingests a minimum infective dose (whatever that is) with its blood meal, the chances of

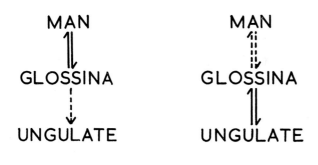

FIG. 3. Transmission 'cycles' of *T. b. gambiense* and *T. b. rhodesiense:* broken lines indicate adventitious parts of the cycles.

a fly becoming infected are very low. Indeed, it often seems surprising that the parasite survives at all—but it does. The reasons for this must be (1) the relatively long time that infected people survive and, because they do not feel too ill, remain available for flies to feed on, and (2) the frequency with which people may be bitten by tsetse, often in quite circumscribed geographical areas (see below).

Amongst the mammals, human beings seem to be one of the more susceptible species to *T. b. gambiense*; their levels of parasitaemia are high enough often enough to ensure transmission of the parasite to its arthropod host. This is not true of the other possible mammalian hosts (mainly ungulates) on which tsetse flies commonly feed (Weitz 1963); in many of these *T. b. gambiense* will produce only, at the most, a fleeting scanty parasitaemia. Thus, although domestic and wild ungulates must sometimes become infected (though this has never been conclusively demonstrated in natural conditions), the ensuing parasitaemia, if any, is apparently not sufficient to allow the parasite to maintain its vertebrate–invertebrate–vertebrate cycle.

The effect of this is that Gambian trypanosomiasis can be maintained only in situations where humans and tsetse come into close and repeated contact (Willett 1963). Without this contact, it is not possible for the parasite to survive; there is no non-human reservoir of *T. b. gambiense*. This does not preclude the (as yet unproven) possibility that men may sometimes be infected by tsetse which acquired the infection from, perhaps, a domestic or wild ungulate or other mammal such as a dog; but it means that the parasite cannot survive where there is no sustained contact between people and tsetse (Fig. 3).

Consequently, the disease is 'peridomestic' in the sense that infection is usually acquired near the victim's home; all members of the family—men, women and children—are at equal risk; and the vector tsetse flies are species which utilize human blood as a major part of their diet—this means, in general, species of the *Glossina palpalis* group which, again in general, inhabit the forested banks of rivers and similar wet places (Fig. 4); hence the association between the distribution of this disease and the region of evergreen hygrophytic forest already mentioned. Other species of *Glossina* can become infected; but if man is not a favourite dietary object, the chances of their inoculating meta-cyclic trypanosomes into an inadequately susceptible species of mammal instead of into another man will be so high that it is very likely that the try-panosome's vital cycle will be broken.

One of the commonest places where adequate contact between humans and these so-called 'riverine' species of tsetse occurs frequently is where people cross rivers or enter them to wash or collect water (Fig. 5). Such sites—fords on paths and roads, village washing or watering places—are classical sites for acquiring *T. b. gambiense* infection. These areas may be of very limited extent; but within them quite small but nevertheless important foci of infection may be built up, with relatively high rates of infection of the tsetse flies.

The Rhodesian disease

The situation is different with this acute form of sleeping sickness. The ability of *T. b. rhodesiense* to multiply to a greater extent in the peripheral blood of a variety of mammals (Soltys 1971) means that it can produce in them levels of parasitaemia adequate to ensure that a feeding tsetse fly will ingest enough trypanosomes to become infected, if the fly is a susceptible individual. (As mentioned earlier, the evidence is that most flies are *not* susceptible individuals.) This higher level of parasitaemia means that, probably, many mammals can support *T. b. rhodesiense* under natural conditions, without the need for the intervention of man. Indeed, the acuteness of the human disease due to this subspecies means that infected persons are relatively soon removed from the

$\rightarrow$

FIG. 4. Riverine habitat of *Glossina palpalis* group; river Gilo near Abol, Illubabor Province, Ethiopia.

FIG. 5. Typical West African region of contact between man and *Glossina palpalis* (Kiyende, Kongo Central Province, Zaire).

FIG. 6. Typical *Glossina morsitans* habitat; wooded savannah with *Acacia* and *Combretum* predominating (near Gambela, Illubabor province, Ethiopia).

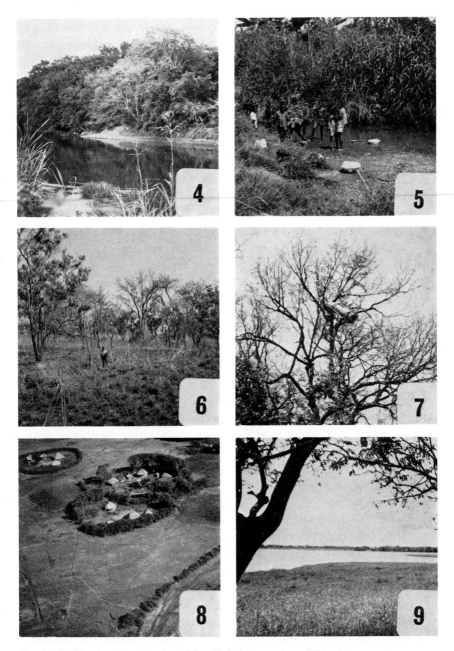

FIG. 7. Beehive in tree; near river Gilo, Illubabor province, Ethiopia.
FIG. 8. Aerial view of homesteads surrounded by *Lantana* thicket in Nyanza district, Kenya (courtesy of Dr B. A. Newton).
FIG. 9. Lake Thatha, Illubabor province, Ethiopia; village of Pinybago on further shore.

'pool' of potential tsetse infectors, either because they feel too ill to leave their homes or, even more effectively, because they die. Thus, although during epidemics man–fly–man transmission undoubtedly occurs, such episodes tend to be self-limiting—because the human reservoir of infection is reduced as just described and, very often, because the surviving population leaves the area. Thus it is likely that, in contrast to *T. b. gambiense*, the Rhodesian parasite could not survive solely in a man–fly–man cycle. The intervention of a non-human host reservoir, in which the infection is less acute but in which the parasitaemia and the attractiveness of the mammal to tsetse are adequate to ensure transmission, may be essential for survival of *T. b. rhodesiense* (Fig. 3).

The consequences of this are that, in general, Rhodesian trypanosomiasis in man is not peridomestic but is associated with areas where wild mammals roam and are fed upon by tsetse species which are often referred to as the 'game' tsetse because of their habit of feeding very largely on 'game' animals (i.e. large ungulates which are hunted for 'sport'). These 'game' tsetse are *Glossina morsitans* and its relatives, species which can withstand a much drier environment than can *G. palpalis*; consequently they inhabit vast areas of East African savannah plains (Fig. 6), which they share with the wild ungulates that provide their main food supply. People may live on these plains in scattered, small communities, but generally their activities tend to drive away the ungulates and the tsetse from the immediate vicinity of their houses. Hence the chances of these people becoming infected with trypanosomes are not high unless they venture out on the plains. Therefore it is mainly the men who are at risk, as they tend to go into the surrounding 'bush' to hunt for food. One of the classically 'high-risk' occupations for acquiring Rhodesian sleeping sickness is that of honey-gathering. Artificial bee-hives (Fig. 7), usually made from hollowed-out logs, are hung in trees in the savannah to attract bees and the latter's nests are then collected and plundered by the honey gatherers, an occupation which exposes them to the bites of tsetse flies as well as the stings of bees, with potentially more disastrous consequences. Another relatively modern occupation which is fast becoming a high-risk one, as far as trypanosomiasis is concerned, is that of tourist; there have been several cases of trypanosomiasis in recent years among tourists visiting the East African game parks.

The only wild ungulate species which have so far been proved conclusively to harbour *T. b. rhodesiense* naturally are *Tragelaphus scriptus* (bushbuck) (Heisch et al. 1958), which are also a favourite food source for tsetse and *Alcelaphus buselaphus* (hartebeest) (Geigy et al. 1971, 1972). It is likely that other species also serve as reservoir hosts, and the fact that none has as yet been definitely incriminated is probably due only to the technical difficulties of positively differentiating *T. b. rhodesiense* from *T. b. brucei*, the subspecies which does not infect man. Domestic ungulates too can serve as hosts. The only positive identifications so far have been from domestic oxen in four different areas of East Africa (Onyango *et al.* 1966; Mwambu & Mayende 1971; Rickman 1971; Geigy *et al.* 1972; Robson *et al.* 1972; Mwambu 1973). Since cattle are grazed often in areas of tsetse-infested bush, tended by herdsmen or boys who are exposed to the bites of the tsetse flies attracted to the cattle, the possible importance of the latter as sources of human infection is obviously worth further investigation.

Thus, whereas with *T. b. gambiense* sustained man–fly contact is needed to maintain the parasite and the infection of man is therefore essential to the parasite's survival, *T. b. rhodesiense* can survive via an ungulate–fly–ungulate cycle and the infection of man is adventitious. For this to occur, an additional element has to be inserted into the cycle—what Apted *et al.* (1963) have called 'sustained triple contact' between the ungulate (or non-human) reservoir host, tsetse flies and man. Man can therefore be regarded as an obligate host of *T. b. gambiense* but only a facultative host of *T. b. rhodesiense*; from the parasite's point of view he may represent a dead end since onward transmission of the parasite to its next (invertebrate) host is less likely to occur from man than it is from a suitable wild ungulate.

It does not necessarily follow that because the tsetse of the *G. morsitans* group and the wild ungulate reservoir hosts of *T. b. rhodesiense* range widely over vast areas of East African savannah the epidemiology of the human disease caused by this parasite is equally diffuse. Recent work in Kenya has led to the suggestion by D. A. T. Baldry and his colleagues (personal communication) that there may be quite limited geographical areas, measurable in square metres rather than square kilometres, where the important 'triple contact' occurs and where men may consequently become infected (see Allsopp 1972, and Allsopp *et al.* 1972).

The mean 'home ranges' of adult *Tragelaphus scriptus* lie between about 25 000 and 50 000 m^2; those of subadult males are rather larger (about 200 000 m^2). Within these ranges the animals tend to hide in thickets during daylight; one calf was observed to stand beneath the same bush for about three hours around noon on each of six consecutive days while its mother fed in a nearby thicket (Allsopp 1970, and personal communication).

If contact with man occurs in such an area, either regularly because the area is close to human habitation (and *Tragelaphus* often lives close to humans) or sporadically because a hunter, honey gatherer or tourist enters one of these areas of bush, and if *T. b. rhodesiense* is already passing around the *Tragelaphus–Glossina* cycle, the chances of a human infection being acquired are considerable. Thus the epidemiology—and epizootiology—of *T. b. rhodesiense* infection may be more focal than has been thought, with hot-spots of infection scattered widely through vast areas of savannah, which may in part explain the paradox, emphasized by Ashcroft (1963), that *T. b. rhodesiense* is apparently less uniformly distributed than *T. b. brucei* in wild mammal populations.

Bradley (1972) has recently attempted to classify parasitic infections in terms of the regulatory mechanisms which control their spread within a host population. Rhodesian human trypanosomiasis (like the Gambian disease) appears to belong to his type 1, 'transmission-regulated', infections, since the incidence of infective vector bites must be very low. In man it probably also belongs to type 2, being controlled partly by the death of the human host (or at least his removal by sickness from that part of the population available to the vector). In ungulates, infection by *T. b. rhodesiense* (and *T. b. brucei*, as well as the human disease caused by *T. b. gambiense*) presumably belongs to Bradley's (1972) type 3, being controlled in part by the hosts' development of non-sterile immunity ('premunition'). Baldry's concept of the existence of hot spots of zoonotic infection, if true, probably represents an enzootic version of the state of affairs described by Bradley (1972) as 'an apparent continuum which may be a collection of microfoci' and illustrated in his Fig. 7—the 'water sources' of Bradley's diagram (which pertains to schistosomiasis) being equivalent to infected *T. scriptus*.

When *T. b. rhodesiense* is transmitted during epidemics via a direct man–fly–man cycle, its association with its usual vectors of the *G. morsitans* group is not necessarily maintained, and flies of the *G. palpalis* group (the usual vectors of *T. b. gambiense*) can maintain the cycle. There is one instance where this has been shown conclusively to occur (Willett 1965). A few years ago an epidemic of Rhodesian sleeping sickness occurred in western Kenya, near the shore of Lake Victoria. During this epidemic, *G. fuscipes* (a close relative of *G. palpalis*) was found to be a vector, and indeed the development of an epidemic situation there was ascribed to the fact that unusually wet weather had enabled *G. fuscipes* to extend its range inland from its usual lake-shore habitat in that region, and to colonize the dense hedges of succulents with which the local residents enclose their homesteads (Fig. 8). This greatly increased the contact between man and *G. fuscipes* in that region and consequently led to a 'Gambian-type' (i.e. peridomestic man–fly–man) epidemic of Rhodesian trypanosomiasis in an area where human infections were usually sporadic and transmitted by *G. pallidipes*, a member of the *G. morsitans* group.

Another probable instance of an epidemic of *T. b. rhodesiense* infection being transmitted by a riverine species of tsetse commonly involved in transmitting *T. b. gambiense* occurred a few years ago in Ethiopia (McConnell *et al.* 1970;

Hutchinson 1971). *T. b. rhodesiense* has apparently only recently reached that country, the northernmost extension of its known range, and a small-scale but quite intense epidemic developed as a result. Some people were undoubtedly infected by game tsetse which had themselves presumably acquired the infection from wild ungulates, but in one particular village on the shore of a lake (Fig. 9; see also Fig. 4) where several people including women and children were infected, presumably peridomestically, the only species of *Glossina* was the riverine *G. tachinoides*, which must almost certainly have been acting as vector (though efforts to demonstrate this, by isolating from these flies a strain of trypanosomes of proven ability to infect man, failed).

In these situations, the epidemiology of the disease more resembled that of the West African form, with peridomestic infection occurring and less marked differences in the infection rates of men, women and children. Both the epidemics were of fairly short duration and represent exceptions to the general situation described above.

ORIGIN AND SPREAD OF THE DISEASES

Probably both subspecies of trypanosomes which infect man in Africa evolved from *T. brucei brucei* or at least from a common ancestral species (Baker 1963). It is likely that *T. b. gambiense* is evolutionarily older than *T. b. rhodesiense*. The evidence suggesting this is as follows: (*i*) *T. b. gambiense* seems better adapted to man, since its lower virulence (i.e. pathogenicity) results in a longer period during which the infected person is available as a source of infection for tsetse flies; it is an unwise parasite which kills its host too soon, especially if it is dependent on a second species of host to ensure its survival. (*ii*) *T. b. gambiense* has become almost if not entirely restricted to man and tsetse and has lost its (presumed) earlier dependence (as *T. b. brucei*) on wild ungulates; this too may suggest a longer period of adaptation to man than that of *T. b. rhodesiense*, which still remains primarily a parasite of ungulates and tsetse. (*iii*) The human disease has been known in West Africa ever since written records were kept—600 years ago, according to Nash (1969), an Arab historian wrote an account of it, and in the days of the slave traders it was well known. In contrast, the first records of acute trypanosomiasis in south-east Africa are surprisingly recent (at the turn of the last century) and its spread northwards can be traced since that time; other conditions such as lack of adequate earlier records and, perhaps, greater population mobility in this century, may however be responsible for this (see Duggan 1970).

If we accept the two premises—that the two African trypanosomes of man

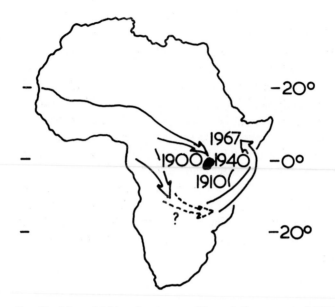

Fig. 10. Map of Africa showing possible evolutionary spread of *T. b. gambiense* and *T. b. rhodesiense*.

evolved from something akin to *T. b. brucei* and that *T. b. gambiense* did so earlier than *T. b. rhodesiense*—there are two main possibilities for their evolutionary origin (Fig. 10): either *T. b. rhodesiense* evolved from *T. b. gambiense*, or both evolved independently from the ancestral species. The evidence for the former view is essentially as follows. There is good evidence that *T. b. gambiense*, long established in West Africa, extended its range east and south-east at the end of the last century, due possibly to the travels of European explorers and their porters—the devastating epidemic of 1900 on the north shore of Lake Victoria may have been due to the carriage of the disease to that region by Stanley's expedition going to the relief of Emin Pasha (Nash 1969). Rhodesian trypanosomiasis was first noted further south-east, in Botswana (Bechuanaland) and southern Rhodesia, at about the same time. It spread north, reaching Tanzania about 1910, southern Kenya about 1930, and the north-eastern shore of Lake Victoria about 1940, where another epidemic developed in more or less the same area as the epidemic caused by *T. b. gambiense* half a century before. The northward spread of the acute disease is apparently still continuing, it having been first encountered in Ethiopia in 1967 (Baker *et al.* 1970). It has been suggested (Willett 1956) that *T. b. rhodesiense* evolved from *T. b. gambiense* when the latter was introduced to the savannah areas of south-east Africa (Botswana etc.) with the concomitant possibility of being transmitted by tsetse of the *G. morsitans* group to wild ungulates as well as to man. The 'virulence' of the parasites might have been increased either in some (unexplained) way by transmission through tsetse of this group or, more probably, as a result of selection of virulent mutants which could survive in an ungulate–fly–ungulate cycle; similar mutants could have been suppressed in the West African ecological situation (man–fly–man cycle) for the reasons already mentioned—that they made men too ill to serve as efficient tsetse infectors.

The second hypothesis—the independent origin from *T. b. brucei* of the two subspecies which are infective to man—seems to me the more probable. On this view, a mutant population arose which was capable of infecting man and whose basic cycle was ungulate–fly–ungulate; after centuries (or more) of association with man, selection pressure would operate towards a reduction in virulence to man in areas where direct man–fly–man transmission was possible (because increased parasitaemic life of infected people increases the chance of transmitting the parasite to a tsetse fly) and, in areas where triple contact (between man, fly and ungulate) was rare, the survival of the trypanosome was better served by this trend than by the retention of sufficient virulence to maintain the ungulate–fly–ungulate cycle. Thus *T. b. gambiense* might have been born. In areas where triple contact was common, as perhaps in the East African savannah, selection pressure might well have favoured the retention of sufficient virulence to maintain the possibility of transmission from ungulate to fly, and this would result in the retention of the 'primitive' (i.e. *T. b. brucei*-like) features of *T. b. rhodesiense*.

Ormerod (1961) has pointed out that the virulence of *T. b. rhodesiense* is positively correlated with its degree of northward spread; the most virulent form of the disease known, probably, is that involved in the recent Ethiopian epidemic (Hutchinson 1971), whereas the most chronic is that occurring in Botswana. Geographically intermediate strains are, in general, also intermediate in virulence. This supports the view that prolonged association with man encourages a reduction in the virulence of the parasite; the northward spread may well have been mediated, on the whole, by the ungulate–fly–ungulate cycle, so that each extension into human populations represented a new introduction to man for the strain of parasites concerned. The extent to which adaptation to man and consequent 'disadaptation' to ungulates (if these characters are in fact inversely correlated) proceeded would depend on a variety of local ecological factors, including the relative proportions of man–fly contact and triple contact, and doubtless many others which are unknown.

Another possibility is a polyphyletic origin for *T. b. rhodesiense*: it may have evolved in different places and at different times by similar mutations among separate populations of *T. b. brucei*. However, the apparently fairly orderly time sequence of the northern spread of the Rhodesian disease (see above) suggests that this polyphyletic hypothesis is unlikely to be generally true.

ACKNOWLEDGEMENTS

I am very grateful to Dr D. A. T. Baldry and Mr R. Allsopp for allowing me to cite their unpublished work, and to Mr G. A. Mewis for printing the photographs. This paper is based on a lecture given at the Bernhardt-Nocht Institut für Schiffs- und Tropenkrankheiten, Hamburg.

References

ALLSOPP, R. (1970) *The Population Dynamics and Social Biology of Bushbuck* (Tragelaphus scriptus *Pallas*), MSc thesis, University of East Africa, Kenya

ALLSOPP, R. (1972) The role of game animals in the maintenance of endemic and enzootic trypanosomiases in the Lambwe Valley, South Nyanza District, Kenya. *Bull. W.H.O.* **47**, 735-746

ALLSOPP, R., BALDRY, D. A. T. & RODRIGUES, C. (1972) The influence of game animals on the distribution and feeding habits of *Glossina pallidipes* in the Lambwe Valley. *Bull. W.H.O.* **47**, 795-809

APTED, F. I. C. (1970) in *The African Trypanosomiases* (Mulligan, H. W. & Potts, W. H., eds.), pp. 645-660, Allen & Unwin, London

APTED, F. I. C., ORMEROD, W. E., SMYLY, D. P., STRONACH, B. W. & SZLAMP, E. L. (1963) A comparative study of the epidemiology of endemic rhodesian sleeping sickness in different parts of Africa. *J. Trop. Med. Hyg.* **66**, 1-16

ASHCROFT, M. T. (1959) A critical review of the epidemiology of human trypanosomiasis in Africa. *Trop. Dis. Bull.* **56**, 1073-1093

ASHCROFT, M. T. (1963) Some biological aspects of the epidemiology of sleeping sickness. *J. Trop. Med. Hyg.* **66**, 133-136

BAKER, J. R. (1963) Speculations on the evolution of the family Trypanosomatidae Doflein, 1901. *Exp. Parasitol.* **13**, 219-233

BAKER, J. R., MCCONNELL, E., KENT, D. C. & HADY, J. (1970) Human trypanosomiasis in Ethiopia. Ecology of Illubabor province and epidemiology in the Baro river area. *Trans. R. Soc. Trop. Med. Hyg.* **64**, 523-530

BRADLEY, D. J. (1972) Regulation of parasite populations. A general theory of the epidemiology and control of paracitic infections. *Trans. R. Soc. Trop. Med. Hyg.* **66**, 697-708

BUXTON, P. A. (1955) *The Natural History of Tsetse Flies*, Lewis, London.

DUGGAN, A. J. (1970) in *The African Trypanosomiases* (Mulligan, H. W. & Potts, W. H., eds.), pp. xli-lxxxviii, Allen & Unwin, London

FORD, J. (1971) *The Role of the Trypanosomiases in African Ecology*, Clarendon Press, Oxford.

GEIGY, R., MWAMBU, P. M. & KAUFFMANN, M. (1971) Sleeping sickness survey in Musoma district, Tanzania. IV. Examination of wild mammals as a potential reservoir for *T. rhodesiense*. *Acta Trop.* **28**, 211-220

GEIGY, R., MWAMBU, P. M. & ONYANGO, R. J. (1972) Additional animal reservoirs of *T. rhodesiense* sleeping sickness. *Acta Trop.* **29**, 199

HEISCH, R. B., MCMAHON, J. P. & MANSON-BAHR, P. E. C. (1958) The isolation of *Trypanosoma rhodesiense* from a bushbuck. *Br. Med. J.* **2**, 1203-1204

HOARE, C. A. (1972) *The Trypanosomes of Mammals*, Blackwell Scientific, Oxford

HUTCHINSON, M. P. (1971) Human trypanosomiasis in Ethiopia. *Ethiop. Med. J.* **9**, 3-69

MCCONNELL, E., HUTCHINSON, M. P. & BAKER, J. R. (1970) Human trypanosomiasis in Ethiopia: the Gilo river area. *Trans R. Soc. Trop. Med. Hyg.* **64**, 683-691

MULLIGAN, H. W. & POTTS, W. H. (eds.) (1970) *The African Trypanosomiases*, Allen & Unwin, London

MWAMBU, P. M. (1973) Importance of cattle as natural reservoir hosts of *T. rhodesiense* and resistance to ethidium (homidium bromide) of *T. brucei* subgroup organisms isolated from cattle. *Trans. R. Soc. Trop. Med. Hyg.* **67**, 286-287.

MWAMBU, P. M. & MAYENDE, J. P. S. (1971) Sleeping sickness survey in Musoma District, Tanzania. III. Survey of cattle for the evidence of *T. rhodesiense* infections. *Acta Trop.* **28**, 206-210

NASH, T. A. M. (1969) *Africa's Bane: The Tsetse Fly*, Collins, London

ONYANGO, R. J., VAN HOEVE, K. & DE RAADT, P. (1966) The epidemiology of *Trypanosoma rhodesiense* sleeping sickness in Alego location, Central Nyanza, Kenya. I. Evidence that cattle may act as reservoir hosts of trypanosomes infective to man. *Trans. R. Soc. Trop. Med. Hyg.* **60**, 175-182

ORMEROD, W. E. (1961) The epidemic spread of Rhodesian sleeping sickness 1908-1960. *Trans. R. Soc. Trop. Med. Hyg.* **55**, 525-538

RICKMAN, L. R. (1971) An evaluation of the blood incubation infectivity test (BIIT) as a method for differentiating *Trypanosoma brucei* from *T. rhodesiense*. *Proc. 13th Meeting Int. Sci. Comm. Tryp. Res.*, Lagos, OAU/STRC Publication no. 105, 67-79

ROBSON, J., RICKMAN, L. R., ALLSOPP, R. & SCOTT, D. (1972) The composition of *Trypanosoma brucei* sub-group in its non-human reservoirs in Lambwe Valley, Kenya, as identified by the blood incubation infectivity test (BIIT); with particular reference to the distribution of *T. rhodesiense*. *Bull. W.H.O.* **46**, 765-770

ROGERS, A., KENYANJUI, E. N. & WIGGWAH, A. K. (1972) A high infection rate of *Trypanosoma brucei* subgroup in *Glossina fuscipes*. *Parasitology* **65**, 143-146

SCOTT, D. (1970) in *The African Trypanosomiases* (Mulligan, H. W. & Potts, W. H., eds.), pp. 614-644, Allen & Unwin, London

SOLTYS, M. A. (1971) Epidemiology of trypanosomiasis in man. *Z. Tropenmed. Parasitol.* **22**, 120-133

WEITZ, B. (1963) The feeding habits of *Glossina*. *Bull. W.H.O.* **28**, 711-729

WILLETT, K. C. (1956) The problem of *Trypanosoma rhodesiense*, its history and distribution, and its relationship to *T. gambiense* and *T. brucei*. *East Afr. Med. J.* **33**, 473-479

WILLETT, K. C. (1963) Some principles of the epidemiology of human trypanosomiasis in Africa. *Bull. W.H.O.* **28**, 645-652

WILLETT, K. C. (1965) Some observations on the recent epidemiology of sleeping sickness in Nyanza region, Kenya, and its relation to the general epidemiology of Gambian and Rhodesian sleeping sickness in Africa. *Trans. R. Soc. Trop. Med. Hyg.* **59**, 374-386

Discussion

Njogu: T. brucei rhodesiense has certainly been moving north over the years and is now reaching northern Uganda and Ethiopia (Onyango 1969). The patients we get at the East African Trypanosomiasis Research Organization (EATRO) Hospital are mainly from around the north-eastern shores of Lake Victoria. They are mostly fishermen and many of them know what the disease is. Since the area is in a fly-belt where no human activity is officially allowed, the disease is probably acquired initially from wild animals but subsequently propagated by human–fly–human contact.

We have been trying to find the underlying causes for the existence of endemic areas, where we detect one or two cases a month, and epidemic areas where we detect, say, 70 cases a month. In a sleeping sickness outbreak in Alego Location, Central Nyanza, Kenya in 1966, we found that the flies *Glossina fuscipes* had an infection rate of 0.31 %, which was higher than normal (EATRO 1965). Even more interesting was the finding that cattle had a high infection rate of 21.2%. Tests on human volunteers implicated these animals as a possible reservoir for the disease (Onyango *et al.* 1966). In 1971, during an epidemic at Busesa, Busoga District, Uganda, the infection rate in the flies was found to be 4.5%, the highest ever recorded for *T. brucei*; 25% of the cattle surveyed were infected with *T. brucei* (Rogers *et al.* 1972). One of these isolates from cattle was found to be positive when tested in a human volunteer (R. J. Onyango & P. M. Mwambu, unpublished results). About two years ago, after some tourists visiting Serengeti National Park in Tanzania were infected with sleeping sickness, we attempted to find the focus of the disease. We found no *T. brucei*-infected flies (Moloo *et al.* 1971). Of the isolates obtained from cattle in the area adjoining the park, one was found to be positive when tested in a volunteer and was in fact very virulent, coming up in about four days. Of the isolates obtained from wild game, however, one from a hartebeest was found to be positive in a volunteer, but it was not virulent as it came up after 30 days (R. Geigy & R. J. Onyango, unpublished results). The cattle appear therefore to be a reservoir for *T. rhodesiense*. We think that the flies transmit trypanosomes from game to cattle and that the infection in man generally comes from cattle, not from game. The focus of the infection at Serengeti National Park must have been the area adjoining the park where people keep cattle. A very complicated picture is now appearing. At our field station at Lugala, South Busoga, Uganda, we detect *T. brucei* in cattle newly introduced into the area within the first 14 days. After about three months *T. brucei* disappears and is replaced by *T. vivax*, which is in turn replaced by *T. congolense*. The *T. brucei* must be in the area, in the flies, because when we introduce new cattle, we again pick up *T. brucei*. We don't know whether it is this low level *T. brucei* that comes up during an epidemic or whether newly introduced cattle in an adjoining area act as a reservoir.

Goodwin: Dr Baker's suggestions about the differences between Gambian and Rhodesian sleeping sickness are interesting and probably correct. But a low level of parasitaemia does not necessarily mean that a tsetse fly can't get at the trypanosomes. The tsetse fly is a pool feeder; it makes a hole in a blood vessel; the blood leaks out and mixes with the tissue fluid and the fly sucks up the lot. In *T. brucei* subgroup infections there are far more trypanosomes in the tissue spaces than there are in the blood.

Lumsden: Hornby (1930) and Ashcroft *et al.* (1959) reported that particular animals were hardly ever parasitaemic but that infected flies regularly fed upon them. The other question is whether the proportion of flies found infected by visual means is a reliable indication of the proportion able to pass on the infection. Ward & Bell (1971) recently reported that they found far more frequent infection when they let flies feed on mice than when they inspected the salivary gland visually. They suggested that this might be due to regurgitation of proventricular forms which might have some infective capability. For a review I wrote recently (Lumsden 1972), I could not find any precise experimental information about when infectivity actually appears. It is reputed to appear only with the metacyclic forms in the salivary glands. Something like Ward & Bell's observation might well explain Dr Njogu's finding that although the infection rates are very low in *Glossina* at Lugala, Uganda, cattle can be shown to be infected with *T. brucei* within a very short time of arriving in the area. It would be useful to have some controlled experiments on the infectivity of hosts to flies. This should be easy now that we have standard, laboratory-bred, tsetse.

Trager: The number of trypanosomes actually ingested by a fly does not necessarily have a bearing on how the infection will develop in the fly. One trypanosome in a good physiological state ingested by a fly may be much more significant than a thousand that are not in the right physiological state to get going in that fly. In malaria, for example, the number of gametocytes taken in by a mosquito is not nearly so important as whether these are physiologically good gametocytes.

Lumsden: Epidemiological pictures as described may often be fascinating and fit in with known movements of human populations. An example is the suggestion that the sleeping sickness epidemic around Lake Victoria in the first few years of the century was touched off by Lugard's transfer of troops from the Lake Albert region to central Uganda in 1896. But in situations of this sort we may not be paying enough attention to the wild animal population. Transmission of the organisms could be going on widely among wild animals, and changing contacts between human and animal populations, natural in developing countries, could produce local epidemics and give a spurious impression of the diseases being transferred about the country by movement of the human populations. It is perhaps significant that the place where the disease was reputed to have been introduced into Uganda by Lugard's troops, the South Busoga area, is precisely the same region in which the disease persists today as an animal-based infection.

Baker: Something of that sort may well account for the apparently recent introduction of human infection into Ethiopia. Ward & Bell's (1971) finding to which you referred, Professor Lumsden, might be explained by the fact that some tsetse develop a very low infection of metacyclic forms in the salivary glands, so that the chance of seeing the parasite is negligible. But presumably one metacyclic trypanosome can infect, so perhaps that is an alternative explanation to the heretical one of suggesting infection by gut forms.

Vickerman: Also, when one extracts the salivary gland to examine it for the presence of trypanosomes, saliva rushes out through the cut duct and metacyclic forms may be lost, so that although the fly appears negative on examination, it could have initiated an infection.

Bray: In your Fig. 10, Dr Baker, does the 1940 point, which is at about the northern end of Lake Victoria, refer to the epidemic that occurred during the Second World War?

Baker: Yes, it is the one that MacKichan (1944) wrote up.

Bray: In that case I would suggest that the other dates you gave also refer to epidemics, not endemics, and this may lead to an error. It may also be that the movement of people bringing them into contact with the enzootic may show up as new cases but in fact the enzootic may have existed there all the time. The apparent northward spread may be based largely on epidemics which result from changed climatic conditions and changed tsetse fly conditions and have nothing to do with the enzootic at all.

Baker: I agree that may be so, but why did it happen in this rather orderly sequence?

Bray: I would suggest that it didn't. The Alego outbreak about 1966 in fact occurred in more or less the same place as the 1940 outbreak. If you had put the Alego outbreak in there as well the 'spread' would in fact have stopped for quite a long time in one place and then jumped to Ethiopia. For all we know there may sooner or later be an epidemic down in Tanzania and you could say that it had gone down south again.

Baker: I was trying to put the date of the first recorded appearance. I am not saying there won't be another epidemic afterwards. I know of no evidence of *T. rhodesiense* being found on the northern shore of Lake Victoria before about 1940.

Bray: All I am really saying is that the evidence you have comes from epidemics which have been reported, whereas the enzootics may have been going on without being noticed.

Baker: That is possible but it is an unproven hypothesis.

Lumsden: On the point about whether the epidemic was of *T. b. rhodesiense* type, it is very difficult to know what was characteristic of the epidemic area.

There has been some suggestion (Buxton 1955) that the epidemic around Lake Victoria at the beginning of the century, which is always reputed to have been due to *T. b. gambiense*, was very virulent in certain places. It could be difficult to separate that from the present *T. b. rhodesiense* situation.

Njogu: On Dr Bray's point about epidemics arising from existing enzootics as a result of altered climatic conditions, and about the evidence of northward movement of *T. rhodesiense* being based on reported epidemics, I would like to point out that our evidence was not based on reported epidemics alone, but also from the normal cases that we have detected. Robertson & Grainge (1960) detected the first two cases to be reported north of the lake shores, in Murchison Falls National Park. Other cases have subsequently been reported in North Uganda and Ethiopia (Onyango 1969). Concerning the spread of epidemics, the evidence points to cattle being involved. John Ford (1970) has found that in Bukedi District, Uganda, epidemics coincide with an increase in cattle exports. The inference is that increased cattle numbers lead to encroachment on fly-belts in the search for pastures. As soon as cattle show signs of illness the owners start selling them. By this time the disease in humans will have changed from endemic to epidemic.

Bowman: Is there any evidence in other trypanosomes of this genetic lability which you imply is present in *T. brucei* so that it leads to *T. b. gambiense* and then to *T. b. rhodesiense*?

Baker: I don't know of any, but the whole salivarian section, especially the *T. brucei* group, seems to be an extremely labile set of organisms at present undergoing very active speciation. Most of the other groups seem to be rather stable.

Bowman: I was indirectly asking whether there was any similarity in Chagas' disease with *T. cruzi*.

Lumsden: There are records of the transference of *Trypanosoma lewisi* from rats into other hosts. It is normally a trypanosome that is narrowly specific for the host species, but there are records of its transference to nutritionally deprived mice. If a previously unsusceptible population became nutritionally deprived, the people might then be infected. This could be a factor in the genesis of epidemics, since transmission would then start within the human population.

Bowman: In developing laboratory strains, we are making use of the genetic lability of the trypanosome. I wonder how far removed these domesticated strains are from the wild type.

Baker: A similar transformation may well have occurred with *T. cruzi*. The *Schizotrypanum* species which infect bats look the same as *T. cruzi* but presumably do not infect man. This might be entirely analogous to the *T. b.*

brucei–T. b. rhodesiense situation. Could a *Schizotrypanum* species suddenly mutate into a strain which infects man and become *T. cruzi*?

Zeledón: It is an open field. Someone has to study this further.

Bray: You are talking about a group of organisms which is apparently able to change its genetic characteristics as well. The same may be true of the relapsing fever organisms, which may move from a rodent host via a tick into man, and then may eventually be taken up by transmission from man to man through the louse. There are apparently serological differences between these forms.

Lumsaen: Is it not likely that the bat isolates are infective to men?

Baker: I would have thought not all of them. At least two species of *Schizotrypanum* are found in bats in England (Baker & Thompson 1971) and there are no cases of Chagas' disease in England as far as I know! If either of these two were infective to man there almost certainly would have been some human cases.

Zeledón: In the Americas we can differentiate *T. vespertilionis* and *T. cruzi* on biological and morphological grounds. *T. vespertilionis* normally would not infect a laboratory animal such as a mouse, and would not evolve in triatomine bugs. On the other hand, strains that behave like *T. cruzi* have been isolated from bats in America. Nevertheless, the two are similar in many other ways.

Martinez-Silva: A similar situation to the one reported by Dr Baker in Africa may occur here in the Americas with *T. cruzi* from the northern and *T. cruzi* from the southern part. Man has been here for some 15 000 years, while the armadillo is considerably older. The different habits of the vectors in the northern part of the western hemisphere may be the reason why man has not been introduced into the transmission cycle. On the other hand the invasion by man of the ecotopes of *T. cruzi* in the southern part led to the increase in virulence produced whenever a new host–parasite situation arises. When standard methods are used it is easy to observe marked differences in behaviour of strains from both parts. With *T. cruzi* isolated from a raccoon in Maryland, we never observed parasitaemia in suckling mice, even when they were injected by the intracerebral route. And yet it is clearly a *T. cruzi* parasite, since it is intracellular and induces strong immunity in mice against a lethal challenge after inoculation of 50 000 parasites. One might speculate that the difference in behaviour is due to the increased virulence produced by the introduction of a new host—man—into the parasite's life cycle.

Goble: The virulence for mice or anything else of these strains doesn't really mean very much. With the Maryland (Patuxent) strain with which you had difficulty in mice, patent infections have been produced in mice and other animals (Walton *et al.* 1958) including dogs (Goble 1961). On the other hand, some strains, which in my hands were avirulent in mice soon after isolation, in someone else's hands might show a completely different picture, depending on how they have been passaged over the years, either in culture or in animals (Norman *et al.* 1959). We know very little about what makes these strains behave one way or another.

Peters: What is *T. cruzi*? As was said earlier, after Professor Lumsden's paper, the organisms that cause the leishmaniases are more or less morphologically indistinguishable. We assume that we can pick out a trypanosome and call it *T. cruzi*. I would not be surprised to find that we are dealing with a complete complex of organisms. We shall only be able to separate them if we apply the same sort of biochemical criteria to isolates from different parts of the world that we are using with *Leishmania*. I presume that this is one of the things that Dr Newton's group is going to work on.

Pulido: With reference to what Professor Lumsden said about *T. cardiodamnum* and the *T. cruzi* visceral type, and to Dr Bowman's question (p. 47), a systematic analysis of the characteristics of the several trypanosomes in different parts of Venezuela or even Brazil will substantiate the fact that they produce quite different pathological results. Perhaps those are the type of markers to which Dr O'Daly was referring (p. 24).

Newton: I think you are right. Some very interesting information is emerging from this type of investigation. We have recently been able to detect significant differences in the DNA composition of various species of trypanosomes, including *T. gambiense* and *T. rhodesiense* (Newton & Burnett 1972). So far we have mainly used the relatively crude technique of buoyant density centrifugation to study differences in base composition; this method will only detect differences of about 1%. In collaboration with Professor P. Borst and Dr M. Steinert we are now developing more sensitive methods based on RNA–DNA and DNA–DNA hybridization, which we hope will detect differences in base sequences in kinetoplast DNA. Preliminary results (Steinert *et al.* 1973) look promising and the work is now being extended to include strains of *T. cruzi* and *Leishmania*.

References

ASHCROFT, M. T., BURTT, E. & FAIRBAIRN, H. (1959) The experimental infection of some African wild animals with *Trypanosoma rhodesiense*, *T. brucei* and *T. congolense*. *Ann. Trop. Med. Parasitol.* **53**, 147-161

BAKER, J. R. & THOMPSON, G. B. (1971) Two species of *Trypanosoma* from British bats. *Trans. R. Soc. Trop. Med. Hyg.* **65**, 427

BUXTON, P. A. (1955) *The Natural History of Tsetse Flies* (London School of Hygiene and Tropical Medicine Memoir No. 10), Lewis, London

EATRO (1965) Epidemiological studies on an outbreak of sleeping sickness in Alego Location in Central Nyanza, Kenya. *East. Afr. Trypanosomiasis Res. Organ. Rep.* 1963/64, p. 54

FORD, J. (1970) *East Afr. Trypanosomiasis Res. Organ. Rep.* p. 4

GOBLE, F. C. (1961) Observations on cross-immunity in experimental Chagas disease in dogs, in *An. Congr. Int. Doen ç Chagas (Rio de J.* 1959), **2**, 603-611

HORNBY, H. E. (1930) Control of animal trypanosomiasis, in *XI Int. Vet. Congr.*, John Bale, Sons & Danielsson, London

LUMSDEN, W. H. R. (1972) Infectivity of salivarian trypanosomes to the mammalian host. *Acta Trop.* **29**, 300-320

MACKICHAN, I. W. (1944) Rhodesian sleeping sickness in eastern Uganda. *Trans. R. Soc. Trop. Med. Hyg.* **38**, 49-60

MOLOO, S. K., STEIGER, R. F., BRUN, R. & BOREHAM, P. F. L. (1971) Sleeping sickness survey in Musoma District, Tanzania. II: The role of *Glossina* in transmission of sleeping sickness. *Acta Trop.* **28**, 189-285

NEWTON, B. A. & BURNETT, J. K. (1972) DNA of Kinetoplastidae: a comparative study, in *Comparative Biochemistry of Parasites* (Van den Bossche, H., ed.), pp. 185-198, Academic Press, New York

NORMAN, L., BROOKE, M. M., ALLAIN, D. S. & GORMAN, G. W. (1959) Morphology and virulence of *Trypanosoma cruzi*-like hemoflagellates isolated from wild mammals in Georgia and Florida. *J. Parasitol.* **45**, 457-463

ONYANGO, R. J. (1969) New concepts in the epidemiology of Rhodesian sleeping sickness. *Bull. W.H.O.* **41**, 815-823

ONYANGO, R. J., VAN HOEVE, K. & DE RAADT, P. (1966) The epidemiology of *Trypanosoma rhodesiense* sleeping sickness in Alego Location, Central Nyanza, Kenya. I: Evidence that cattle may act as a reservoir host of trypanosomes infective to man. *Trans. R. Soc. Trop. Med. Hyg.* **60**, 175-182

ROBERTSON, D. H. H. & GRAINGE, E. B. (1960) Cases of *T. rhodesiense* sleeping sickness from Murchison Falls National Park. *East Afr. Trypanosomiasis Res. Organ. Rep.* 1959, p. 31

ROGERS, A., KENYANJUI, E. N. F. & WIGGWAH, A. K. (1972) A high infection rate of *Trypanosoma brucei* subgroup in *Glossina fuscipes*. *Parasitology* **65**, 143-146

STEINERT, M., VAN ASSEL, S., BORST, P., MOL, J. N. M., KLEISEN, C. M. & NEWTON, B. A. (1973) Specific detection of kinetoplast DNA in cytological preparations of trypanosomes by hybridization with complementary RNA. *Exp. Cell Res.* **76**, 175-185

WALTON, B. C., BAUMAN, P. M., DIAMOND, L. S. & HERMAN, C. M. (1958) The isolation and identification of *Trypanosoma cruzi* from raccoons in Maryland. *Am. J. Trop. Med. Hyg.* **7**, 603-610

WARD, R. A. & BELL, L. H. (1971) Transmission of *Trypanosoma brucei* by colonized *Glossina austeni* and *G. morsitans*. *Trans. R. Soc. Trop. Med. Hyg.* **65**, 236-237

Epidemiology, modes of transmission and reservoir hosts of Chagas' disease

RODRIGO ZELEDÓN

Department of Parasitology, University of Costa Rica, and Louisiana State University International Center for Medical Research and Training (LSU-ICMRT), San José, Costa Rica

Abstract American trypanosomiasis is primarily a domestic infection. Its epidemiology is determined by the triatomine vectors involved, the wild and synanthropic reservoirs, and socioeconomic problems, particularly housing. Climate influences the distribution and infection indices of vectors as well as the rate of transmission, and possibly the degree of parasitaemia and pathological changes. Besides the classical contaminative mechanism of transmission by the insect, two other modalities, transfusional and transplacental, are becoming increasingly important. Among animals, several modes of transmission have also been suggested. Of the approximately 92 known species of triatomines of the New World, some 36 have been found associated with human dwellings but only one-third of these are epidemiologically important as vectors. Their importance varies with factors related to the insect (geographical distribution, adaptability to the house, aggressiveness, vectorial capacity, anthropophilism, potential reproductive index), and related to the human environment (type of construction, sanitary conditions of the house, educational level of the inhabitants, climate, natural enemies and competitors). About 150 species of wild mammals from seven orders have been incriminated as reservoir hosts of *Trypanosoma cruzi*. Some of these animals frequent inhabited areas (vectors associated with them may enter human dwellings), so establishing a link between the wild and domestic cycles of the zoonosis.

Chagas' disease, originally an infection of wild mammals of the American continent, with apparently multiple foci, became a zoonosis when the reduviid insect vectors adapted to human dwellings. The disease in man extends from the United States to Argentina and Chile. Autochthonous cases, demonstrated parasitologically, have been reported in all countries except British Honduras, Guiana, Surinam and the Caribbean Islands. A conservative estimate of the prevalence of the infection made by WHO in 1960, based on serological data, indicates that about seven million people were then infected. Not less than 35 million people are exposed to the infection in the New World.

It is important to bear in mind that the 'iceberg phenomenon' applies to Chagas' disease. Only about 1% of those infected present enough clinical symptoms to attract the attention of the physician (Rosenbaum & Cerisola 1961). Since in most instances the 'acute' period will have a mild or silent course and symptoms may appear only after several years, it is understandable why, in some countries, the disease is still underestimated or neglected as a public health problem.

While many patients remain asymptomatic for many years or during their entire lives, Chagas' cardiopathy is the most significant clinical form of the chronic phase. One of its main electrocardiographic manifestations, a complete right bundle-branch block, when present in a young individual from an endemic area, is considered of great epidemiological significance by cardiologists (Laranja et al. 1948; Rosenbaum 1964; Puigbó et al. 1966).

In spite of apparent geographical differences in the magnitude of the pathological lesions, chronic Chagas' disease constitutes in some areas the most frequent cause of heart disease in general (Rosenbaum & Cerisola 1961; Pifano & Guerrero 1963; Puigbó et al. 1966; Kloetzel & Dias 1968). In an urban area of Ribeirão Preto, São Paulo, Brazil, in the group aged 15–74 years 13% of all deaths over a two-year period were attributable to Chagas' disease; in those aged 25–44 years, Chagas' disease was the cause of 29% and 22% of male and female deaths, respectively (Puffer & Griffith 1967).

Lesions of the digestive tract, due to destruction of parasympathetic nerve cells according to Köberle (1970), are common in certain areas of Brazil and have also been reported in Argentina and Chile (Rezende 1968). They appear to be rare in other areas or countries, for reasons that are not yet well understood.

VECTORS

Species

About 100 species and several complexes of subspecies of triatomine bugs have been described so far, most of them (about 92) being found in the Americas. The subfamily Triatominae (family Reduviidae) can be divided into four tribes and 15 genera (this varies according to different authors), as follows:

Tribe Bolboderini
    Genera: *Bolbodera* (1 sp.), *Belminus* (3 spp.), *Parabelminus* (1 sp.) and
        Microtriatoma (2 spp.)

Tribe Rhodnini
   Genera: *Rhodnius* (10 spp.) and *Psammolestes* (3 spp.)

Tribe Cavernicolini
   Genus: *Cavernicola* (1 sp.)

Tribe Triatomini
   Genera: *Triatoma* (approx. 58 spp.), *Panstrongylus* (12 spp.), *Eratyrus* (2 spp.),
         Neotriatoma (1 sp.), *Dipetalogaster* (1 sp.), *Nesotriatoma* (1 sp.),
         Paratriatoma (1 sp.), and *Linshcosteus* (1 sp.).

Only one exotic genus (*Linshcosteus*) and six species (*T. migrans, T. bouvieri, T. pugasi* and *L. carnifex* [Oriental region]; *T. leopoldi, T. amicitae* and *T. migrans* [Australian region]) are found outside the American continent. The cosmopolitan *T. rubrofasciata* has been found in practically every continent (Usinger 1944; Lent 1951, 1953, 1960, 1962).

About 53 species of triatomines have been found naturally infected with *Trypanosoma (Schizotrypanum) cruzi*, but only about 36 are associated with human dwellings. However, no more than a dozen species are epidemiologically important in the transmission of the disease to man.

Life cycle

The length of the reproductive cycle varies markedly among the various species of triatomine. In some species the cycle normally takes five months or even less (*R. prolixus, T. infestans*) under laboratory conditions, so that two full cycles a year can be predicted under favourable natural conditions (Buxton 1930; Perlowagora-Szumlewicz 1953; Hack 1955): in fact, field observations in Brazil suggest that *T. infestans* produces two generations a year (Dias 1955a). In other species, development from egg to adult takes about a year (*T. dimidiata, P. megistus, T. sordida, T. brasiliensis*) but it may also take two years or even more (Usinger 1944; Dias 1955b; Zeledón *et al.* 1970a). Various factors may affect this cycle, such as temperature and the frequency with which the insect takes its blood meal. In natural conditions the lack of aggressiveness of some species and their resistance to starvation for several months are also responsible for longer cycles. The number of eggs deposited by a female during her lifetime averages around 300 for *P. megistus, R. prolixus* and *T. infestans*, 700 for *T. sanguisuga* and 1000 for *T. dimidiata* (Neiva 1910; Uribe 1926; Hack 1955; Hays 1965; Zeledón *et al.* 1970b).

Habits and ecology of the vectors

Triatomine bugs are of sylvatic origin and their degree of adaptation to human habitation varies from one species to another. Some species live exclusively or preferentially in intimate contact with wild animals and never or seldom have contact with man. For example, in North America *Paratriatoma hirsuta* and some members of the *T. protracta* complex are commonly found in nests of rodents of the genus *Neotoma*; in South America, species of *Psammolestes* and *T. delpontei* are found in birds' nests; *Panstrongylus geniculatus* is found in armadillo burrows, while *Cavernicola pilosa* is associated with bats. Some of these, and other species that are also commonly found in natural ecotopes in association with different animals, are common visitors to human habitations, particularly at night when they are attracted by lights. They may or may not breed successfully in their new environment. A few have become so well adapted to the domestic ecotope that today in some areas it is not easy to find them represented in their original natural habitats. Several other species should be considered as having reached different levels of this process of adaptation to human dwellings with different degrees of success, and yet are still well represented in wild ecotopes. Observations in different countries suggest that some species, or even individuals of the same species from different areas, are one or more steps behind in this dynamic and continuous phenomenon of adaptation to human dwellings. Finally, some triatomines are assiduous visitors to houses only in the adult stage but they do not seem to thrive there.

The domiciliary species shelter during the day in areas of houses, depending on the species, which include cracks and walls, roofs and floors, dark corners, mattresses or objects accumulated beneath beds or behind wallpaper or pictures.

Among the important epidemiological factors influencing adaptation and propagation of these insects in human habitations are the following:

(1) Entomological factors: physiological adaptability; alimentary eclecticism; natural aggressiveness; duration of life cycle; biotic potential; protective mechanisms.

(2) Anthropocentric and environmental factors: sanitary conditions in houses; type of construction; educational level of the inhabitants; climatic conditions; natural enemies and competitors.

On this basis, and taking into consideration the practical limitations of a changing dynamic phenomenon, not always with well defined limits, we may classify these insects according to their present relation to human dwellings as follows:

(a) *Insects well adapted to houses, with a very long relationship with man (several centuries), relatively few natural ecotopes and commonly subject to passive dissemination by man himself.* The best example of this adaptation is *T. infestans,* followed by *R. prolixus.* The former species is extremely well adapted to human dwellings, can reach very high densities inside houses (Dias & Zeledón 1955) and occupies a large territory in South America, from around 45° S in southern Argentina, to Lima, Perú in the west and Pernambuco, Brazil in the east. *T. infestans* was introduced by man into these latter areas, the northern limits for the species. Its great adaptability to different conditions (high humidity seems to be the only limiting factor in its distribution) suggests that it will soon spread to other areas. Its preference for man and a few domestic animals has been shown repeatedly by precipitin tests (Correa & Aguiar 1952; Mayer & Alcaraz 1955; Barretto 1968). *R. prolixus,* a common species also highly adapted to human dwellings, is found from northern South America to Mexico. Curiously enough its distribution is interrupted in Panama and most of Costa Rica. In Venezuela, it has been found in natural ecotopes in palm trees, sometimes associated with a migratory bird (*Mycteria americana*) in whose feathers it is possible to find eggs and small nymphs (Gamboa 1962, 1963). Since these birds migrate seasonally to northern areas of Central America they may carry *R. prolixus* to these sites, which may explain its interrupted distribution. Man is the favourite prey, as we have shown by precipitin tests (C. Ponce *et al.,* unpublished data). Though *R. prolixus* prefers thatched roofs of palm or grass where it is camouflaged by its colour, it also breeds well in cane or similar material used for partitions. In Venezuela Gamboa (1963) observed that newly thatched palm huts already contained *Rhodnius* before their human tenants moved in. In houses, *Rhodnius* is very often, like *T. infestans,* numbered in the thousands (Gómez-Núñez 1963).

(b) *Insects adapted or still in the process of adaptation to human habitation, with many natural ecotopes.* In this category we find several species, some of which have been moderately successful in adapting to domiciliary conditions but are in a transitional phase, for they are still found in numerous natural ecotopes. Some species, such as *T. dimidiata, T. sordida* and *P. megistus,* are already widespread in different territories. *T. dimidiata* is found from Mexico to Ecuador, although it does not seem to reach high densities in houses, probably partly because of its long cycle and lack of aggressiveness (Zeledón *et al.* 1970a). Whereas in Ecuador this species exhibits a marked preference for rat blood even inside houses (Arzube 1966), in Costa Rica it more often bites man: the population of insects surrounding houses showed human blood almost as often as that of dogs (the most popular outdoor host), indicating that the insects belong to the same population as that inside the houses (Zeledón et al. 1973).

T. sordida is found in Bolivia, Argentina and Brazil, mainly in peridomiciliary areas, and is a good candidate for replacing T. infestans once this domiciliary species has been exterminated by insecticides (a similar phenomenon is taking place in Venezuela with T. maculata and R. prolixus). P. megistus occupies an important portion of Brazilian territory. Pessôa (1962) advanced the hypothesis that domiciliary and wild forms are genetic variants of the same species produced by mutation of the latter form and he argues that in some areas P. megistus seems unable to adapt itself to conditions in houses. There are several arguments against this hypothesis, such as the eclectic feeding habits of most of these insects (euryphagia) and the ease with which wild strains can be bred in the laboratory, which would indicate a great capacity for adaptation to synanthropic conditions. The difficulty of P. megistus in becoming adapted to human dwellings in some areas is partly because this species requires high relative humidities for breeding, which would explain its limited distribution in Brazilian territory (Deane & Deane 1957; Aragão 1961; Lucena 1970). In our laboratory in Costa Rica we had to increase the humidity of the breeding boxes for this species (and also for Rhodnius pallescens from Panama). In general, relative humidities below 60% (temperatures of 21–28°C) are deleterious for these stenohydric species.

Other examples in this category are: T. phyllosoma, T. maculata, T. carrioni, T. guasayana, T. patagonica, T. brasiliensis, T. rufrofasciata, P. chinai, P. lignarius, P. rufotuberculatus and R. pallescens.

(c) Essentially wild insects, attempting adaptation to human dwellings. In some cases a few nymphs have been found inside houses. Here we include, as examples, some North American species or subspecies such as T. protracta protracta, T. sanguisuga, T. rubida uhleri, T. lecticularius and the South American T. platensis, T. rubrovaria and R. neglectus. All these species still seem to be a step further behind than those of category (b) in their adaptation processes. Occasionally their nymphs are found in houses and it is possible that their relationship with man does not go as far back as that of the other species. In general, the type of house construction and the degree of education of the people, for the North American species, are factors that work against the establishment of an intimate relationship between these insects and man.

(d) Essentially wild insects, whose adults are occasionally found in or around houses, attracted by lights, but apparently unable to thrive in the artificial ecotope. Species whose adults could be found in or around houses and which seem to have difficulty in adapting to this artificial habitat are exemplified by *P. geniculatus*, *E. cuspidatus*, *T. vitticeps*, *T. spinolai*, *T. eratyrusiforme*, *T. nitida*, *P. lutzi*, and a few species of *Rhodnius*. Some of these cannot be maintained in the laboratory indefinitely (Lent & Jurberg 1967, 1969; R. Zeledón, unpublished data). It is not clear whether this is due to a highly specialized food niche (stenophagia) or to the loss of certain symbionts in the laboratory, or to both factors.

(*e*) *Totally wild insects, with habits that will probably make their adaptation to human dwellings difficult and indefinite survival in the laboratory unlikely.* In this category we have different examples, represented by members of the genera: *Psammolestes*, *Cavernicola*, *Microtriatoma*, *Belminus*, *Parabelminus* and *Dipetalogaster*. We know practically nothing about the behaviour and biology of these species but their frequent association with certain hosts and the specific habitats of at least some of them suggest that they are more exacting in some of their biological requirements than the other species.

Transmission by insect

The hypothesis of transmission of *T. cruzi* through the bite of the insect ('anterior transmission') was held for several years after Chagas' discovery, in spite of the fact that Brumpt (1912, 1913*a*) had found metacyclic trypanosomes in the posterior intestine of the insect and had proved their infective capacity. Today it is well established that when the insect contains metacyclic trypanosomes the excreta are the common vehicle of contamination of the mammal, and that trypanosomes can easily penetrate the mucosae and the skin once the natural barriers have been broken by wounds, excoriations, abrasions, punctures and so on.

Whether metacyclic trypanosomes are capable of invading the intact skin is still a moot question. Since data in the literature are contradictory we decided to study the subject in the laboratory. It now seems evident that, at least in mice, under certain conditions metacyclic trypanosomes can occasionally penetrate the intact skin but that blood or culture trypanosomes cannot (R. Zeledón & M. Trejos, unpublished data). Since transmission of *T. cruzi* is of the contaminative and not of the inoculative type, and since the intact skin offers a natural barrier against metacyclic trypanosomes, the possibly irritative character of the saliva could play a significant role in the mechanism of infection. Marked immediate reactions with intense itching, urticaria and erythema have been reported with some species (Africa 1934; Wood 1950; Zeledón

1953; Lumbreras *et al.* 1959; Dias 1968). This immediate reaction is species-specific and indicative of previous sensitization (Zeledón 1953), as confirmed by new xenodiagnostic tests in an endemic area of Chagas' disease in Costa Rica: specimens of *T. dimidiata* (the only species present in the area) feeding on one arm of patients commonly produced an immediate intense itching and urticaria or erythema, or both, while *T. infestans* or *R. prolixus* on the other arm produced no discomfort. Thus this immediate reaction in the sensitive patient may be of significance in the autoinoculation of the parasite.

Transmission without any apparent contact with the insect might be due to the abundance of insects in the rafters or ceilings of houses, when faeces may drop in the eyes or mouth when a person looks up or is sleeping. One such case was described by Romaña in Argentina (1963) and another possible case by C. Ponce *et al.* (unpublished) in Honduras. The frequency and incidence of these cases, particularly in areas heavily infested with *T. infestans* or *R. prolixus*, should be further investigated.

The frequency of the 'eye sign' or 'Romaña sign' seems to vary in different geographical areas, perhaps depending on the insect species. Some species may prefer to bite the face rather than other parts of the human body. For example, *T. infestans* has a marked thermotropism which is less evident in *Rhodnius prolixus* and even less so in *T. dimidiata*. This last species, for example, can feed on the tail of a mouse, which has a temperature of approximately 23°C, whereas hungry *T. infestans* do not easily detect this source but tend to search for their food in the warmer body (R. Zeledón, unpublished). Some species, such as *T. infestans*, are particularly attracted to the face of the victim by the warm air and carbon dioxide exhaled during respiration, as experimentally demonstrated in *T. infestans* by Wiesinger (1956).

Another possible route of penetration is the mouth, when faeces are deposited near the lips. That this is a feasible mode of transmission has been amply proved experimentally with insect trypanosomes (Cardoso 1938; Mayer 1961; Diaz-Ungría *et al.* 1967; R. Zeledón & M. Trejos, unpublished), while infection with blood forms is not always successful in mice (Nattan-Larrier, 1921a; R. Zeledón & M. Trejos, unpublished). Dias (1936) reported that the habit of eating the insect is common among cats and armadillos and we have observed it in dogs. Other mammals such as rats and opossums (*Didelphis* spp.) eat insects avidly in the laboratory, which may explain their high incidence of *T. cruzi* infection in several areas. Furthermore, these and other animals can acquire the infection simply by licking their fur, which is contaminated with insect faeces. Although the importance of oral spread of the parasite in nature is not known, it is apparently a common mechanism of transmission among reservoir hosts and probably in man, as postulated by Brumpt (1913*b*).

When the efficacy of the insect as a vector is being evaluated, the time between a blood meal and defaecation is of utmost importance. Not all triatomines defaecate during or immediately after feeding (Wood 1951); the North American species *T. rubida uhleri* defaecates more rapidly than do *T. protracta*, *T. recurva* (= *T. longipes*) or *Paratriatoma hirsuta*. Dias (1956) confirmed this and also claimed that several South American species are potentially more efficient vectors than the North American *T. protracta*. Pippin (1970) observed that the percentage of defaecations within two minutes after feeding was considerably higher for all stages of *R. prolixus* than for *T. sanguisuga texana* and *T. gerstaeckeri*. Adult males of the latter two species did not defaecate in that period and *R. prolixus* females defaecated more often than the males. In our experiments (R. Zeledón *et al.*, unpublished), we observed that even though the results may vary with sex and instar, *R. prolixus* defaecates sooner and more often within ten minutes after feeding than *T. infestans* and *T. dimidiata*; females defaecate more often than males in the three species, and generally the percentage of *T. dimidiata* that defaecates within this period is lower than in the other two species (Figs. 1, 2).

The aggressiveness of the insect should also be taken into consideration; for example, we found that *T. dimidiata* is very timid in its feeding habits in the laboratory, whereas *T. infestans* and *R. prolixus* are very aggressive.

The ability of these insects to produce infective forms in the faeces is important. Differences between various species may be observed in Wood's (1960) postulated 'infectivity index' (number of metacyclic forms/number of non-metacyclic forms). The factors that intervene in morphogenesis may not be present to the same extent in all species, thus affecting transmission of the parasite; or the intestinal tract of different species of insects may not offer the same physiological conditions to a particular strain of *T. cruzi*. In this respect Dias (1940*a*) first called attention to the greater susceptibility of Brazilian insects to local strains of *T. cruzi* in contrast to the lower susceptibility of *R. prolixus* from Venezuela. The opposite was true when a Venezuelan strain of *T. cruzi* was in use. Ryckman (1965) claims that in North American triatomines infected with North American strains of *T. cruzi* infections are heavier than with South American strains, or *vice versa*. Within the last seven years we have observed (R. Zeledón *et al.*, unpublished), in people from an endemic area of Costa Rica, a few positive cases which were detected only by xenodiagnoses with the local species, *T. dimidiata*, and not with the exotic *R. prolixus* or *T. infestans*. More recently, Cerisola *et al.* (1971), performing xenodiagnoses for three patients with chronic Chagas' disease in Argentina, found

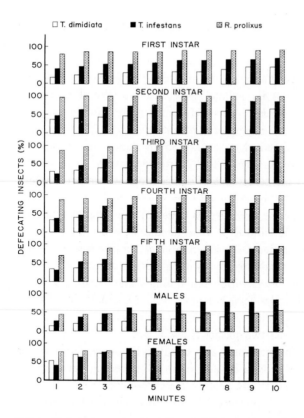

Fig. 1. Cumulative percentage of nymphal instars and adults of three species of triatomines defaecating after a blood meal, based on the first defaecation of 30 individuals in each case.

that the local species of *T. infestans* was more susceptible to the infection, followed by *T. phyllosoma pallidipennis* and *R. prolixus*. Three other exotic species (*T. dimidiata*, *P. herreri* [= *P. lignarius*], *R. pallescens* and another strain of *R. prolixus*) were not infected by blood from these patients.

Blood polymorphism of the trypanosomes has important implications in the development of the parasite and its ultimate transmission by the insect. This polymorphism was observed by Chagas (1909, 1911a), Brumpt (1912) and Mayer & Rocha Lima (1914), but it was not until recently that, as knowledge of the biology of the group increased, physiological implications were attributed to this phenomenon. Da Silva (1959) and Brener (1971) believe that only the stumpy blood forms are capable of infecting the insect. Brener also observed that many insects feeding on vertebrates with predominantly thin blood forms did not acquire the infection. Although several arthropods other than triatomines are easily infected experimentally with *T. cruzi*, and although

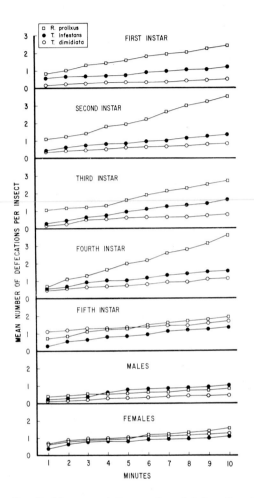

FIG. 2. Mean cumulative number of defaecations in nymphs and adults of three species of triatomines after a blood meal, based on 30 individuals in each case.

bed bugs (*Cimex*), ticks (*Rhipicephalus*, *Amblyomma*) and house flies have occasionally been found naturally infected, their importance as *T. cruzi* vectors in nature has not been established (Pessôa 1958; Neiva 1913; Pinto 1920; Pifano 1941; Diaz-Ungría *et al.* 1967). These are unusual findings and only the triatomine should be considered epidemiologically important in the transmission of the disease.

Although transmission from one insect to another seems unlikely in nature, this should be considered because of its theoretical importance in the perpetuation of the parasite species in the absence of a vertebrate host. Coprophagy in *R. prolixus*, the only species in which it has been confirmed, was first observed by Brumpt (1914). This phenomenon is, however, uncommon and unlikely as a major mode of transmission among insects (Dias 1936; Phillips 1960). Cannibalism or the ability of an insect to suck blood from a companion could be another method of infection. Transmission by this method has been observed in laboratory conditions a few times in South American species (Dias 1936; Phillips 1960); it could not be demonstrated in two North American species (Pippin 1970). Either coprophagy or cannibalism may have been responsible for the infection when groups of *R. prolixus* nymphs were maintained in the same container (Marinkelle 1965). In a similar experiment, Székely *et al.* (1971) were unable to demonstrate transmission among *T. infestans* individuals. Further research would be necessary to clarify the role of these two mechanisms in the perpetuation of the trypanosome among insects of this group, but there is no good support for the idea that these mechanisms could play an epidemiologically important role in natural conditions.

LIVING CONDITIONS, HUMAN HABITS AND CLIMATIC FACTORS

It is well known that Chagas' disease occurs principally in rural areas and that it is closely related to low socioeconomic conditions in endemic zones. Dirty poorly lit houses, built of adobe, mud or cane, with numerous cracks in the walls or partitions and with a large number of accumulated household objects, afford excellent shelter and breeding places for species of *Triatoma* and *Panstrongylus*. *Rhodnius* in general prefers thatched roofs of palm leaves or grass. In certain places such as Costa Rica *Triatoma dimidiata* is frequently found in and around houses with earthen floors or in houses raised above the ground and open underneath: the nymphs can cover themselves with earth and thus stay hidden from predators or other enemies (Zeledón *et al.* 1969, 1973). In Chile, infected *T. infestans* at all stages of development have been found in long-distance passenger trains (Neghme *et al.* 1960).

The tendency of some species to invade buildings in large cities and in rural areas in the process of urbanization warrants comment. This phenomenon is linked to socioeconomic circumstances among certain sectors of modern Latin American cities. Examples of such invasions are those of *T. dimidiata* in the Central American capitals and in Guayaquil, Ecuador; *T. infestans* in some areas of Uruguay and other South American countries; *T. rubrofasciata* in Recife, Belem and Salvador on the coast of Brazil; *P. megistus* is also found in Salvador, Brazil.

Woodpiles near houses provide shelter for species that are still adapting to the domestic or peridomestic environment. In Costa Rica, *T. dimidiata* is commonly found with opossums in hollow trees and is passively brought into the house in lumber or firewood. Opossum blood (and sometimes that of other animals) is not difficult to find in the stomachs of both adult insects and nymphs captured in woodpiles or in and around houses, strongly suggesting an important link between the wild and domestic cycles of the trypanosome, the wild cycle being represented by *T. dimidiata* and the opossum, and the domestic by the same insect and man or other domestic or synanthropic animals, or both (Zeledón *et al.* 1970c, 1973).

The custom of keeping domestic animals such as chickens, pigs, goats or cattle in or near the house often means that large numbers of triatomines that may be associated with these animals can easily invade the living quarters. An interesting situation occurs in Bolivia and southwestern Peru, where guinea pigs are reared inside houses as a food source. The infection rates in these animals varies from 25 to 60%; thus they are the most important animal reservoir in the epidemiology of the disease in these countries (Herrer 1959; Torrico 1959).

Climate may affect not only the distribution of the vector insects but also transmission of the disease. In countries with clearly marked seasons the number of acute cases of the disease increases during spring and summer. Some observations on animals indicate that high environmental temperatures produce lower parasitaemias (Kolodny 1940; Franca-Rodríguez & Mackinnon 1962). Furthermore, at 37°C mice survive ten times longer than control groups and have no parasites in the heart or signs of myocarditis (Trejos *et al.* 1965). Marinkelle & Rodríguez (1968), who have confirmed some of these observations, have also suggested that 'healthy carriers' of *T. cruzi* are more common among people who live in warm climates. Environmental temperature may also influence the infection rates of the insects and, in consequence, the incidence of the disease. Wood (1954) observed that lower temperatures (22–23°C) retard while higher ones (28–34.5°C) increase the number of metacyclic trypanosomes in infected adult *T. protracta*. Neves (1971) claims that at temperatures below 15°C *T. cruzi* does not evolve in *T. infestans*; at between 15 and 22°C no metacyclic forms are produced; and at 36–37°C both epimastigotes and trypomastigotes are absent or scarce. He found that the optimum range for production of metacyclic forms was between 23 and 27°C.

Some species such as *T. infestans* have a great adaptive capacity, behaving like eurythermal and euryhydric species, although *T. infestans* prefers a warm and not too humid climate. *T. brasiliensis* has a marked preference for dry, semi-arid areas (Lucena 1970). *T. dimidiata* appears to prefer dry but not too warm climates and lives almost exclusively along the Pacific coast from Ecuador to Mexico but also penetrates into the mountain chains of Central America. Other species, as already mentioned, prefer moist climates and in general do not tolerate relative humidities of less than 60%. This is true of *R. pallescens* in Panama and *P. megistus* in South America.

OTHER MECHANISMS OF TRANSMISSION

Transmission of the disease by blood transfusion is rapidly increasing. Mazza *et al.* (1936) were the first to call attention to this as a possible mechanism of transmission of Chagas' disease in Argentina. Dias (1945) in Brazil indicated the danger of accepting infected donors, suggesting that they be excluded from blood banks. In 1949 Pellegrino found the first donors who were serologically positive for Chagas' disease, and in 1952 Freitas *et al.* concluded that about 2% of potential donors in São Paulo were infected. At the same time they found positive proof, both parasitologically and serologically, of transmission through blood transfusion in two cases. Nussenzweig *et al.* (1955) demonstrated that the trypanosome can live for several weeks in refrigerated blood without losing its infectivity; that infection is easily achieved, as confirmed in three further cases; and that gentian violet added to the blood in a concentration of 1:4000 killed the trypanosomes within 24 hours without affecting the blood or the recipient. Subsequently, new cases have been reported from Argentina (Cerisola *et al.* 1964), Venezuela (Salazar *et al.* 1962) and El Salvador (Peñalver *et al.* 1965). In 1968, Cerisola found that among more than 50 000 blood donors in Buenos Aires who had probably emigrated from endemic areas of the country, almost 6% were serological reactors. This and other serological data from blood banks in different countries indicate that a serious problem exists. Transmission of Chagas' disease through transfusions, at least in some areas, is probably more common than we realize at present, in spite of possible limitations as suggested by Rohwedder (1969).

Another mechanism of transmission is via a damaged placenta. Carlos Chagas (1911*b*) was the first to suspect this mechanism in an infected infant. In 1916 he also reported finding the infection in at least 14 children under one year of age, most of them from mothers with Chagas' disease or with symptoms attributable to the disease. The intrauterine passage of *T. cruzi* was later confirmed in guinea pigs (Nattan-Larrier 1921*b*, 1928) and in dogs (Villela 1923; Campos 1928) with chagasic endometritis and placentitis. More recently, chagasic placentitis and fetal death have been reported in monkeys of the genus *Saguinus* (Lushbaugh *et al.* 1969). This is a well-known phenomenon in human beings, in whom chagasic placentitis can be an important cause of abortion;

congenital infection of the child, usually born prematurely, is quite frequent. The subject has recently been reviewed by Howard (1962) in Chile and by Bittencourt (1968) in Brazil. The first evidence of transplacental transmission in humans was observed by Dao (1949) in Venezuela and since then a few dozen cases of importance have been reported from Chile, Argentina, Brazil and Venezuela. Bittencourt (1968) believes that infection of the fetus by the mother is more frequent than previously believed, since she found an incidence of 2.66% and 1.29% respectively in 296 and 232 fetal and newborn autopsies taken at random in two maternity hospitals in Salvador, Bahia, Brazil. Howard (1962) reported that, in a clinic for premature children in Chile, one child with Chagas' disease was found among every 200 infants admitted weighing less than 2 kg. Bittencourt (1968) adds that even when a mother has given birth to infected fetuses, she can eventually give birth to a healthy child. More recently, Bittencourt et al. (1972) concluded that the overall incidence of congenital transmission in 500 deliveries studied in Bahia was 2% and when the mothers had Chagas' disease this rate increased to 10.5%; they suggest that similar studies should be done in other endemic areas, with stillbirths, neonatal deaths and placentas, as well as macerated fetuses, being examined. Careful observations on larger groups of mothers from endemic areas will be necessary if a more accurate estimate of the frequency of transplacental transmission is to be obtained. Lactogenic infection is another possible method of transmission that deserves further study. The presence of trypanosomes in the milk of guinea pigs has been reported, by Nattan-Larrier (1913), and more recently in mice by Disko & Krampitz (1971). Mazza et al. (1936) suggested this mode of transmission after they had found trypanosomes in the blood of an Argentinian infant aged three months, born apparently normal; trypanosomes were found in the mother's milk. They also observed the infection in suckling puppies, presumably infected in the same way.

Triatomines were apparently absent in the microepidemic of Chagas' disease in Teutonia, Rio Grande do Sul, Brazil, in which several deaths occurred. Seventeen people acquired the disease at practically the same time and the only thing they had in common was that they were either employed by a rural agricultural school or took their meals there (Guimarães et al. 1968; Silva et al. 1968). Since no insect vectors were found nearby, and the patients had no lesions of primary infection, it was concluded that the infection may have been transmitted through food contaminated by faeces or urine of infected Didelphis spp. found in the vicinity. Shaw et al. (1969) reported what seem to be the first four cases of autochthonous Chagas' disease in Belem, Pará, Brazil, all from the same house, in which no triatomine insects were found. They too suggested that infection might have been acquired orally through contaminated material.

Further observations will be necessary to clarify these points.

Transmission between individual animals of the same or different species is also possible by several routes. Dias (1940*b*) experimentally demonstrated that cats can become infected by eating parasitized mice. In this way, cats, and possibly dogs, could acquire the infection from household rodents and other small wild animals.

McKeever *et al.* (1958) and Olsen *et al.* (1964) isolated *T. cruzi* from the urine of *D. marsupialis*, suggesting that transmission between animals of the same species could be effected through the urine or during mating. The same may happen in raccoons (*Procyon lotor*), since Walton *et al.* (1958) found several infected animals in Maryland, USA, without being able to find the vectors. This brings to mind that Vianna (1911) found *T. cruzi* in the testicles, semen and spermatozoids of infected guinea pigs. In our laboratory, on one occasion, we observed *T. cruzi* in the urine of a mouse and in several instances we confirmed parasitism of the testicles and sperm tubes of mice by tissue forms (amastigotes) of the parasite. We also reported parasitism of the epithelium of the bladder in mice (Bice & Zeledón 1970). Infection with blood trypanosomes through the vagina of female mice has been demonstrated experimentally (Nattan-Larrier 1921*c*). Transplacental transmission seems possible in acutely infected pregnant mice (Apt *et al.* 1968). This mechanism and transmission through the mother's milk should be investigated among wild reservoir hosts.

RESERVOIRS

Dogs and cats are important domestic reservoirs of *T. cruzi*, especially in those areas where *T. infestans* is the principal vector of the disease. Freitas (1950) in Brazil found, by xenodiagnosis, 28.15 and 19.7% infection in 563 dogs and 492 cats, respectively. Neghme & Schenone (1960) in Chile found 9.1% positive cases among 3321 dogs and 11.9% among 1805 cats examined by the same method. Naturally infected dogs and cats have been found in several other countries. The importance of guinea pigs as intradomestic reservoirs in Bolivia and Peru has already been mentioned.

In Panama and Costa Rica the common rat (*Rattus rattus*) appears to be the main domiciliary reservoir. In the former country 57 out of 100 animals were infected (Edgcomb & Johnson 1970), and in an endemic area of Costa Rica 30.6% of 121 rats were infected (R. Zeledón *et al.*, unpublished).

About 150 species or subspecies of sylvatic reservoirs belonging to seven different orders have already been identified as naturally infected with *T. cruzi* or '*T. cruzi*-like' trypanosomes: Marsupialia, Chiroptera, Rodentia,

Lagomorpha, Edentata, Carnivora and Primates (Deane 1964; Barretto 1964).

Some of the sylvatic reservoirs, because of their habits, play an important role in linking the sylvatic and the domestic cycles, in which man is one of the victims. Species and subspecies of *Didelphis* are probably the most important sylvatic reservoirs on the American continent, since the common opossum is a highly prolific animal, with a great adaptive capacity; it is widely distributed from Argentina to the United States and its indices of *T. cruzi* infection are generally quite high (Barretto *et al.* 1964). Apart from the fact that it shows parasitaemia for a long time (possibly throughout its entire life), this marsupial lives in close association with several triatomine species on which it feeds, assuring its continued infection. Nevertheless, parasitaemia of long duration is probably due to the lack of adequate immunological mechanisms in these animals. We have shown persistent positive xenodiagnoses in captive animals that have not been reinfected for periods of over two years (Zeledón *et al.* 1970c) (Fig. 3). In some areas, armadillos constitute important reservoirs, with high indices of infection. Furthermore, one triatomine frequently associated with these animals, *P. geniculatus*, is readily attracted to human habitations by lights, as already mentioned. The part played by other wild reservoirs in the domestic cycle of *T. cruzi* needs to be more accurately assessed (see Fig. 4).

The variety of reservoir hosts and insect vectors involved in the transmission of the trypanosome appears to explain, in evolutionary terms, the variations that are evident among the strains of the parasite. In general, when a 'cruzi-like' trypanosome is found in a wild animal it is identified as *T. cruzi* when it can fulfil a few criteria such as having the typical morphological features and measurements of *T. cruzi*, having its ability to infect laboratory animals, producing amastigotes in a mammalian host, and growing or reproducing easily in common conventional cultures and in triatomine bugs.

CONCLUSION

Although much information on different aspects of American trypanosomiasis has been gathered, particularly within the last two decades, our knowledge of the disease still has many gaps and obscure points.

The difference in the seriousness of the disease in different areas of the New World provides an interesting challenge for researchers. Some of these variations could be due to the lack of strict standardization of working methods, particularly in the selection of population groups to be studied. Nevertheless, the available data indicate that there are marked differences in the character-

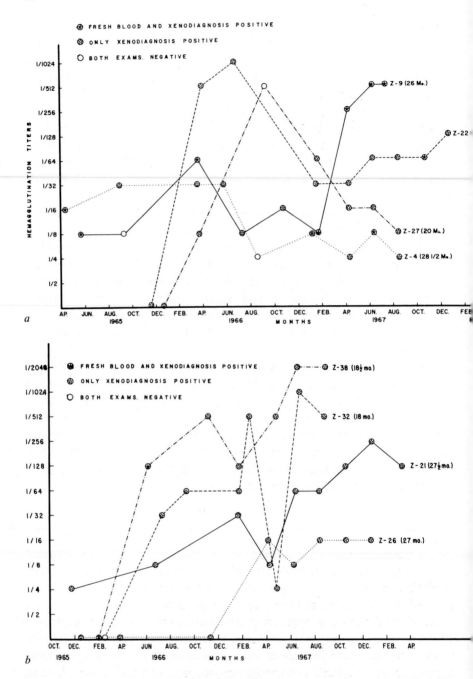

FIG. 3a, b. Serial xenodiagnoses and haemagglutination titres in 8 opossums *(Didelphis marsupialis)* over periods of 18 to 28.5 months after arrival in the laboratory.

WILD CYCLES

DOMICILIARY CYCLES

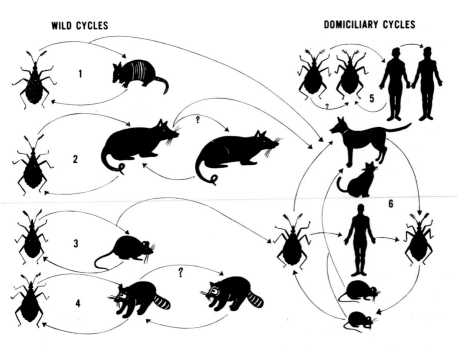

FIG. 4. Wild and domestic cycles of Chagas' disease—modalities and relationships. (1) *P. geniculatus* is often associated with armadillos; adults enter houses, attracted by lights. (2) Opossums (*Didelphis* spp.) are associated with several triatomines and both marsupials and insects visit human dwellings. (3) Rats and other rodents are associated with insects that also fly to houses. (4) Raccoons may be associated with triatomines but, as with opossums, they may transmit *T. cruzi* among themselves without participation of the insect. (5) In the absence of domestic animals there is a cycle between the insect and man. Transmission from one insect to another has been suggested and transmission from man to man is a fact, both transplacentally and transfusionally. (6) Other domestic animals might participate in the cycle and some of them may become infected by eating small rodents.

istics of the disease, for instance in the degree to which it produces cardio-myopathy in areas of Chile or the southern part of Brazil (Schenone & Niedmann 1957; Brant *et al.* 1957) as compared with other places in the latter country and Argentina (Brasil 1968; Rosenbaum 1964) where *T. infestans* is a common vector. On the other hand, gross alterations in the digestive tract, very common in some areas of Brazil (Rezende 1968), seem to be rare or lacking in other areas or countries. To attribute all these differences only to the peculiar characteristics of the strain of the parasite in a particular region seems to be an oversimplification. Nutritional, hormonal, immunological and climatic factors, acting either separately or in conjunction, deserve more attention. Also, comparative studies on strains from different geographical areas, under well standardized conditions (stabilates), are very desirable.

In some areas, the high densities of triatomines in houses suggest that the inhabitants are subject to continuous reinfection; repeated parasitaemia or exposure to new exogenous antigenic challenges may have something to do with the pathological changes in the host.

The application of mathematical models, such as the 'reversible catalytic model' put forward by da Silva (1969), to the epidemiology of Chagas' disease might be useful in the description of the kinetics of the different sources of infection in different endemic areas.

Reliable population estimates and quantitative data on population dynamics, particularly life budget analyses, are necessary to the understanding of some aspects of the transmission and control of the disease. The use of statistical analysis and computer models based on laboratory or field data, as reported recently by Rabinovich (1972) for *T. infestans*, should be extended to other species. Basic laboratory studies on the vectors and reservoirs, completed with quantitative ecological information in the field, are of great importance to a better understanding of the epidemiological factors involved in the natural history of the disease in different geographical areas. Some studies show or suggest important differences between the vectors in their association with man, in relation to the different types of human dwellings, dispersal of the insects within a house, their vectorial capacity and their host preference indices. More information is needed on these aspects, especially under natural conditions. Radioactively tagged material has been shown by D'Ascoli & Gómez-Núñez (1966) to be useful for studies of the dispersal of the insects from a wild habitat to a domestic one and their relationship with the food chain of this new biotope. The method described by Gómez-Núñez (1965) for evaluating the density of insects in a house, based on practical and theoretical principles, also seems promising for this purpose. We still lack information on those physiological factors in the vectors that control the development of the parasite. Basic information is needed about the physiological and biochemical characteristics of the intestinal tract of the triatomines and on the factors that influence development and transformation of the flagellate, as well as on the physiological factors governing adaptation of insects to human dwellings. The basic physiological factors that make insects respond differently to the different stimuli that lead them to a given host should also be assessed more accurately.

Besides the normal mechanism of transmission by the insect, two other modes, the transfusional and transplacental, may be epidemiologically important in the maintenance of the disease. Careful evaluations of the importance of these two mechanisms should be carried out in different countries.

Finally, it is of great importance in the epidemiology of the disease that uniform methods of surveillance should be devised, particularly of the prevalence of the disease in man and for all factors related to vectors and reservoirs.

ACKNOWLEDGEMENTS

This work was supported in part by U.S. Public Health Service Research Grants AI-05938 and TW00148 from the National Institute of Allergy and Infectious Diseases, and by a WHO grant.

References

AFRICA, C. M. (1934) Three cases of poisonous insect bite involving *Triatoma rubrofasciata*. *Philipp. J. Sci.* **53**, 169-176

✕ APT, W., NÁQUIRA, C. & STROZZI, L. (1968) Transmisión congénita del *Trypanosoma cruzi*. III: En ratones con infección aguda y crónica. *Bol. Chil. Parasitol.* **23**, 15-19

ARAGÃO, M. B. (1961) Aspectos climáticos da doença de Chagas II. Area de occurrência do *Panstrongylus megistus* (Burmeister, 1835). *Rev. Bras. Malariol. Doencas Trop.* **13**, 171-193

ARZUBE, R. M. (1966) Investigación de la fuente alimenticia del *T. dimidiata* Latr., 1811 (Hemiptera, Reduviidae), mediante la reacción de precipitina. *Rev. Ecuat. Hig. Med. Trop.* **23**, 137-152

BARRETTO, M. P. (1964) Reservatórios do *Trypanosoma cruzi* nas américas. *Rev. Bras. Malariol. Doencas Trop.* **16**, 527-552

BARRETTO, M. P. (1968) Estudos sôbre reservatorios e vectores silvestres do '*Trypanosoma cruzi*'. XXXI: Observações sôbre a associação entre reservatórios e vectores, com especial referência à região Nordeste do Estado de São Paulo. *Rev. Bras. Biol.* **28**, 481-494

BARRETTO, M. P., SIQUEIRA, A. F., CORRÊA, F. M. A., FERRIOLLI FILHO, F. & CARVALHEIRO, J. R. (1964) Estudos sôbre reservatórios e vectores silvestres do '*Trypanosoma cruzi*'. VII: Investigações sôbre à infecção natural de gambas por tripanosomos semelhantes ao *T. cruzi. Rev. Bras. Biol.* **24**, 289-300

BICE, D. E. & ZELEDÓN, R. (1970) Comparison of infectivity of strains of *Trypanosoma cruzi* (Chagas, 1909), *J. Parasitol.* **56**, 663-670

BITTENCOURT, A. L. (1968) Transmissão congênita da doença de Chagas, in *Doença de Chagas* (Cançado, J. R., ed.), pp. 100-129, Imprensa Oficial, Belo Horizonte, Brazil

BITTENCOURT, A. L., BARBOSA, H. S., ROCHA, T., SODRÉ, I. & SODRÉ, A. (1972) Incidencia da transmissão congênita da doença de Chagas em partos prematuros na maternidade Tsylla Balbino (Salvador, Bahía). *Rev. Inst. Med. Trop. São Paulo* **14**, 131-134

BRANT, T. C., LARANJA, F. S., BUSTAMANTE, F. M. DE & MELO, A. L. (1957) Dados sorológicos e electrocardiográficos obtidos em populaçoes não seleccionadas de zonas endemicas de doença de Chagas no Estado do Rio Grande do Sul. *Rev. Bras. Malariol. Doencas Trop.* **9**, 141-148

BRASIL, A. (1968) Cardiopatia chagásica crónica, in *Doença de Chagas* (Cançado, J. R., ed.), pp. 481-500, Imprensa Oficial, Belo Horizonte, Brazil

BRENER, Z. (1971) Life cycle of *Trypanosoma cruzi*. *Rev. Inst. Med. Trop. São Paulo* **13**, 171-178

BRUMPT, E. (1912) Le *Trypanosoma cruzi* évolue chez *Conorhinus megistus*, *Cimex lectularius*, *Cimex boueti* et *Ornithodorus moubata*. Cycle évolutif de ce parasite. *Bull. Soc. Pathol. Exot.* **5**, 360-364

BRUMPT, E. (1913a) Evolution de *Trypanosoma lewisi, duttoni, nabiasi, blanchardi*, chez les puces et les punaises. Transmission par les déjections. Comparaison avec *T. cruzi*. *Bull. Soc. Pathol. Exot.* **6**, 167-172

BRUMPT, E. (1913*b*) Immunité partielle dans les infections à *Trypanosoma cruzi*, transmission de ce trypanosome par *Cimex rotundatus*. Rôle régulateur des hôtes intermédiaires. Passage à travers la peau. *Bull. Soc. Pathol. Exot.* **6**, 172-176

BRUMPT, E. (1914) Importance du cannibalisme et de le coprophagie chez les Réduvidés hématophages (*Rhodnius, Triatoma*) pour le conservation des Trypanosomes pathogènes en dehors de l'hôte vertébré. *Bull. Soc. Pathol. Exot.* **7**, 702-705

BUXTON, P. A. (1930) The biology of a blood sucking bug *Rhodnius prolixus*. *Trans. R. Entomol. Soc. Lond.* **78**, 227-236

CAMPOS, E. DE S. (1928) Transmissão intrauterina do *Trypanosoma cruzi* na infecção experimental do cão. *An. Fac. Med. Univ. São Paulo* **3**, 35-39

CARDOSO, F. A. (1938) Sur le mécanisme de la transmission de la maladie de Chagas. *Ann. Parasitol. Hum. Comp.* **16**, 341-349

CERISOLA, J. A., LAZZARI, J. D. & DI CARLETO, C. A. (1964) El peligro de la transmisión de la infección chagásica por la transfusión de sangre en la ciudad de Buenos Aires. *Bol. Inf. Dir. Enferm. Transm. Minist. Asist. Soc. Salubr. Publica*, pp. 3-12

X CERISOLA, J. A. (1968) Epidemiología de la enfermedad de Chagas en zonas de alta endemicidad, in *VIII Int. Congr. Trop. Med. Malar.* Teheran, 12 pp. (mimeogr.)

X CERISOLA, J. A., ROHWEDDER, R. W. & PRADO, C. E. DEL (1971) Rendimiento del xenodiagnóstico en la infección chagásica crónica humana utilizando ninfas de diferentes especies de triatominos. *Bol. Chil. Parasitol.* **26**, 57-58

CHAGAS, C. (1909) Nova tripanosomiase humana. Estudos sôbre a morfología e o ciclo evolutivo do *Schizotrypanum cruzi* n. gen., n. sp., ajente etiolójico de nova entidade morbida do homen. *Mem. Inst. Oswaldo Cruz Rio de J.* **1**, 159-218

CHAGAS, C. (1911*a*) Le cycle de '*Schizotrypanum cruzi*' chez l'homme et les animaux de laboratoire. *Bull. Soc. Pathol. Exot.* **4**, 467-471

CHAGAS, C. (1911*b*) Nova entidade morbida do homen. Resumo geral dos estudos etiológicos e clínicos. *Mem. Inst. Oswaldo Cruz Rio de J.* **3**, 219-275

CHAGAS, C. (1916) Tripanosomiase americana. Forma aguda da moléstia. *Mem. Inst. Oswaldo Cruz Rio de J.* **8**, 37-69

CORRÊA, R. R. & AGUIAR, A. A. (1952) O teste de precipitina na identificação da fonte alimentar do *Triatoma infestans* (Hemiptera, Reduviidae). *Arq. Hig. Saude Publica (São Paulo)* **17**, 3-8

DAO, L. (1949) Otros casos de enfermedad de Chagas en el Estado Guárico (Venezuela). Formas agudas y crónicas. Observación sobre enfermedad de Chagas congénita. *Rev. Policlin. Caracas* **18**, 17-32

X D'ASCOLI, A. & GÓMEZ-NÚÑEZ, J. C. (1966) Notas sobre los medios de dispersión del *Rhodnius prolixus* Stål. *Acta Cient. Venez.* **17**, 22-25

DEANE, L. M. (1964) Animal reservoirs of *Trypanosoma cruzi* in Brazil. *Rev. Bras. Malariol. Doencas Trop.* **16**, 27-48

DEANE, L. M. & DEANE, M. P. (1957) Notas sôbre transmissores e reservatórios do *Trypanosoma cruzi* no Noroeste do Estado do Ceará. *Rev. Bras. Malariol. Doencas Trop.* **9**, 577-595

DIAS, E. (1936) Xenodiagnóstico e algumas verificações epidemiológicas na moléstia de Chagas, in *IX Reun. Soc. Argent. Patol. Reg. Norte* **1**, 89-119

DIAS, E. (1940*a*) Xenodiagnósticos seriados em cães infectados com amostras venezuelanas de *Schizotrypanum cruzi*. *Bras.-Med.* **54**, 859-861

DIAS, E. (1940*b*) Transmissão do '*Schizotrypanum cruzi*' entre vertebrados, por vía digestiva. *Bras.-Med.* **54**, 775

DIAS, E. (1945) *Um Ensaio de Profilaxia de Molestia de Chagas*, Imprensa Nacional, Rio de Janeiro

DIAS, E. (1955*a*) Variações mensais da incidência das formas evolutivas do *Triatoma infestans* e do *Panstrongylus megistus* no Municipio de Bambuí, Estado de Minas Gerais. *Mem. Inst. Oswaldo Cruz Rio de J.* **53**, 457-472

DIAS, E. (1955*b*) Notas sobre o tempo de evolução de algumas espécies de triatomíneos em laboratorio. *Rev. Bras. Biol.* **15**, 157-158

DIAS, E. (1956) Observações sôbre eliminação de dejeções e tempo de sucção em alguns triatomíneos sul-americanos. *Mem. Inst. Oswaldo Cruz Rio de J.* **54**, 115-124

DIAS, E. & ZELEDÓN, R. (1955) Infestação domiciliaria em grau extremo por *Triatoma infestans*. *Mem. Inst. Oswaldo Cruz Rio de J.* **53**, 473-486

DIAS, J. C. P. (1968) Manifestações cutâneas na prática do xenodiagnostico. *Rev. Bras. Malariol. Doenças Trop.* **20**, 247-257

DIAZ-UNGRÍA, C., YÉPES, M. S. & TORRES-ARTIGAS, R. (1967) La vía bucal en la transmissión de las tripanosomiasis animales. *Bol. Acad. Cienc. Fis. Mat. Nat. (Caracas)* **27**, 33-50

DISKO, R. & KRAMPITZ, H. E. (1971) Das Auftreten von *Trypanosoma cruzi* in der Milch infizierter Mäuse. *Z. Tropenmed. Parasitol.* **22**, 56-66

EDGCOMB, J. H. & JOHNSON, C. M. (1970) Natural infection of *Rattus rattus* by *Trypanosoma cruzi* in Panama. *Am. J. Trop. Med. Hyg.* **19**, 767-769

FRANCA-RODRÍGUEZ, M. E. & MACKINNON, J. E. (1962) Efecto de la temperatura ambiental sobre la infección por *Trypanosoma cruzi*. *An. Fac. Med. Montev.* **47**, 310-313

FREITAS, J. L. P. DE (1950) Observações sôbre xenodiagnósticos practicados em reservatorios domésticos e silvestres do *Trypanosoma cruzi* em uma localidade endémica da moléstia de Chagas no estado de São Paulo. *Hospital (Rio de J.)* **38**, 521-529

FREITAS, J. L. P. DE, BIANCALANA, A., AMATO NETO, V., NUSSENZWEIG, V., SONNTAG, R. & BARRETO, J. G. (1952) Molestia de Chagas em bancos de sangue na capital de São Paulo. *Hospital (Rio de J.)* **41**, 229-236

GAMBOA, J. (1962) Dispersión de *Rhodnius prolixus* en Venezuela. *Bol. Inf. Dir. Malariol. Saneam. Amb.* **3**, 262-272.

GAMBOA, J. (1963) Comprobación de *Rhodnius prolixus* extradomiciliario en Venezuela (Comunicación preliminar). *Bol. Ofic. Sanit. Panamer.* **54**, 18-25

GÓMEZ-NÚÑEZ, J. C. (1963) Notas sobre la ecología del *Rhodnius prolixus*. *Bol. Inf. Dir. Malariol. Saneam. Amb.* **3**, 330-335

GÓMEZ-NÚÑEZ, J. C. (1965) Desarrollo de un nuevo método para evaluar la infestación intradomiciliaria por *Rhodnius prolixus*. *Acta Cient. Venez.* **16**, 26-31

GUIMARÃES, F. N., SILVA, N. N. DA, CLAUSELL, D. T., MELLO, A. L. DE, RAPONE, T., SNELL, T. & RODRÍGUEZ, N. (1968) Um surto epidemico de doença de Chagas de provável transmissão digestiva, ocorrido em Teutonia (Estrela, Rio Grande do Sul). *Hospital (Rio de J.)* **73**, 1767-1804

HACK, W. H. (1955) Estudios sobre la biología del *Triatoma infestans* (Klug, 1834) (Hem., Reduviidae). *An. Inst. Med. Reg. Tucumán* **4**, 125-147

HAYS, K. L. (1965) The frequency and magnitude of intraspecific parasitism in *Triatoma sanguisuga* (Leconte) (Hemiptera). *Ecology* **46**, 875-877

HERRER, A. (1959) La enfermedad de Chagas en el Perú. Breve revisión de los conocimientos adquiridos hasta 1958. *Rev. Goiana Med.* **5**, 389-409

HOWARD, J. E. (1962) *La Enfermedad de Chagas Congénita*, Universidad de Chile

KLOETZEL, K. & DIAS, J. C. P. (1968) Mortality in Chagas' disease: life-table for the period 1949-1967 in an unselected population. *Rev. Inst. Med. Trop. São Paulo* **10**, 5-8

KÖBERLE, F. (1970) The causation and importance of nervous lesions in American trypanosomiasis. *Bull. W.H.O.* **42**, 739-743

KOLODNY, M. H. (1940) The effect of environmental temperature upon experimental trypanosomiasis *(T. cruzi)* of rats. *Am. J. Hyg.* **32**, (sect. c), 21-23

LARANJA, F. S., DIAS, E. & NOBREGA, G. (1948) O electrocardiograma na cardiopatía crônica da doença de Chagas. *Bras.-Med.* **62**, 51-52

LENT, H. (1951) Triatominae das Regiões Oriental, Australiana, Etiopica e Paleartica, com descrição de uma nova especie (Hemiptera, Reduviidae). *Rev. Bras. Biol.* **11**, 425-429

Lent, H. (1953) Nova especie de *Triatoma* da Região Oriental (Hemiptera, Reduviidae). *Rev. Bras. Biol.* **13**, 315-319

Lent, H. (1960) Sôbre dois pretensos redúvideos hematofagos africanos do género '*Panstrongylus*' Berg, 1879 (Reduviidae, Triatominae). *Rev. Bras. Biol.* **20**, 163-170

Lent, H. (1962) Estado atual dos estudos sobre os transmissores da Doença de Chagas (Relatório). *An. Congr. Int. Doença Chagas* **3**, 739-760

Lent, H. & Jurberg, J. (1967) Algumas informações sobre '*Triatoma spinolai*' Porter, 1934, com um estudo sobre as genitalias externas (Hemiptera, Reduviidae). *Rev. Bras. Biol.* **27**, 273-288

Lent, H. & Jurberg, J. (1969) Observações sôbre o ciclo evolutivo, em laboratorio, do *Panstrongylus geniculatus* (Latreille, 1811) (Hemiptera, Reduviidae, Triatominae). *An. Acad. Bras. Cienc.* **41**, 125-131

Lucena, D. T. de (1970) Estudos sôbre à Doença de Chagas no Nordeste do Brasil. *Rev. Bras. Malariol. Doencas Trop.* **22**, 3-173

Lumbreras, H., Flores, W. & Escallón, A. (1959) Allergische Reaktionen auf Stiche von Reduviiden und ihre Bedeutung bei der Chagaskrankheit. *Z. Tropenmed. Parasitol.* **10**, 6-19

Lushbaugh, C. C., Humason, G. & Gengozian, N. (1969) Intrauterine death from congenital Chagas' disease in laboratory-bred marmosets *(Saguinus fuscicollis lagonotus)*. *Am. J. Trop. Med. Hyg.* **18**, 662-665

Marinkelle, C. J. (1965) Direct transmission of *Trypanosoma cruzi* between individuals of *Rhodnius prolixus* Stål. *Rev. Biol. Trop.* **13**, 55-58

Marinkelle, C. J. & Rodríguez, E. (1968) The influence of environmental temperature on the pathogenicity of *Trypanosoma cruzi* in mice. *Exp. Parasitol.* **23**, 260-263

Mayer, H. F. (1961) Infección experimental con *Trypanosoma cruzi* por vía digestiva. *An. Inst. Med. Reg. Tucumán* **5**, 43-48

Mayer, H. F. & Alcaraz, I. L. (1955) Estudios relacionados con las fuentes alimentarias de *Triatoma infestans* (Hem., Reduviidae). *An. Inst. Med. Reg.* **4**, 195-201

Mayer, M. M. & Rocha Lima, H. da (1914) Zum Verhaltem von *Schizotrypanum cruzi* in Warmblütern und Arthropoden. *Arch. Schiffs- & Tropenhyg.* **18**, 101-136

Mazza, S., Montaña, A., Benitez, C. & Janzi, E. Z. (1936) Investigaciones sobre la enfermedad de Chagas. VI: Transmisión del *Schizotrypanum cruzi* al niño por leche de la madre con enfermedad de Chagas. *MEPRA* (Argentina), Publ. 28, 41-53

McKeever, S., Gorman, G. W. & Norman, L. (1958) Occurrence of a *Trypanosoma cruzi*-like organism in some mammals from southwestern Georgia and northwestern Florida. *J. Parasitol.* **44**, 583-587

Nattan-Larrier, L. (1913) Sur le passage des trypanosomes dans le lait. *Rev. Pathol. Comp. Hyg. Gén.* **3**, 282-285

Nattan-Larrier, L. (1921a) Infections à trypanosomes et voies de pénétration des virus. *Bull. Soc. Pathol. Exot.* **14**, 537-542

Nattan-Larrier, L. (1921b) Hérédité des infections expérimentales à *Schizotrypanum cruzi*. *Bull. Soc. Pathol. Exot.* **14**, 232-238

Nattan-Larrier, L. (1921c) La schizotrypanosomiase américaine peut-elle être transmise par contagion génitale. *C. R. Séances Soc. Biol. Fil.* **84**, 773-775

Nattan-Larrier, L. (1928) L'hérédité de la maladie de Chagas. *Bull. Acad. Méd. (Paris)* **99**, 98-99

Neghme, A. & Schenone, H. (1960) Resumen de veinte años de investigación sobre la enfermedad de Chagas en Chile. *Rev. Med. Chile* **88**, 82-93

Neghme, A., Schenone, H., Reyes, H., Carrasco, J. & Alfaro, E. (1960) Hallazgo de *Triatoma infestans* en vagones de ferrocarril. *Bol. Chil. Parasitol.* **15**, 86-87

Neiva, A. (1910) Informações sôbre a biolojia do *Conorhinus megistus* Burm. *Mem. Inst. Oswaldo Cruz Rio de J.* **2**, 206-212

Neiva, A. (1913) Transmissão do *Trypanosoma cruzi* pelo *Rhipicephalus sanguineus* (Latr.). *Bras.-Med.* **27**, 498

NEVES, D. P. (1971) Influencia da temperatura na evolução do *Trypanosoma cruzi* em triatomíneos. *Rev. Inst. Med. Trop. São Paulo* **13**, 155-161

NUSSENZWEIG, V., AMATO NETO, V., FREITAS, J. L. P. DE, SONNTAG, R. & BIANCALANA, A. (1955) Moléstia de Chagas em bancos de sangue. *Rev. Hosp. Clin. Fac. Med. Univ. São Paulo* **10**, 265-283

OLSEN, P. F., SHOEMAKER, J. P., TURNER, H. F. & HAYS, K. L. (1964) Incidence of *Trypanosoma cruzi* (Chagas) in wild vectors and reservoirs in East-Central Alabama. *J. Parasitol.* **50**, 599-603

PELLEGRINO, J. (1949) Transmissão da doença de Chagas pela transfusão de sangue. Primeiras comprovacões sorologicas em doadores e em candidatos a doadores de sangue. *Rev. Bras. Med.* **6**, 297-301

PEÑALVER, L. M., RODRÍGUEZ, M. I., BLOCH, M. & SANCHO, G. (1965) Tripanosomiasis en El Salvador. *Arch. Col. Med. El Salv.* **18**, 97-134

PERLOWAGORA-SZUMLEWICZ, A. (1953) Ciclo evolutivo do *Triatoma infestans* em condições de laboratorio. *Rev. Bras. Malariol. Doencas Trop.* **5**, 35-47

PESSÔA, S. B. (1958) *Parasitología Medica*, 5th edn, Livraria Ed. Guanabara, Rio de Janeiro

PESSÔA, S. B. (1962) Domiciliação dos triatomíneos e epidemiología da doença de Chagas. *Arq. Hig. Saúde Publica (São Paulo)* **27**, 161-171

PHILLIPS, N. R. (1960) Experimental studies on the quantitative transmission of *Trypanosoma cruzi*: aspects of the rearing, maintenance and testing of vector material, and of the origin and course of infection in the vector. *Ann. Trop. Med. Parasitol.* **54**, 397-414

PIFANO, F. (1941) Parasitismo natural de *Amblyomma longyrostre* Koch, 1844 por *Schizotrypanum cruzi* Chagas, 1909. *Gac. Med. Caracas* **48**, 288-289

PIFANO, F. C. & GUERRERO, L. (1963) Campaña contra la enfermedad de Chagas en Venezuela. Aspectos metodológicos, encuestas epidemiológicas de reconocimiento en escala nacional e investigación científica. *Bol. Ofic. Sanit. Panamer.* **54**, 396-411

PINTO, C. (1920) Sôbre à transmissão do *Trypanosoma cruzi* (Chagas, 1909) do tatú ão cobayo pela picada de Ixodides. *Arch. Parana. Med.* **1**, 165-170

PIPPIN, W. F. (1970) The biology and vector capability of *Triatoma sanguisuga texana* Usinger and *Triatoma gerstaeckeri* (Stål) compared with *Rhodnius prolixus* (Stål) (Hemiptera: Triatominae). *J. Med. Entomol.* **7**, 30-45

PUFFER, R. R. & GRIFFITH, G. W. (1967) Patterns of urban mortality. *Pan. Am. Health Organ. Sci. Publ.* no. 151

PUIGBÓ, J. J., NAVA-RHODE, J. R., GARCÍA-BARRIOS, H., SUÁREZ, J. A. & GIL-YÉPEZ, C. (1966) Clinical and epidemiological study of chronic heart involvement in Chagas' disease. *Bull. W.H.O.* **34**, 655-669

RABINOVICH, J. E. (1972) Vital statistics of Triatominae (Hemiptera: Reduviidae) under laboratory conditions. I: *Triatoma infestans* Klug. *J. Med. Entomol.* **9**, 351-370

REZENDE, J. M. DE (1968) Manifestações digestivas da molestia de Chagas, in *Doença de Chagas* (Cançado, J. R., ed.), pp. 442-480, Imprensa Oficial, Belo Horizonte, Brazil

ROHWEDDER, R. W. (1969) Infección chagásica en dadores de sangre y las probabilidades de transmitirla por medio de la transfusión. *Bol. Chil. Parasitol.* **24**, 88-93

ROMAÑA, C. (1963) *Enfermedad de Chagas*, Lopez Libreros, Buenos Aires

ROSENBAUM, M. B. (1964) Chagasic myocardiopathy. *Prog. Cardiovasc. Dis.* **7**, 199-225

ROSENBAUM, M. B. & CERISOLA, J. A. (1961) Epidemiología de la enfermedad de Chagas en la República Argentina. *Hospital (Rio de J.)* **60**, 55-100

RYCKMAN, R. E. (1965) Epizootiology of *Trypanosoma cruzi* in southwestern North America. Part V: Host parasite specificity between *Trypanosoma cruzi* and Triatominae (Kinetoplastida: Trypanosomatidae) (Hemiptera: Triatominae). *J. Med. Entomol.* **2**, 96-99

SALAZAR, J., ARENDS, T. & MAEKELT, G. A. (1962) Comprobación en Venezuela de la transmisión del *Schizotrypanum cruzi* por transfusión de sangre. *Arch. Venez. Med. Trop. Parasitol. Med.* **4**, 355-364

SCHENONE, H. & NIEDMANN, G. (1957) Nuevos aportes al estudio de la cardiopatía chagásica crónica en Chile. *Bol. Chil. Parasitol.* **12**, 2-7

SHAW, J. J., LAINSON, R. & FRAIHA, H. (1969) Considerações sobre a epidemiologia dos primeiros casos autóctones de doença de Chagas registrados em Belem, Para, Brasil. *Rev. Saúde Publica* **3**, 153-157

SILVA, G. R. DA (1969) Sôbre o modelo catalítico reversivel aplicado ao estudo da cinética da infecção chagásica. *Rev. Saúde Publica* **3**, 23-29

SILVA, L. H. P. DA (1959) Observações sôbre o ciclo evolutivo do *Trypanosoma cruzi*. *Rev. Inst. Med. Trop. São Paulo* **1**, 99-118

SILVA, N. N., CLAUSELL, D. T., NÓLIBOS, H., MELLO, A. L. DE, OSSANAI, J., RAPONE, T. & SNELL, T. (1968) Surto epidémico de doença de Chagas com provável contaminação oral. *Rev. Inst. Med. Trop. São Paulo* **10**, 265-276

SZÉKELY, R., ROJO, M. & REYES, H. (1971) Estudio sobre transmisión directa de *Trypanosoma cruzi* entre ninfas de *Triatoma infestans*. *Bol. Chil. Parasitol.* **26**, 17-19

TORRICO, R. A. (1959) Enfermedad de Chagas en Bolivia. *Rev. Goiana Med.* **5**, 375-387

TREJOS, A., URQUILLA, M. A. DE & PAREDES, A. R. (1965) Influence of environmental temperature on the evolution of experimental Chagas' disease in mice. *Prog. Protozool. (Abstr. II Int. Conf. Protozool.)* p. 144, I.C.S. no. 91, Excerpta Medica, Amsterdam

URIBE, C. (1926) On the biology and life history of *Rhodnius prolixus* Stähl. *J. Parasitol.* **13**, 129-136

USINGER, R. L. (1944) The triatominae of North and Central America and the West Indies and their public health significance. *Public Health Bull. (U.S. Public Health Serv.)*, no. 288

VIANNA, G. (1911) Contribuição para o estudo da anatomia patolojica da 'molestia de Carlos Chagas'. *Mem. Inst. Oswaldo Cruz Rio de J.* **3**, 276-294

VILLELA, E. (1923) A transmissão intra-uterina da molestia de Chagas. Encephalite congênita pelo *Trypanosoma cruzi* (Nota previa). *Folha Med.* **4**, 41-43

WALTON, B. C., BAUMAN, P. M., DIAMOND, L. S. & HERMAN, C. M. (1958) The isolation and identification of *Trypanosoma cruzi* from raccoons in Maryland. *Am. J. Trop. Med. Hyg.* **7**, 603-610

WIESINGER, D. (1956) Die Bedeutung der Umweltfaktoren für den Saugakt von *Triatoma infestans*. *Acta Trop.* **13**, 97-141

WOOD, S. F. (1950) Allergic sensitivity to the saliva of the western cone-nosed bug. *Bull. S. Calif. Acad. Sci.* **49**, 71-74

WOOD, S. F. (1951) Importance of feeding and defecation times of insect vectors in transmission of Chagas' disease. *J. Econ. Entomol.* **44**, 52-54

WOOD, S. F. (1954) Environmental temperature as a factor in development of *Trypanosoma cruzi* in *Triatoma protracta*. *Exp. Parasitol.* **3**, 227-233

WOOD, S. F. (1960) A potential infectivity index for *Triatoma* harboring *Trypanosoma cruzi* Chagas. *Exp. Parasitol.* **10**, 356-365

WORLD HEALTH ORGANIZATION (1960) *Chagas' disease. Report of a Study Group.* W.H.O. Tech. Rep. Ser. no. 202

ZELEDÓN, R. (1953) Manifestaciones alérgicas consecuentes a la picada de triatomas (Hemiptera, Reduviidae). *Rev. Biol. Trop.* **1**, 17-20

ZELEDÓN, R., ZÚÑIGA, A. & SWARTZWELDER, J. C. (1969) The camouflage of *Triatoma dimidiata* and the epidemiology of Chagas' disease in Costa Rica. *Bol. Chil. Parasitol.* **24**, 106-108

ZELEDÓN, R., GUARDIA, V. M., ZÚÑIGA, A. & SWARTZWELDER, J. C. (1970a) Biology and ethology of *Triatoma dimidiata* (Latreille, 1811). I: Life cycle, amount of blood ingested, resistance to starvation and size of adults. *J. Med. Entomol.* **7**, 313-319

ZELEDÓN, R., GUARDIA, V. M., ZÚÑIGA, A. & SWARTZWELDER, J. C. (1970b) Biology and ethology of *Triatoma dimidiata* (Latreille, 1811). II: Life span of adults and fecundity and fertility of females. *J. Med. Entomol.* **7**, 462-469

ZELEDÓN, R., SOLANO, G., SÁENZ, G. & SWARTZWELDER, J. C. (1970c) Wild reservoirs of

Trypanosoma cruzi with special mention of the opossum, *Didelphis marsupialis*, and its role in the epidemiology of Chagas' disease in an endemic area of Costa Rica. *J. Parasitol.* **56**, 38

ZELEDÓN, R., SOLANO, G., ZÚÑIGA, A. & SWARTZWELDER, J. C. (1973) Biology and ethology of *Triatoma dimidiata* (Latreille, 1811). III: Habitat and blood sources. *J. Med. Entomol.* **10**, 363-370

Discussion

Pifano: I would like to present some results from field investigations of natural infection, by *Schizotrypanum cruzi*, of wild animals living in the palm tree *Attalea humboldtiana* in the Naranjos valley, Carabobo State, Venezuela. The infection is maintained by the wild ecological system of *Rhodnius prolixus*, which became adapted to huts ('ranchos') when people began to use the palm tree in the construction of the roofs. The area is one where *R. prolixus* is the main vector and the epidemiology here is not necessarily the same as in other regions where the biology of the vectors is different.

Forty-five palm trees were studied in relation to their microclimate and to the capture of triatomids and wild animals in the biotope, so that the ecological relationships might be better understood. Colonies of *R. prolixus* were found in 40 palm trees (88.88%), and in three trees they were in association with *Triatoma maculata*. Of 465 samples, 427 were *R. prolixus* (92.22%) and 36 *T. maculata* (7.78%). In 435 samples of *R. prolixus*, 238 (51.40%) had trypanosomes in the intestinal lumen; 207 of these (86.99%) had *S. cruzi*, 26 had *Trypanosoma rangeli* (10.92%) and five (2.10%) had both *S. cruzi* and *T. rangeli*. Of the 36 *T. maculata*, five were infected with *S. cruzi* (16.66%).

The source of food of the triatomids captured in the palm trees was investigated with the precipitin test, using the serum of rabbits previously injected with blood from animals that live in the palm trees, especially *Didelphis marsupialis* ('rabipelado'), *Calluromys philander* ('comadreja'), *Rattus rattus frugivorus* ('rata de monte'), *Oecomys (Oryzomys) concolor* ('ratón montañero'), lizards and birds. Of the 278 samples of *R. prolixus* investigated, 68 were positive in response to the blood of *C. philander* (24.42%), 66 to the blood of *D. marsupialis* (20.10%), 34 to the blood of *O. (O.) concolor* (12.23%), 22 to the blood of the lizard (7.94%), 16 to the blood of birds (5.79%), 12 to the blood of *R.r. frugivorus* (4.30%) and none to human blood (0%). In some samples the precipitin test showed combined sources of feeding.

Two hundred and fourteen animals captured in the palm trees were investigated by xenodiagnostic tests and blood cultures which showed that 116 (54.20%) were infected with trypanosomes, including: 52 *D. marsupialis* out of

70 examined (74.28%); 60 *C. philander* out of 139 examined (43.23%); three *O. (O.) concolor* out oft hree examined (100%) and one *R.r. frugivorus* out of two examined (50%). The distribution of the types of trypanosomes among these animals was as follows: of 52 *D. marsupialis*, 45 had *S. cruzi* (86.53%), five had *T. rangeli* (9.61%) and two had both *S. cruzi* and *T. rangeli* (3.84%). Of 139 *C. philander*, 60 had *S. cruzi* (43.23%). The three *O. (O.) concolor* all had *S. cruzi* and of the two *R.r. frugivorus* one had *S. cruzi*. When laboratory animals were inoculated with blood or intestinal material of *R. prolixus* used in the xenodiagnostic test, a strain of *S. cruzi* which we called *Calluromys LNX* was isolated from the *C. philander*. This strain has a high virulence and infectivity and is cardiotrophic.

These results show that in the palm tree the ecological relationship between *R. prolixus* and its feeding sources, especially *D. marsupialis* and *C. philander*, is stable and permits the existence of zoonotic foci transferable to the rural medium by man when he uses the palm tree for building his huts. The wild ecosystem of *R. prolixus* is perfectly adapted to the hut, in which it transmits the infection to man and domestic animals. Transference of Chagas' disease from its wild natural foci to rural human communities is further ensured by the incursion of *D. marsupialis* into the houses. This animal has epidemiological importance since it can live in the palm tree roofs of the huts and act as a source of food for *R. prolixus* in its domestic ecosystem. The degree of parasitaemia is low but the parasite remains in the blood for long periods. This makes the animal an important source of *S. cruzi* for domestic and wild triatomids. In consequence, the enzootic potential of *S. cruzi* through *Rhodnius–Didelphis* is increased and the epidemiological chain is reinforced.

The Naranjaros valley has many small villages in between forests of palm trees, with a total population of 2000 people who work in agriculture and cattle raising. Complement fixation tests with *S. cruzi* as the antigen, xenodiagnosis, clinical and electrocardiographic examinations were carried out. Of the 1000 people aged between ten and 43 years who were examined, 709 showed a positive complement fixation test (70.9%) and 213 (21.3%) were positive in xenodiagnostic tests. The behaviour of the parasite was studied in 219 people by means of blood cultures and periodic xenodiagnosis and the appearance of myocardial damage was measured over several years. Among these 219 people, 128 showed trypanosomes in the blood (58.44%): 126 had *S. cruzi* (98.43%) and two *T. rangeli* (1.56). In the first cardiovascular survey, 17% presented with chronic myocarditis and seven years later 39.4% had chronic myocarditis.

Thirty-eight dogs in the area were also examined by means of xenodiagnosis and blood cultures and 16 (42.10%) had trypanosomes: ten had *S. cruzi* (62.50%), two *T. rangeli* (12.50%) and four (25%) had both *S. cruzi* and *T. rangeli*.

The finding that out of 219 people with positive complement fixation tests, 128 (58.44%) had trypanosomes in the peripheral blood points to the importance of man as a source of infection in the domestic ecosystem of *R. prolixus*. This, and the high degree of natural infection of *R. prolixus* captured in the rural houses, are elements that make the Naranjaros valley an endemic one. The dog is also an important epidemiological factor.

Lumsden: Do the skin hypersensitivity reactions seen with *Triatoma dimidiata* affect the acquisition of infection, Professor Zeledón?

Zeledón: There is no clear evidence that they play an important role. On occasions the insect may defaecate two or three inches away from the place where it has bitten, and when a person has been sensitized to the saliva of the insect, itching starts immediately. For xenodiagnosis we use three boxes, each holding ten insects of three different species. If we put the box with *T. dimidiata* on the right arm and the other two boxes with *T. infestans* or *Rhodnius prolixus* (exotic species) on the left arm, the person immediately feels the itching only in the right arm. So I believe that this hypersensitivity reaction, which is species-specific, sometimes plays an important role in the auto-inoculation of the parasite.

Lumsden: Wasn't there a suggestion that the people in Teutonia had been dosed with corticosteroids (Haase & De Lima 1967; Di Primio 1965), which may have brought to light a subclinical infection with *T. cruzi* which they all had?

Zeledón: Yes, perhaps something else may have been involved in that microepidemic and I want to leave a big question mark there.

Bowman: Your suggestion that blood transfusions increase the risk of infection is interesting. Is it possible to use blood safely after it has been stored for seven to ten days to let *T. cruzi* die off?

Zeledón: The trypanosomes can survive for months in the refrigerator and remain quite infective. In some areas of Argentina, the complement fixation test indicates that up to 70% of donors may harbour parasites in their blood. There, they now add crystal violet, 1:4000, to the blood in order to sterilize it and there is very little risk to the person being transfused.

Maekelt: One problem for blood banks is that apparently healthy people may have trypanosomes in their blood for many years. We have seen some people who had lived for more than 23 years outside the endemic zones and yet were still positive on xenodiagnosis. Another problem, as already mentioned, is that trypomastigotes survive in samples of stored blood. Many years ago Sullivan (1944) showed that trypanosomes may survive in citrated blood for more than 300 days. We found we could recover added epimastigotes from stored blood after more than three weeks, which indicates that refrigerated blood may be an excellent culture medium (Maekelt & Hidalgo 1958).

Skin hypersensitivity is a serious problem with *R. prolixus*. In follow-up studies using xenodiagnosis we saw not only local skin reactions but also spreading of cutaneous hypersensitivity over wide areas. This occurs especially when we use 40, 80 or more bugs for xenodiagnosis in follow-up studies. In one case we observed a very serious clinical picture of a general hypersensitivity reaction, with bronchospasm, glottal oedema, bronchial asthma and cerebral oedema. Thus, the use of *R. prolixus* for xenodiagnosis in follow-up studies is not recommended. We can avoid these hypersensitivity reactions by using *T. infestans*, with which we have never seen any reactions, or by using *R. prolixus* for so-called 'artificial xenodiagnosis', practised with citrated venous blood in a beaker closed by a dialysis membrane.

Goble: If the medium is sterile, such as in a blood culture or something of that sort, I believe the organism will last not only for months but actually for years. Many of us must have put blood cultures at the back of a desk and found living parasites in them after at least a couple of years (Price *et al.* 1964). These are culture forms but if one puts bloodstream forms into a supportive medium, one will eventually have culture forms anyway.

Baker: Packchanian (1943) has recorded that cultures of *T. cruzi* lasted up to six years.

Professor Zeledón, you suggested that some mammalian reservoir hosts may become infected by eating bugs. This route of infection may be much more important than has previously been thought. For example, lions in Africa may become infected by eating other infected mammals (Baker 1968). Certainly with some trypanosomes of birds, the host can become infected by eating the vector (Baker 1956; Cotton 1970). Has this been conclusively shown for *T. cruzi*?

Zeledón: Insect forms easily infect mammals that eat them. We have observed many times in the laboratory that opossums eat these insects avidly, and so do cats and dogs. Blood forms and insect forms differ greatly in their infectivity by mouth. In current experiments we are having problems in infecting dogs and mice with blood forms by mouth, although with metacyclic forms it is very easy. We are now trying to quantitate this.

In my paper I suggest that the annual migration of *Mycteria americana* from Venezuela to Central America may explain the gap in the geographical distribution of *R. prolixus*. I wonder if this makes sense, or has anyone another hypothesis?

Maekelt: Why is *R. prolixus* *not* found south of the equator? If I understand it correctly, *M. americana* migrates not to Central America but to the south, that means to the northern part of Brazil. If that is so, it should be easier to find *R. prolixus* south of the equator, for instance in the northern part of Brazil, than in Central America.

Zeledón: I read the literature before I was tempted to suggest that Central America was infested by *R. prolixus* from the South American focus. I found that *M. americana* migrations range from northern Brazil to Central America. In fact *R. prolixus* has been found wild in northern Brazil.

Peters: In the United States it is almost routine now that if a small outbreak of malaria occurs, one immediately tries to establish whether the people affected happen to be drug addicts who are sharing needles. Has any outbreak of Chagas' disease been found to be due to sharing of needles among drug addicts, or has this even been taken into consideration in these rather odd outbreaks?

Newton: We should certainly bear that possibility in mind.

Maekelt: Seroepidemiological surveys in Venezuela have shown that in seven different rural endemic zones from 1% to 55% of the apparently healthy non-selected population were carriers of *T. cruzi* antibodies (6110 [41.3%] of 14 753 people from 11 zones gave positive reactions in complement fixation tests). An increasing prevalence of carriers was found with age, ranging from 15.1% of those aged 5–14 years (459 out of 3014) up to 78.7% of those aged 35–44 years (1050 of 1343) (Maekelt 1971). Seroepidemiological surveys showed that the minimum prevalence (calculated on the basis of a three-time standard deviation) of *T. cruzi* antibody carriers (17 066 apparently healthy soldiers aged 18–20 years) was as follows: 12–17% in soldiers from the states of Portuguesa, Cojedes, Yaracuy and Carabobo, 5–10% in those from the states of Lara, Trujillo, Guárico, Aragua, Miranda, Anzoátegui and Sucre, and 2–5% in those from the states of Táchira, Mérida, Falcón and Monagas (Mora 1964).

These results on the prevalence of *T. cruzi* antibody carriers accord with the degree of infestation of houses with the main transmitting vector, *Rhodnius prolixus*, and with the areas where bugs are most highly infected with *T. cruzi*.

It is to be expected that the epidemiological data related to the prevalence of *T. cruzi* infection in man will change in the course of time, due to population migration and dynamics, and especially to the prophylactic sanitary measures taken against the transmitting vector.

The study of the soldiers mentioned above was performed during the years 1960–1962 (Mora 1964). Follow-up surveys in 1963–1969 showed that the prevalence of carriers hardly changed, remaining at 4.5–5% (Maekelt 1970).

T. cruzi humoral antibodies and *T. cruzi* infection persist in the human body for a long time, as we have shown by standardized follow-up studies (Maekelt 1969). Control of Chagas' disease will result mainly from effective sanitary measures taken to control the vectors, and one would expect children from their first year of life to benefit first, since they will no longer be exposed to primary infections.

We will not expect a lowering of *T. cruzi* antibody carriers among the Venezuelan soldiers aged 18–20 years, until this year, 1973, since effective residual insecticides (dieldrin and gamexan) have only been used since 1952.

The prevalence of *T. cruzi* antibody carriers among apparently healthy blood donors, representing groups over 20 years of age, has not yet diminished and has remained almost unchanged for the last 20 years. Thus, from 1963 to 1969, more than 500 000 blood donors were examined by the complement fixation test; *T. cruzi* antibody prevalence ranged from 3.5 to 5%. The prevalence of carriers also remained unchanged in the blood banks of different geographical locations: 9–13% of the donors at the Blood Bank in Valencia, which is in a highly endemic area of Chagas' disease, showed *T. cruzi* antibodies, while in Maracaibo, situated in a low endemic area, only 1.7% to 2.8% of blood donors showed *T. cruzi* antibodies (Maekelt 1970).

Lumsden: I wanted to add a little to the earlier discussion on the possibility of transmission of infection by ingestion. Wilkes (1972), recently a student of mine, did comparative titrations of the same suspensions of trypanosomes by different routes in mice. He compared, for instance, abraded skin and unabraded skin, instillation into the conjunctiva, into the nose and so on. Unabraded skin was very resistant while intranasal instillation was very infective, giving titres nearly as high as one gets by direct intraperitoneal inoculation. With *T. brucei* organisms infectivity was not quite as high but it was still one of the most infective routes. Much less infectivity than was expected was found by conjunctival instillation or instillation into the mouth, and these results seem to be related to the low tonicity of saliva. The extremely high infectivities found by intranasal instillation have made us very cautious. We avoid things like laminar flow cabinets for handling the organisms and adopt the greatest precautions. Aerosol formation and inhalation may well account for some of the otherwise unaccountable laboratory infections.

Maekelt: One problem is the infectivity of the different developmental stages of *T. cruzi* in mammals and man, but another is the infectivity of trypomastigotes of *T. cruzi* in different species of reduviid bugs. Recently, R. W. Rohwedder, J. A. Cerisola and C. E. del Prado (1972, personal communication) put the same number (four specimens) of seven different species (*T. infestans*, *T. pallidipennis*, *T. dimidiata*, *P. herreri*, *R. prolixus*, *R. prolixus zeledon* and *R. pallescens*) of the same nymph-stage for xenodiagnosis together on three patients. Positive xenodiagnosis was much higher in the Argentine species of *T. infestans* (10/12) than in the other species (e.g. *R. prolixus* from Venezuela, 2/11). This study should be repeated in other countries to indicate which species of triatomid bugs are most readily infected with local strains of *T. cruzi*.

Zeledón: At the Teheran Congress on Tropical Medicine in 1968 I reported (unpublished) that in a survey in Costa Rica we found a group of patients with positive xenodiagnoses that were revealed only by the local species, *T. dimidiata*; two exotic species, *R. prolixus* and *T. infestans*, gave negative tests in the same people. Cerisola *et al.* (1971*a*) confirmed this in Argentina, using Panamanian and Argentinian bugs. It is certainly important to know that some species of bugs may be more susceptible to some local strains of *T. cruzi* and to learn why this is so.

Tonn: *T. rangeli* is a common parasite found in triatomids in Venezuela. In one state in Malariology Zone 7 of the Ministry of Health, over 5000 triatomids, mostly *R. prolixus*, were examined in 1972. About 150 triatomids were positive for trypanosomes, with nine infested with *T. cruzi* only, 70 infected with both *T. cruzi* and *T. rangeli*, and 75 with only *T. rangeli*. In xenodiagnoses done over several years within this Malariology Zone, a high percentage of the individuals tested were infected with both parasites (monthly unpublished reports of Malariology Zone 7). Under these conditions, where does *T. rangeli* fit into the epidemiological picture?

Zeledón: From the epidemiological standpoint there is no problem, since *T. rangeli* can be clearly differentiated from *T. cruzi*. The cycle of *T. rangeli* in *Rhodnius* is quite different from that of *T. cruzi*. Also the transmission of *T. rangeli* is much more effective, because it is done by direct inoculation. In my opinion, metacyclic forms are produced only in the salivary glands but Dr Cecil Hoare still thinks that metacyclic forms could be produced in the hindgut of *Rhodnius*. In his excellent book (1972) he has reproduced a diagram I sent him, but he has slightly modified it to include a metacyclic form in the hindgut that I didn't put there! In any event, *T. rangeli* is biologically and morphologically quite different from *T. cruzi*.

Maekelt: Do you get *no* contamination with blastocrithidiae?

Zeledón: Blastocrithidiae have been reported only from *T. infestans* (Cerisola *et al.* 1971*b*). In natural conditions *T. rangeli* and *T. cruzi* are probably found only in *Rhodnius*, the only contrary report being one from Marinkelle (1965) in Colombia. Anyway, with some experience, *T. rangeli* and *T. cruzi* can be separated rather easily and there is no problem in knowing which is which.

Tonn: I don't think there is a problem in that respect, but where does *T. rangeli* fit when there are dual infections in man? Does it affect the serology or the pathology, or is it a separate entity not only in epidemiology but in pathology as well?

Zeledón: People infected with *T. rangeli* alone give a negative complement fixation test for Chagas' disease and we admit that *T. rangeli* does not produce any evidence of disease. Several years ago, the late Emmanuel Dias raised the very important point that some of the regional differences in pathology in Chagas' disease could arise through repeated reinfections, which might be more common in areas where a particular insect occurs in large numbers in houses. In those cases, reinfection would occur very easily. What does this new injection of live flagellates or antigens have to do with pathological changes, or with the destruction of neurons, or with the pathological consequences? I am talking now of reinfections with *T. cruzi*, but could *T. rangeli* interfere somehow with this process?

Maekelt: Of 224 individuals infected only with *T. rangeli* and who had no *T. cruzi* in their blood and no *T. cruzi* antibodies, 15 (6.7%) showed electrocardiographic (ECG) alterations, which is not significantly different from the 231 (4.4%) of 5251 individuals without any trypanosome infection who showed ECG changes (Maekelt 1970). This statistical evaluation supports the clinical data which may confirm the non-pathogenicity of *T. rangeli* infection in man.

However, 258 (72%) of 357 individuals infected with *T. cruzi* alone (positive xenodiagnosis) and with specific *T. cruzi* antibodies showed ECG changes, and this is 16.5 times more than the non-infected controls (Maekelt 1970).

Zeledón: I was trying to discover what would happen in a person with a mixed infection, that is one who already has Chagas' disease and then receives repeated injections of *T. rangeli* antigens. I wonder whether the immunological mechanism has anything to do with the pathological lesions.

Baker: Today we have heard about three main types of epidemiology. One might sum up the differences by saying that in the African salivarian trypanosomes the 'pick-up' of the parasite by the vector is very inefficient, but once it has been picked up the transfer back to the mammal is probably quite efficient. In leishmaniasis perhaps it is fair to say that the pick-up of the parasite is efficient but its return to the mammal is rather inefficient. In Chagas' disease, both pick-up and transmission, given the right combination of hosts, can be highly efficient.

References

BAKER, J. R. (1956) Studies on *Trypanosoma avium* Danilewsky, 1885. II. Transmission by *Ornithomyia avicularia* L. *Parasitology* **46**, 321-334

BAKER, J. R. (1968) Trypanosomes of wild mammals in the neighbourhood of the Serengeti National Park. *Symp. Zool. Soc. Lond.* **24**, 147-158

CERISOLA, J. A., ROHWEDDER, R. W. & PRADO, C. E. DEL (1971a) Rendimiento del xenodiagnóstico en la infección chagásica crónica humana utilizando ninfas de diferentes especies de triatóminos. *Bol. Chil. Parasitol.* **26**, 57-58

CERISOLA, J. A., PRADO, C. E. DEL, ROHWEDDER, R. W. & BOZZINI, J. P. (1971b) *Blasto-crithidia triatomae* n. sp. found in *Triatomo infestans* from Argentina. *J. Protozool.* **18**, 503-506

COTTON, T. D. (1970) A life cycle study of *Trypanosoma macfiei*, a natural hemoflagellate parasite of canaries *(Serinus canarius)*. *J. Parasitol.* **56** (4), 63

DI PRIMIO, R. (1965) Doença em Teutonia. *An. Fac. Med. Porto Alegre*, **25**, 17-46

HAASE, H. B. & DE LIMA, G. M. (1967) Microepidemia de molestia de Chagas em Teutonia, Rio Grande do Sul. *Hospital (Rio de J.)* **72**, 229-238

HOARE, C. A. (1972) *The Trypanosomes of Mammals*, Blackwell Scientific Publications, Oxford

MAEKELT, G. A. (1969) Evaluación clínica y serológica de la droga Bay-2502 en pacientes con infección chagásica. *Bol. Chil. Parasitol.* **24**, 96

MAEKELT, G. A. (1970) Seroepidemiology of Chagas disease, *J. Parasitol.* **56** (4) 557 (summary only)

MAEKELT, G. A. (1971) Die Serodiagnose der Trypanosomiasen, insbesondere der Chagas-krankheit, in *Kongressbericht über die II Tagung der Österreichischen Gesellschaft für Tropenmedizin und der IV Tagung der Deutschen Tropenmedizinischen Gesellschaft e.V. 1969 vom 21 bis 23. April in Salzburg und in Bad Reichenhall* (Flamm, H. & Mohr, W., eds.), pp. 111-121, Hansisches Verlagskontor H. Scheffler, Lübeck

MAEKELT, G. A. & HIDALGO, V. (1958) Estudio sobre el tiempo de sobrevivencia del *Schizo-trypanum cruzi* a temperatura bajas. *Bol. Lab. Clin. 'Luis Razetti'* **3**, 17-28

MARINKELLE, C. J. (1965) Direct transmission of *Trypanosoma cruzi* between individuals of *Rhodnius prolixus* Stål. *Rev. Biol. Trop.* **13**, 55-58

MORA, R. (1964) Estudio epidemiológico sobre las infecciones chagásicas entre los donantes de sangre de las Fuerzas Armadas de Venezuela. *Arch. Venez. Med. Trop. Parasitol. Med.* **3**, 125-131

PACKCHANIAN, A. (1943) On the viability of various species of *Trypanosoma* and *Leishmania* cultures. *J. Parasitol.* **29**, 275-277

PRICE, D. L., CHAFFE, E. F. & WINSLOW, D. J. (1964) Viability, infectivity, and pathogenicity of cultural forms of a strain of *Trypanosoma cruzi* isolated from a raccoon in Maryland. *J. Parasitol.* **50** (3), 19

SULLIVAN, T. D. (1944) Viability of *Trypanosoma cruzi* in citrated blood stored at room temperature. *J. Parasitol.* **30**, 200

WILKES, R. W. (1972) Interactions of trypanosomes with tissue surfaces and secretions of their vertebrate hosts. Ph.D. thesis, University of London

Epidemiology of leishmaniasis: some reflections on causation

R. S. BRAY

Wellcome Parasitology Unit No. 2, Institute of Pathobiology, Haile Sellassie I University, Addis Ababa*

Disease is embedded in the environment of man
(Stallones 1972)

Abstract A 'web' of causation is presented for zoonotic leishmaniasis as exemplified by cutaneous leishmaniasis of the Ethiopian highlands which involves the *Phlebotomus longipes* group, rock hyraxes, *Leishmania* and man. The following factors are discussed both in relation to Ethiopian cutaneous leishmaniasis and to similar factors in other areas of zoonotic leishmaniasis:
    Man: occupation, defence of home or health, crop growing, shade for coffee;
    Sandfly: temperature, humidity, species, food preferences;
    Hyrax: habitat, immunity.
    These factors are cross-linked to the places and times at which man is in contact with sandflies which are themselves in contact with rock hyraxes and leishmaniae.
    Events are then followed via the immunity and other conditions of man and the attack rate to the acquisition of active leishmanial infection in man.

To say that oriental sore is caused by *Leishmania tropica* is far too confining a statement to anyone interested in epidemiology. Oriental sore is also caused by the bite of a sandfly, by proximity to a reservoir host, by the way man fits into the ecosystem of sandfly and reservoir host, by the immune reaction of man, and possibly by his nutritional, viraemic or temperature states. One could go on.

MacMahon & Pugh (1970) have written of the 'web of causation' which is an essential study in the epidemiology of disease. When the Pavlovsky school speak of natural foci or natural nidality of disease or when the Meyer/Audy group speak of landscape epidemiology, they employ this interlocking net of

---

* Present address: MRC Laboratories, Fajara, nr Bathurst, The Gambia.

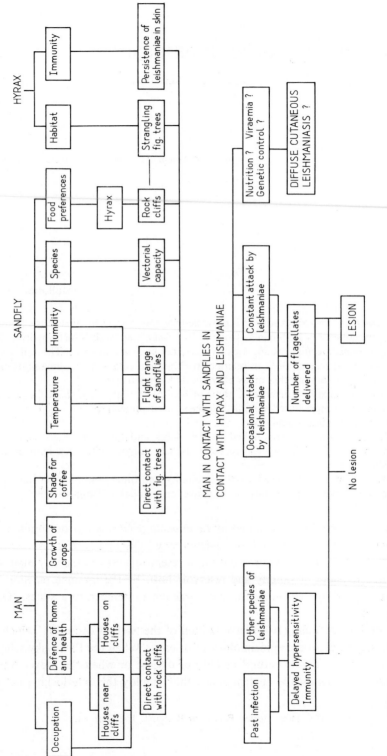

Fig. 1. Web of causation of leishmaniasis in the Ethiopian highlands.

causation. A partial reconstruction of such a web in one situation where leishmaniasis occurs should help to show the number of features in the eco-system which may play a part. Stallones (1972) has pointed to the existence of an equal web of effects but here I wish to take the story only as far as the ap-pearance of a skin lesion of leishmaniasis in the Ethiopian highlands. I shall first present this diagrammatically (Fig. 1) and then discuss some of the causes and effects, primarily in zoonotic cutaneous leishmaniasis of Ethiopia but also with reference to similar situations elsewhere. Finally I shall examine how each cause exerts its effect and how similar causes exert their effects in other areas of leishmaniasis.

MAN

(1) *Occupation.* In parts of Ethiopia where the cliff-face with its infected hyrax and sandflies is the focal point of infection (Ashford *et al.* 1973) the oc-cupation of herding is probably important. The children aged 4–14 years, both male and female, who herd the goats and sheep are frequently at the cliff face, and the goats in particular graze on the steep slopes of the gorges. It is this age group which is most affected by cutaneous leishmaniasis. In south-west Ethiopia coffee growing is important in bringing man into contact with infected hyraxes. In Kenya herding and contact with termite hills and their population of *Phlebotomus martini* are important in the acquisition of kala azar (Manson-Bahr & Southgate 1964). In British Honduras (Belize) one is in some danger from cutaneous leishmaniasis if one lies down and disturbs the forest floor at 0700 h, according to Williams (1970).

(2) *Defence of home and health.* In Ethiopia traditional ideas of defence against both attack and lowland disease cause huts to be built halfway up the slopes of the gorges of the river systems. Frequently these are built on the slope or talus just under a cliff face. There tends to be a focal distribution of cutaneous leishmaniasis in such huts immediately under the cliff face.

Notions of defence, fear of the unhealthy lake shore below and possibly other reasons have contributed to one village in southern Ethiopia being located on a rock cliff and rock fall area inhabited by hyrax. In this village the in-cidence of old and new cutaneous leishmaniasis is about 40% compared to 1.5% in villages near but not on cliff faces. In the former no particular activity is needed for people to acquire cutaneous leishmaniasis, and babies are infected, while in the latter areas the cliff face must be visited for a person to acquire the disease.

In another context, ideas of cool or efficient or aesthetic house-building become significant because of the proclivity of many phlebotomine sandfly species for resting and possibly breeding in cracks in masonry or in the crevices between bricks or stones. So in Calcutta kala azar and sandflies used to predominate in masonry houses as compared to bamboo huts (Napier 1926). In Artuf in former Palestine the houses had whitewashed masonry walls and sandflies and cutaneous leishmaniasis occurred, while in the Arab village some 100 metres away the huts were of mud construction with no sandflies and cutaneous leishmaniasis was absent (Adler & Theodore 1925). In southern Ethiopia sandflies can be caught in walled tin-roofed houses in which cooking fires are not lit but never in bamboo huts in which cooking fires are lit. Baghdadi houses have flat roofs and the inhabitants like to sleep on them in summer, thereby meeting the bite of infected *Phlebotomus sergenti* (Adler & Theodore 1929).

(3) *Crop growing.* In some areas of Ethiopia the taluses of the steep-sided and terraced gorges are cultivated right up to the cliff face, so that tending the crops may take man to the cliff face at dusk when sandflies are most likely to be active. In Panama a newly made road led to strip-cultivation and cutting of the forest and this appeared to be the direct cause of an outbreak of cutaneous leishmaniasis in the newly arrived farmers. When crops began to be produced after two years of cultivation, transmission died out, presumably as the reservoir host and its attendant sandflies emigrated.

(4) *Shade for coffee.* In south-west Ethiopia large strangling fig trees (*Ficus vasta*) are left standing to provide shade for the growth of coffee (see Fig. 2). Where there are no cliffs these fig trees provide a suitable habitat for the rock hyrax and for *P. longipes* and *Leishmania*, and so become a focal point of cutaneous leishmaniasis.

Thus in Ethiopia these various causes lead man into contact with the natural foci of cutaneous leishmaniasis, a cliff face or a strangling fig tree. In Turkmenistan when new land was brought under cultivation man came in contact with the gerbil burrows harbouring *Leishmania*-infected rodents and sandflies capable of biting man (Petresčeva 1971). In the Americas the mahogany cutters, the chicle gatherers and the wild-rubber tappers come in contact with infected cricetid rodents and their sandflies in the forests—another natural, if diffuse, focus of cutaneous leishmaniasis (Lainson & Strangways-Dixon 1963).

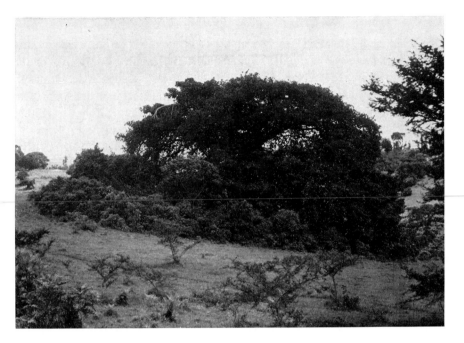

FIG. 2. *Ficus vasta*, the large strangling fig tree of south-west Ethiopia, shading coffee and harbouring hyrax.

SANDFLY

(1) *Temperature and humidity*. Both these conditions have a profound effect on larval development, breeding cycle, flight range and ability to feed of sandflies (Adler & Theodore 1957; Lewis 1971). Considerable fluctuations in these variables such as occur in the Middle East cause large numbers of biting sandflies to be present in the summer months (July to September) and virtually none from December to April (Adler & Theodore 1929; Pringle 1957). Thus infected dogs in Baghdad are numerous in November to May but absent from May to September (Chadwick & McHattie 1927) and transmission to both dogs and man is confined to the summer months (Bray *et al*. 1967).

Seasonal variability may spring from many sources. Just as accountants tend to show significant rises in serum cholesterol that correspond to critical dates in the fiscal calendar (Frideman *et al*. 1958), so does *P. langeroni orientalis*, the vector of kala azar in the Sudan, reach its highest numbers just before the wet season as the rains wash out its breeding and resting sites (Dietlein 1964; Quate 1964), and the peak incidence of kala azar is some eight months later, in

December and January (Van Peenan & Reid 1963). There are hardly any seasonal fluctuations in numbers or feeding habits among *P. longipes* of the temperate Ethiopian highlands, where there are few seasonal fluctuations in temperature, or among the sandflies of the tropical rain forest belt of Amazonia, which has constant high humidity and little change in temperature. In neither place is there a seasonal incidence of cutaneous leishmaniasis.

In Central Ethiopia at 2600 m the temperature is so low that *P. longipes* does not venture far from its habitat in hyrax-inhabited cliff faces and man is rarely infected with cutaneous leishmaniasis (0.9%). At 2000 m in Southern Ethiopia the related *P. pedifer* flies freely from hyrax habitats about a village at dusk and freely bites man, who is frequently infected (10.7%). At 2200 m, between these two habitats, *P. longipes* moves fairly freely but appears to breed over a wide area not confined to hyrax habitats, and it uses cattle as a blood source. Man is very rarely infected ($< 0.50\%$). It was the great Venezuelan parasitologist and epidemiologist Felix Pifano who noted that *Phlebotomus* leaves its habitat when the ambient temperature and humidity approach those of its micro-habitat (Pifano *et al.* 1960).

(2) *Species*. Obviously the species of sandfly must be capable of infection with the relevant species of *Leishmania* and of being infected heavily in the anterior portions of the alimentary tract, particularly at the end of the proboscis itself. In the Sudan Heyneman (1963) showed that *L. donovani* heavily infected both *P. papatasi* and *P. langeroni orientalis* but the infection in *P. papatasi* progressively died out and never infected the anterior parts of the midgut with any great concentration, while in *P. l. orientalis* the infection became progressively greater and was exceptionally heavy in the anterior end of the midgut.

Adler *et al.* (1938) showed that Palestinian strains of *L. tropica* readily and heavily infected *P. papatasi* from Palestine but Cretan strains of *L. tropica* only poorly infected *P. papatasi* of both Palestine and Crete. Hindle (1931) showed that Chinese strains of *L. donovani* grew in *P. chinensis* and *P. mongolensis* much more readily than Indian strains.

(3) *Food preferences*. In zoonotic leishmaniasis—and it should be stressed that most human leishmaniasis is zoonotic—an essential feature is that the sandfly, which normally feeds on the reservoir host and maintains the enzootic between reservoir hosts, feeds readily on man. Thus in Ethiopia where *P. longipes* feeds primarily on rock hyrax it will feed readily on man (and cattle) if and when the occasion arises. *P. l. orientalis* live in the acacia-balanites woodlands away from human habitation and its primary hosts

must be non-human; man is bitten only accidentally but none the less avidly.

A species of sandfly maintains an enzootic among pi-dogs in Senegalese villages but apparently this species does not bite man; otherwise, with such a domestic reservoir 70% infected with leishmania, human leishmaniasis would be common in Senegal, which it is not (Ranque *et al.* 1971). *Lutzomyia flaviscutellata* rarely bites man, though it maintains most effectively an enzootic among forest rodents (Shaw & Lainson 1968). This enzootic is caused by the fast-growing *L. mexicana amazonensis*. The slow-growing *L. braziliensis braziliensis* is transmitted by several sandflies of the *Lu. intermedia* and *Psychodopygus* groups which bite man readily. Hence *L. b. braziliensis* is probably a good deal more widespread among human intruders into the Amazonian forests than is *L. m. amazonensis* (Lainson & Shaw 1972).

Some sandflies, normally reluctant to feed on man, may do so if disturbed and Williams (1970) maintains that *Lu. olmeca* transmits *L. m. mexicana* in Belize to an appreciable degree by being disturbed from its resting site on the ground among forest litter between 0600 and 0800 h. In Surinam *Lu. anduzei* also bites when disturbed (Wijers & Linger 1966) and it is said to be unwise to urinate on forest tree buttresses, a resting place of *Lu. anduzei*, as the consequent lesion upon the exposed penis tends to argue an aetiology other than resting sandflies. Other sandflies have divided loyalties and are dangerous vectors. *P. papatasi* in the Isfahan area of Iran shows an equal liking for the burrows of the reservoir host (gerbils) and human habitations, and an equal liking for gerbil and human blood. They are therefore efficient transmitters of cutaneous leishmaniasis from gerbils to man (Nadim *et al.* 1968).

Still other sandflies, such as *P. argentipes* in Bengal, lived in human habitations, fed largely on man and were able to effect the man-to-man transmission of the kala azar of Bengal and the classic epidemics of middle and west Bengal and the Brahmaputra valley of Assam. It is worth mentioning that these epidemics displayed the cyclical periodicity (between 10 and 15 years) of a typical man-to-man epidemic rather than the non-periodical focal type of increase typical of a reservoir-based endemic.

RESERVOIR HOST

(1) *Habitat.* A reservoir can only act as such if its habitat also provides a habitat for sandflies which can then feed readily on it. The sandfly must be attracted to the reservoir host of course, but if the macroclimate or microclimate of the reservoir habitat is not suitable for the sandfly then no enzootic will be set up as the fly will not feed. If the temperature and humidity are

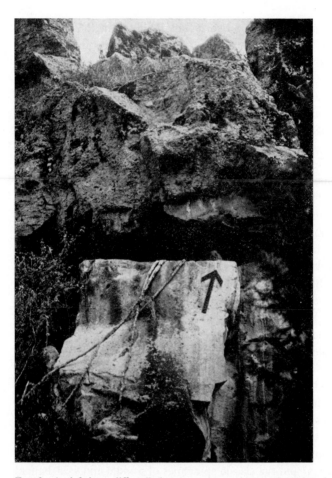

FIG. 3. A cleft in a cliff wall showing a hyrax (arrowed) and its habitat.

'right' then the habitat may be a whole forest. But in harsher conditions the common habitat may be strictly confined.

Thus rock hyraxes in Ethiopia at 2600 m live in deep fissures or caves in the cliff faces of the tremendous gorge systems (see Fig. 3), and deep in these fissures the microclimate becomes warm, humid and stable enough for the resting, feeding and breeding of *P. longipes*. In the slightly milder climate of south-west Ethiopia at 2200 m, where there are no rock-cliffs, the rock hyrax has found an alternative habitat in the enormous strangling fig trees which eventually kill their host trees and so become hollow inside. As the coffee trees and other vegetation provide shelter from the wind and increase the humidity these fig trees also become a suitable habitat for *P. longipes*.

In the arid open areas of Soviet Asia and Iran the reservoir is a burrowing animal (gerbils) and their burrows provide suitable microclimates for *P. caucasicus* and *P. papatasi* (up to 65% infected), which are the two major vectors. In the complex burrows of *Rhombomys opimus*, the great gerbil (up to 100% infected), as many as 500 larvae or pupae of sandflies may be recovered from a single nesting chamber where the humidity is 75–90% and the temperature no higher than 25°C (Petreshcheva *et al.*, undated; Petrescčeva 1971). Equally the termite hills of the Kitui area of Kenya with their many chambers and burrows provide excellent shelter for *P. martini*, the vector of kala azar (Minter 1963), though here the existence of a cohabiting reservoir is doubtful.

On the subject of reservoir hosts, it is time we buried the somewhat anthropocentric notion that Middle Asia is the 'home of leishmaniasis' (Pringle 1957; Lysenko 1971), as it is difficult to believe that hyraxes in Ethiopia, cricetid rodents in Mexico and Brazil, murine rodents in Senegal and sloths and kinkajous in Panama all derived their leishmaniasis from Turkmenistan or Balkh.

(2) *Immunity*. A reservoir host cannot show either innate immunity to leishmaniasis or acute acquired immunity which eradicates the disease quickly. Nor can it show the sort of susceptibility possessed by hamsters to *L. donovani* or *L. m. amazonensis*, which leads to death. In the Ethiopian highlands a hyrax is bitten by an infected sandfly about every three days (Ashford *et al.* 1973), yet many of the hyraxes found to be infected have been fully grown adults. This would seem to argue a very incomplete immune reaction to leishmaniasis, borne out by the apparent lack of delayed hypersensitivity to leishmanin among infected hyrax populations. However the infection in the hyrax is apparently confined to the skin, largely to the very tip of the nose, which is where the sandfly most often bites. Some host reaction would seem to confine the development and distribution of the leishmaniasis to the site of original infection and thus to the most likely point for the next sandfly to bite.

Somewhat the same story holds for the great gerbil in Turkmenistan, where the ears of the gerbil can remain infected for up to two years and sandflies can thus be continuously infected from their favourite site for feeding (Sidorova 1962). On the other hand the cricetid reservoirs of New World cutaneous leishmaniasis seem to recover from the infection and show delayed hypersensitivity. Presumably in animals with a lifespan measured only in months and infection rates of up to 100%, the turn-over of leishmania is rapid and constant and immunity has little effect upon the enzootic.

Lack of immunity combined with extensive infection of the dermis also occurs with *L. infantum* in dogs, which appear unable to control the infection and show nodules and ulcers containing numerous *Leishmania* all over the body surface. These areas also become depilated and this makes it easier for the sandflies to feed, as hair is a formidable barrier for them.

We have arrived at a situation where man is in contact with the enzootic of reservoir, sandfly and leishmania. Other factors now come into play.

MAN

(1) *Past infection.* If a person has had a past infection with the same strain of *Leishmania* it is generally assumed that he will have complete resistance to reinfection. However this is not always the case. Heyneman (1971) reports Davydov as having recorded a reinfection rate as high as 10%. Rahim & Tatar (1966) have noted cases of reinfection seemingly with the same strain. In the village (see p. 89) in southern Ethiopia where about 40% of the population has old or new lesions and no other comparable endemic centre exists in the area, delayed hypersensitivity is frequently lost between 10 and 15 years after spontaneous cure of cutaneous leishmaniasis. We do not know whether this means that susceptibility to the same strain is regained but at least two cases of reinfection are known (M. P. Hutchinson, personal communication). This may argue that the *Leishmania* of Ethiopian cutaneous leishmaniasis is less immunogenic in that the clone of lymphocytes caused to multiply in response to leishmanial antigen may produce fewer memory cells or produce them for a shorter time, or even that it contains antigens with a deleterious effect upon memory cells. It seems that delayed hypersensitivity is less easily lost in the Middle East and it is also known that Iraqi *Leishmania* contains more antigens than Ethiopian *Leishmania* (Bray & Rahim 1969), and Ethiopian *Leishmania* is apparently able to suppress lymphocyte activation or reaction, or both, under certain conditions.

Past infection does not necessarily mean past infection with full symptoms. Almost every area where leishmaniasis is known has yielded a higher incidence of delayed hypersensitivity to leishmanin than can be accounted for by evidence of overt infection. It must be assumed that both kala azar and cutaneous leishmaniasis can be acquired and cured spontaneously before the full array of symptoms appear.

(2) *Other species of Leishmania.* In at least one area (in Kenya) a very high incidence of delayed hypersensitivity reactions has been recorded in the absence of known human leishmaniasis (Southgate & Orieto 1967). It was assumed that in this case the subjects had contracted an ephemeral infection with lizard leishmaniasis and had acquired a genus-specific delayed hypersensitivity without

symptoms. These subjects were immune to infection with *L. donovani* (Manson-Bahr & Heisch 1961; Southgate & Manson-Bahr 1967; Southgate 1967).

(3) *Nutrition; viraemia; genetic control.* I mention here only three of the conditions which might influence the form taken by leishmanial infection in man.

There is increasing evidence that the state of nutrition of the host may have a profound effect on the immune capacity of the host. One theory postulated to explain the occurrence of diffuse cutaneous leishmaniasis (a disease shared by Ethiopia and Venezuela) is that an event supervenes which weakens or eliminates the cellular immune reaction long enough for the parasite to multiply enough for sufficient antigen to reach the lymph nodes, where either a high zone tolerance to the antigen dose is produced or the clone of lymphocytes responsible for the effective immune reaction is actually killed off. Malnutrition is a state that lasts long enough to allow such a multiplication.

Hoogstraal & Heyneman (1969) have suggested that 'the general good health enjoyed by' the American NAMRU-3 personnel in the Sudan who suffered only skin lesions on naturally acquiring *L. donovani* infection may have contributed towards their lack of general visceral involvement. However of three infected American Embassy personnel in the Sudan two had visceral involvement so it seems doubtful that good health or good nutrition can easily be adduced as an explanation, unless it is claimed that conditions in the US Navy are far better than for the US State Department.

Another possible mechanism for the 'turn off' of the cellular immune system is a viraemia, which is known experimentally to depress delayed hypersensitivity and its correlates greatly (Wheelock *et al.* 1971). I feel that no viraemia could exert its effect long enough to allow leishmania to proliferate to a point where excess leishmanial antigen could turn off the immune system. Two unrelated facts here are that Bryceson (1970) found that measles caused considerable regression of the lesions of diffuse cutaneous leishmaniasis in Ethiopia, and that an influenza epidemic immediately preceded an epidemic of kala azar in Assam (Napier & Das Gupta 1931)—although I would put more emphasis on the climatic alteration which also preceded that epidemic.

Finally, an outside event may not be necessary to explain the onset of diffuse cutaneous leishmaniasis. A large number of injected promastigotes of a strain genetically determined to be more virulent to the clone of lymphocytes multiplying to deal with it (the strains in Ethiopia and Venezuela) may occasionally multiply and produce paralysing or killing antigens faster than the proliferating lymphocyte clone and thereby neutralize or destroy it. This clone may also be at some disadvantage in terms of activation, proliferation or effect in some genetically deficient individuals in the population, though there is no evidence for this.

SANDFLY

(1) *Occasional or constant attack by infected sandflies.* There is some evidence that in epidemic conditions such as existed in the great outbreaks of kala azar in Assam, *L. donovani* increased in virulence and the number of organisms per fly increased. This could be critical in the production of many more proboscis infections in the fly and thus many more transmissions (Shortt 1945).

Equally, in the enzootic situation it is possible that the higher the incidence in both reservoir and sandfly the more virulent the organism is to man and the more flies have proboscis infections. However in a stable zoonotic condition there should be no difference in the number of lesions or their severity per person, whether few or many people are infected.

(2) *Number of promastigotes delivered.* This factor is obviously critical. In most cases an infected sandfly probably delivers no promastigotes into the skin of a vertebrate. If very few promastigotes are delivered all the parasites may die in attempting to reach and penetrate a histiocyte. Even if the parasite enters a histiocyte it may still be lysed there if its anti-lysosome mechanism functions faultily. If only a very few parasites enter histiocytes and transform successfully into amastigotes, they may still activate an immune reaction which mobilizes and deals with them before they multiply and occupy sufficient space to become a noticeable papule or ulcer, or before they invade the viscera to multiply further and cause fully fledged kala azar. The number of organisms may also be important in diffuse cutaneous leishmaniasis, as already explained.

The factors governing the numbers of promastigotes in a sandfly that are capable of being delivered to the skin of a vertebrate, and the mechanism or mechanisms which cause them to be deposited in the skin, remain completely unknown and, to my mind, constitute the most important gap in our knowledge of this disease. The salivary duct joins the food channel so anteriorly that the passage of saliva could be of little assistance. It is possible that an unsuccessful probe when blood is not taken up might be the infecting occasion, as when the pumps cease to operate the general subsidence of the walls of the pharynx might carry pharyngeal contents forward into the wound.

References

ADLER, S. & THEODORE, O. (1925) The experimental transmission of cutaneous leishmaniasis to man from *Phlebotomus papatasi. Ann. Trop. Med. Parasitol.* **19**, 365-371

ADLER, S. & THEODORE, O. (1929) The distribution of sandflies and leishmaniasis in Palestine, Syria and Mesopotamia. *Ann. Trop. Med. Parasitol.* **23**, 269-306

ADLER, S. & THEODORE, O. (1957) Transmission of disease agents by phlebotomine sandflies. *Ann. Rev. Entomol.* **2**, 203-226

ADLER, S., THEODORE, O. & WITENBURG, G. (1938) Investigations on Mediterranean Kala-azar. XI. A study of leishmaniasis in Canea (Crete). *Proc. R. Soc. Lond. B. Biol. Sci.* **125**, 491-516

ASHFORD, R. W., BRAY, M. A., HUTCHINSON, M. P. & BRAY, R. S. (1973). The epidemiology of cutaneous leishmaniasis in Ethiopia. *Trans. R. Soc. Trop. Med. Hyg.* **67**, 568-601

BRAY, R. S. & RAHIM, G. A. F. (1969) Studies on the immunology and serology of leishmaniasis. VII. Serotypes of *Leishmania tropica. Trans. R. Soc. Trop. Med. Hyg.* **63**, 383-387

BRAY, R. S., RAHIM, G. A. F. & TAJ-EL-DIN, S. (1967) The present state of leishmaniasis in Iraq. *Protozoology.* **2**, 171-186

BRYCESON, A. D. M. (1970) Diffuse cutaneous leishmaniasis in Ethiopia. II. Treatment. *Trans. R. Soc. Trop. Med. Hyg.* **64**, 369-379

CHADWICK, C. R. & McHATTIE, C. (1927) Notes on cutaneous leishmaniasis of dogs in Iraq. *Trans. R. Soc. Trop. Med. Hyg.* **20**, 422-432

DIETLEIN, D. R. (1964) Leishmaniasis in the Sudan Republic. 16. Seasonal incidence of *Phlebotomus* species (Diptera: Psychodidae) in an Upper Nile Province town and village. *Ann. Entomol. Soc. Am.* **57**, 243-246

FRIDEMAN, M., ROSEMAN, R. H. & CARROLL, V. (1958) Changes in the serum cholesterol and blood clotting time in men subjected to cyclic variations of occupational stress. *Circulation,* **17**, 852-861

HEYNEMAN, D. (1963) Leishmaniasis in the Sudan Republic. 12: Comparison of experimental *Leishmania donovani* infection in *Phlebotomus papatasi* (Diptera: Psychodidae) with natural infections found in man-baited *P. orientalis* captured in a kala-azar endemic region of the Sudan. *Am. J. Trop. Med. Hyg.* **12**, 725-740

HEYNEMAN, D. (1971) Immunology of leishmaniasis. *Bull. W.H.O.* **44**, 499-514

HINDLE, E. (1931) The development of various strains of *Leishmania* in Chinese sandflies. *Proc. R. Soc. Lond. B Biol. Sci.* **108**, 366-383

HOOGSTRAAL, H. & HEYNEMAN, D. (1969) Leishmaniasis in the Sudan Republic. 30. Final epidemiological report. *Am. J. Trop. Med. Hyg.* **18**, 1091-1210

LAINSON, R. & SHAW, J. J. (1972) Leishmaniasis of the New World: taxonomic problems. *Br. Med. Bull.* **28**, 44-48

LAINSON, R. & STRANGWAYS-DIXON, J. (1963) *Leishmania mexicana:* the epidemiology of dermal leishmaniasis in British Honduras. *Trans. R. Soc. Trop. Med. Hyg.* **57**, 242-265

LEWIS, D. J. (1971) Phlebotomid sandflies. *Bull. W.H.O.* **44**, 535-551

LYSENKO, A. JA. (1971) Distribution of leishmaniasis in the Old World. *Bull. W.H.O.* **44**, 515-520

MACMAHON, B. & PUGH, T. F. (1970) *Epidemiology: Principles and Methods*, Little Brown, Boston

MANSON-BAHR, P. E. C. & HEISCH, R. B. (1961) Transient infection of man with a *Leishmania (L. adleri)* of lizards. *Ann. Trop. Med. Parasitol.* **55**, 381-382

MANSON-BAHR, P. E. C. & SOUTHGATE, B. A. (1964) Recent research on kala-azar in East Africa. *J. Trop. Med. Hyg.* **67**, 79-84

MINTER, D. M. (1963) Studies on the vector of kala-azar in Kenya. III: Distributional evidence. *Ann. Trop. Med. Parasitol.* **57**, 19-23

NADIM, A., MESGHALI, A. & AMINI, H. (1968) Epidemiology of cutaneous leishmaniasis in the Isfahan province of Iran. III. The vector. *Trans. R. Soc. Trop. Med. Hyg.* **62**, 543-549

NAPIER, L. E. (1926) A comparative study of the environment associated with kala-azar prevalence in Calcutta. *Indian J. Med. Res.* **12**, 755-772

NAPIER, L. E. & DAS GUPTA, C. R. (1931) An epidemiological investigation of kala-azar in a rural area in Bengal. *Indian J. Med. Res.* **19**, 295-341

PETRESČEVA, P. A. (1971) The natural focality of leishmaniasis in the USSR. *Bull. W.H.O.* **44**, 567-576

PETRESHCHEVA, P., ZASUKIN, D. & SAFYANOVA, V. (undated) in *Human Diseases with Natural Foci* (Pavlovsky, Y. N., ed.), pp. 286-346, Foreign Languages Publishing House, Moscow

PIFANO, F., ORITZ, I. & ALVAREZ, A. (1960) La ecologia en condiciones naturales y de laboratorio, de algunas especies de Phlebotomus de la region de Guatopo, Estado Miranda, Venezuela. *Arch. Venez. Med. Trop. Parasitol. Med.* **3**, 63-71

PRINGLE, G. (1957) Oriental sore in Iraq; historical and epidemiological problems. *Bull. Endem. Dis.* **2**, 41-76

QUATE, L. W. (1964) Phlebotomus sandflies of the Paloich area in the Sudan (Diptera: Psychodidae). *J. Med. Entomol.* **1**, 213-268

RAHIM, G. F. & TATAR, I. H. (1966) Oriental sore in Iraq. *Bull. Endem. Dis.* **8**, 29-52

RANQUE, PH., BUSINERAS, J. & ABBONENC, E. (1971) Acquisitions récentes sur l'épidémiologie de la leishmaniose au Senegal. *C. R. I Multicolloq. Eur. Parasitol., Rennes*, pp. 170-172, Faculté de Médecine & Pharmacie, Rennes

SHAW, J. J. & LAINSON, R. (1968) Leishmaniasis in Brazil. II: Observations on enzootic rodent leishmaniasis in the lower Amazon region, the feeding habits of the vector *Lutzomyia flaviscutellata* in reference to man, rodents and other animals. *Trans. R. Soc. Trop. Med. Hyg.* **62**, 396-405

SHORTT, H. E. (1945) Discussion following: Recent research on kala-azar in India. *Trans. R. Soc. Trop. Med. Hyg.* **39**, 37-39

SIDOROVA, G. A. (1962) On the epidemiology and epizootology of cutaneous leishmaniasis of the rural type in the Karshinsk Oasis in the Uzbek SSR. V: On the duration of *Leishmania* infection in *Rhombomys opimus* Licht, under natural conditions (in Russian). *Med. Parazitol. Parazit. Bolezn.* **31**, 412-414

SOUTHGATE, B. A. (1967) Studies on the epidemiology of East African leishmaniasis. 5: *Leishmania adleri* and natural immunity. *J. Trop. Med. Hyg.* **70**, 33-36

SOUTHGATE, B. A. & MANSON-BAHR, P. E. C. (1967) Studies on the epidemiology of East African leishmaniasis. 4: The significance of the positive leishmanin test. *J. Trop. Med. Hyg.* **70**, 29-33.

SOUTHGATE, B. A. & ORIETO, B. V. D. (1967) Studies in the epidemiology of East African leishmaniasis. 3: Immunity as a determinant of geographical distribution. *J. Trop. Med. Hyg.* **70**, 1-4

STALLONES, R. S. (1972) Environment, ecology and epidemiology. *W.H.O. Chron.* **26**, 294-298

VAN PEENAN, P. F. D. & REID, T. P. (1963) Leishmaniasis in the Sudan Republic. 15. An outbreak of kala-azar in the Khor Falus area, Upper Nile Province. *J. Trop. Med. Hyg.* **66**, 252-254

WHEELOCK, E. F., TOY, S. T. & STJERNHOLM, R. L. (1971) Interaction of viruses with human lymphocytes, in *Progress in Immunology* (Amos, B., ed.), pp. 787-801, Academic Press, New York

WIJERS, D. J. B. & LINGER, R. (1966) Man-biting sandflies in Surinam (Dutch Guiana): *Phlebotomus anduzei* as a possible vector of *Leishmania braziliensis*. *Ann. Trop. Med. Parasitol.* **60**, 501-508

WILLIAMS, P. (1970) Phlebotomus sandflies and leishmaniasis in British Honduras (Belize). *Trans. R. Soc. Trop. Med. Hyg.* **64**, 317-368

Discussion

Baker: Is it really known that anterior station development and transmission by bite is essential for all transmission of *Leishmania*?

Bray: To the best of my knowledge, every sandfly which has been shown fairly conclusively to be responsible for zoonosis has been one in which progressive anterior station development occurred. Adler (1964) suggested that one form of kala azar, produced by *Leishmania donovani*, was transmitted when a fly such as *Phlebotomus argentipes* was crushed, but that another form, produced by *Leishmania infantum*, with the reservoir in the dog, was probably transmitted by bite. That theory has been lost now, partly because very little work has been done on infantile kala azar in recent years.

Newton: So far in our discussions we haven't heard much about the role of direct inoculation in the transmission of African trypanosomes but under certain circumstances it can be important. Can *Leishmania* be transmitted by other flies, simply by direct inoculation?

Bray: It is certainly possible. With some of the larger biting flies (*Stomoxys*, tabanids) transmission can be shown in this manner in the laboratory, as Lainson & Southgate (1965) showed. Berberian (1966) long contended that in the Middle East some *Leishmania tropica* was transmitted by *Stomoxys*, but I think that practically all leishmaniasis is transmitted by *Phlebotomus*, and most of it by biting.

Lumsden: What proportion of *Phlebotomus* get infected if they are fed on different cases? Do a higher proportion become infected if there are large numbers of *Leishmania* in the skin, for example in diffuse cutaneous leishmaniasis? They must then be picking up infected macrophages at the same time as they are taking blood. How much is known about the intake of cells by *Phlebotomus*?

Bray: All the sandflies we dissected appear to take up mostly red cells, with just a few leucocytes; but there is no evidence that whole mammalian macrophages are taken up. The pick-up of infection is extremely efficient. With what are obviously very few flagellates in the nose of about 25% of hyraxes, the infection rate in sandflies is high, between 3 and 15%, and this is in a very short-lived insect. In a fresh blood meal, quite often we are able to find one or two flagellates immediately, very shortly after the actual feed. We have evidence that the delivery is as inefficient as pick-up is efficient. We also have some evidence indicating that infected flies have a higher death rate, which is quite interesting.

Pifano: Do you agree with the classification of *Leishmania* species proposed by Lainson & Shaw (1972)?

Bray: Broadly, yes. The leishmania of the New World need constant taxonomic revision and I would say that this was what Lainson & Shaw (1972) have done. This revision helps us to understand the situation better now, but it doesn't mean that in three or four years you or I, or Lainson and Shaw, will not change this classification. I would disagree with it only about *Leishmania pifanoi* in that I don't believe that the organisms causing diffuse cutaneous leishmaniasis differ in any way from those causing normal cutaneous leishmaniasis in either Ethiopia or Venezuela.

Pifano: When you find *Leishmania* in ulcerations in man, what name do you give to the parasite? Hamsters inoculated with strains isolated from patients with leishmaniasis of the same clinical characteristics sometimes show lesions like those produced by the 'Pifanoi complex' and sometimes like those produced by *L. braziliensis*.

Bray: This is the sort of question that Lainson & Shaw (1972) were trying to resolve by classifying Brazilian *Leishmania* into *L. mexicana* and into *L. braziliensis*. It is of course quite possible that in man the lesions, particularly the early lesions, of these two forms look exactly the same. I wouldn't dream of giving a name to the organism in any situation which was new to me. Its behaviour in a hamster does not help, because I would, like Professor Peters, ask 'What is a hamster?' I would want to see what the buoyant density of the parasite's DNA was and what its enzyme systems were. I would also want to apply to it the serological techniques which we have used for a number of Old World species. Only in a homogeneous situation such as that in Ethiopia would I give the parasite a new name. In our paper (Bray *et al.* 1973) we call our organism *Leishmania aethiopica* and this is based on serological grounds, on the buoyant density of DNA, on the chemotherapy, and lastly and least on its clinical manifestations.

Peters: Professor A. Zuckerman's group have worked on the immunological relations between various Middle East strains of *Leishmania* and have concluded that the clinical classification means very little (Schnur *et al.* 1972). Whatever sort of clinical lesion the parasite comes from, it could still be one of a number of serological types of organism.

Bray: Professor Zuckerman is looking at only one or two antigens and the fact that one or two antigens don't reflect the clinical entity is hardly surprising.

Peters: No, but it is a fragment of extra evidence which is beginning to fit in with the biochemical classification that other people are coming up with now.

Zeledón: The anterior development of leishmania may be a little different in the *L. braziliensis* complex. As shown by Johnson & Hertig (1970) at the Gorgas Memorial Laboratory, Panama, and as also seems to be the case in Costa Rica, there is development of flagellates in the midgut and even in the hindgut, which these workers, and ourselves, could consider to be *L. braziliensis* in the broad sense. I quite agree on the interpretation of the diffuse type of leishmaniasis; a case was recently described in Mexico too. Has anybody looked at the possibility that in man some sort of impairment of T lymphocytes may occur and that as a consequence a leishmanial infection tends to produce the diffuse picture?

Bray: In patients with diffuse cutaneous leishmaniasis T lymphocytes are incompetent in relation to leishmanial antigens. But to the best of our knowledge, from just a few experiments, the T cells are competent in relation to other antigens. They react to a tuberculin test, for example. And Dr J. Convit (personal communication) showed that patients with diffuse cutaneous leishmaniasis reacted normally to schistosomal antigen and to lepromin antigen.

Maekelt: Do you know what the infection rate is in the population living in endemic zones in Africa? This is important when the prevalence and distribution of the clinical forms of leishmaniasis in different zones are being considered. Dr Pifano's epidemiological study (1962) with skin tests in Venezuela indicated that many subclinical cases of leishmanial infection must exist.

Bray: I was attempting to indicate this without actually stating it when I said that obviously a condition can occur where promastigotes convert inside the macrophage and presumably begin to grow, but then the body mounts an immunological reaction against them and wipes them out before a clinical sign occurs. In these conditions delayed hypersensitivity probably would occur and one would see it in a patient who had never shown any clinical signs of the disease. This is pure hypothesis. All we know for sure is that the rates of delayed hypersensitivity are always higher than the rates of known clinical disease.

Zeledón: Recently we isolated, in culture, a strain of *Leishmania braziliensis* from a Costa Rican sandfly. I injected a human volunteer with a very small inoculum of this culture. This person was originally Montenegro-negative and he eventually developed a tiny lesion that healed spontaneously in a few months, making him strongly Montenegro-positive. A few months after the lesion had healed, I injected him again with a larger dose of the same strain and injected myself with the same amount. He responded against this new challenge as if it were a new Montenegro test, indicating that he was quite immune. I developed a typical lesion on my arm.

Baker: You apparently suggested that the strains that cause diffuse cutaneous leishmaniasis may have particular antigens that tend to produce tolerance, Dr Bray. I think Professor Kerdel-Vegas said in London that he had found that strains of *Leishmania* isolated from patients with diffuse cutaneous leishmaniasis and injected into hamsters and mice produced rather more florid lesions of different types (see Convit & Kerdel-Vegas 1965), and that these differences remained for at least two or three passages in the animals. These two things might be related. If there are some slight differences in the antigens of strains, these might be reflected in the behaviour of the parasite in the hamsters and mice.

Bray: Florid lesions were certainly a feature of that work, but it is a question of more florid than what? Lainson & Shaw's (1972) work seems to show that diffuse cutaneous leishmaniasis in Brazil is always due to *L. mexicana amazonensis* whereas the more usual infection in man is due to *L. braziliensis*. If one inoculates organisms from a patient with diffuse cutaneous leishmaniasis into a hamster, one will certainly get very florid lesions of the *L. mexicana* type. With organisms from a patient with espundia, practically no lesions will be seen, because they produce the *L. braziliensis* type of lesion. So the lesion has to be more florid than its real equivalent, not its apparent equivalent, to be significant taxonomically. That is, a single lesion in Brazil may be due to *L. m. amazonensis* or *L. b. braziliensis*. If the organisms are inoculated into a hamster different lesions will appear. Equally different sequelae will appear in man.

Pifano: In neotropical regions I believe that the same species of *Leishmania* can produce different types of lesions, and that the same lesion can be produced by different strains of *Leishmania*. I believe that the organism we call *L. braziliensis* represents an aetiological complex, consisting of biologically different species, varieties or strains.

Trager: Dr Bray, in the promastigotes in the heavily infected sandfly, where the organisms are in the anterior station, could certain of these organisms be the ones that can initiate infection, although perhaps the majority cannot?

Bray: We have no evidence on this, except that if culture forms which are presumably the same are inoculated either *in vivo* or into a tissue culture, the 'take' is about 0.01 of that seen if amastigotes had been used. We do not know whether that is because one particular promastigote is suitable for invasion of the cell, or whether that is the normal death rate under the conditions. Adler considered this problem over at least 20 years but came to no conclusion (Adler 1964).

Trager: We have some indication (J. Keithly, unpublished) that in cultures of *L. donovani* there is a stage in development when infectivity seems to be maximal in proportion to the number of organisms present. There might be a similar situation in the fly.

Lumsden: With trypanosomes, there are certain situations in which the infectivity of a trypanosome suspension (measured in ID_{63}) is much less than the actual concentration of organisms in it. Yet all the organisms are active, motile. There might well be a parallel between this situation and the *Leishmania* one.

Bray: In support of Dr Trager, the sandfly, particularly an infected one, does not live very long and if it is going to deliver the infection it had probably better do it quickly. So there might be an evolutionary argument for thinking that the *Leishmania* would be best prepared for infecting a vertebrate host about three days after their ingestion by the sandfly.

References

ADLER, S. (1964) Leishmania. *Adv. Parasitol.* **2**, 35-96

BERBERIAN, D. A. (1966) Mechanical transmission of *Leishmania. Trans. R. Soc. Trop. Med. Hyg.* **60**, 277-278

BRAY, R. S., ASHFORD, R. W. & BRAY, M. A. (1973) The parasite causing cutaneous leishmaniasis in Ethiopia. *Trans. R. Soc. Trop. Med. Hyg.* **67**, 345-348.

CONVIT, J. & KERDEL-VEGAS, F. (1965) Disseminated cutaneous leishmaniasis. *Arch. Dermatol.* **91**, 439-447

JOHNSON, P. T. & HERTIG, M. (1970) Behavior of *Leishmania* in Panamanian phlebotomine sandflies fed on infected animals. *Exp. Parasitol.* **27**, 281-300

LAINSON, R. & SHAW, J. J. (1972) Leishmaniasis of the New World: taxonomic problems. *Br. Med. Bull.* **28**, 44-48

LAINSON, R. & SOUTHGATE, B. A. (1965) Mechanical transmission of *Leishmania mexicana* by *Stomoxys calcitrans. Trans. R. Soc. Trop. Med. Hyg.* **59**, 716

PIFANO, F. (1962) La evaluación de la leishmaniasis tegumentaria americana en el Valle de Aroa, Estado Yaracuy, Venezuela, mediante el índice alérgico (intradermoreacción con antígeno de *Leishmania braziliensis*). *Arch. Venezol. Med. Trop. Parasitol. Med.* **4** (2), 25-36

SCHNUR, L. F., ZUCKERMAN, A. & GREENBLATT, C. L. (1972) Leishmanial serotypes as distinguished by the gel diffusion of factors excreted *in vitro* and *in vivo. Isr. J. Med. Sci.* **8**, 932-942

The African scene: mechanisms of pathogenesis in trypanosomiasis

L. G. GOODWIN

Nuffield Institute of Comparative Medicine, The Zoological Society of London

Abstract Trypanosomes of the *Trypanosoma* (*Trypanozoon*) *brucei* subgroup, including those that cause African sleeping sickness in man, live mainly in the connective tissues of the host. The lesions they cause are brought about in part by the metabolic activity of the organisms, but it is likely that most of the damage to the host results from allergic responses to successive antigenic variants of the parasite.

The infection also causes immunosuppression; the ability of the host to raise antibodies to other antigens is impaired, rendering it susceptible to intercurrent infections. *T. vivax* and *T. congolense*, the important trypanosomes of domestic stock in Africa, live mainly in the bloodstream; their pathogenic effects are also related to the immunological responses of the host. An understanding of the pathogenic processes may contribute towards improved methods of treatment.

Trypanosomiasis has much the same hold on the African continent today as it had at the beginning of the century. The distribution of the disease changes from time to time as efforts are made to control it, but village populations in the Congo basin are still decimated by epidemics of sleeping sickness and the ancient endemic foci, such as Gboko in Nigeria, still remain. Wars still generate refugees to drift across the country and establish new centres of endemicity. The only really novel part of the picture is the appearance of the luxury hotels that have sprung up like mushrooms to cope with the flood of international tourists to the game reserves. Many have been built in the heart of the tsetse bush and some of them are dangerous places to work in or to visit. Human trypanosomiasis has been added to the list of African exports.

It is still impossible to keep most breeds of domestic cattle, sheep or goats in about four million square miles of territory south of the Sahara because of trypanosomiasis. Most African governments are too poor, their basic veterinary services too sparse and the degree of cooperation with their neighbours too primitive to make a lasting impression on this immense problem, although we now have the knowledge—given the necessary finance, manpower and cooperation—needed to control the fly and the trypanosome in man and his domestic stock. Complete eradication would be unlikely, even if all the tsetse were to die; *Trypanosoma vivax* is transmitted quite effectively on the South American continent by biting flies that act as mechanical vectors.

Much has been learned about the biology of the tsetse fly and the nature and behaviour of the various species of trypanosome parasites, but relatively little advance has been made in the study of the pathology of the diseases caused by trypanosomes or, of recent years, in the provision of new medicaments for prevention and cure. The dearth of recent studies in pathology is due in part to the excellence of the observations made by the early workers in the field. After one has read the works of Mott, Laveran, Peruzzi and others, written during the first 30 years of the century, it may appear that there is little more to be done. But this is not so. Serious gaps exist in our knowledge of the histopathology of natural trypanosome infections in man and animals, domestic and wild (Ormerod 1970; Goodwin 1970; Losos & Ikede 1972). And it is high time that attempts were made to fit together what we already know of the morphological, metabolic and immunological behaviour of trypanosomes and the effects that they have on their hosts. A better understanding of pathogenesis might help to provide better methods of prophylaxis and treatment.

PATHOLOGICAL EFFECTS OF TRYPANOSOMES OF THE TRYPANOSOMA (TRYPANOZOON) BRUCEI SUBGROUP

The *T. brucei* subgroup, which includes the parasites of human sleeping sickness, is characterized by a predilection for living in connective tissue. This was fully understood by early investigators but in recent years has tended to be overlooked. Except in laboratory rats and mice, parasitaemia is no guide to the number of parasites in the host's body; organisms may be scanty or apparently absent from the bloodstream, while swarming in the tissue spaces. There is so far no evidence that trypanosomes in the tissue spaces differ in any way from those in the blood. The pathogenesis is complex and the cause of death is still somewhat obscure. Damage to the tissues is brought about perhaps through the metabolic activities of the trypanosomes, more certainly through the repeated insults offered by the emergence of successive trypanosome variants and the attempts made to suppress them by the host's defence mechanisms. Antigen–antibody reactions are accompanied by activation of plasminogen, the release of pharmacologically active substances such as kinins, changes in the state of the blood-clotting mechanisms and deposition of immune complexes in the kidney and other organs; all of these can cause harmful effects. In addition, the host's ability to raise an immune response to antigens other than trypanosomes is impaired and there is an increased hazard from concurrent viral, bacterial and helminthic infections.

An overwhelming parasitaemia may kill the host very quickly; an effective antibody response may bring about complete cure, with lasting immunity to local variants. More often, a balance is established between host and parasite and there is a tendency for local lesions to be repaired and for physiological disturbances to be corrected. The balance, more or less precarious, can be upset by stress or by intercurrent infection at any time.

Trypanosome motility

Although their movement is unceasing, there is no evidence that the activity of trypanosomes is in itself damaging to the tissues of the host. It is difficult to see any advantage to the parasite from 'this unforgiving work, this grey unresting industry. What aim, what future does it mark?' (Slater 1946). Non-motile protozoa—leishmania, plasmodia, coccidia—manage perfectly well without this obsessive restlessness. *T. vivax*, with its apparently purposeful movement, seems to have no advantage over *T. congolense* or *T. brucei*, which are more sluggish, apparently aimless, and share the same vectors. In spite of its activity, there is some doubt as to whether *T. vivax* ever manages to leave the blood vessels and enter the tissues. Trypanosomal movement would appear to be one of nature's throw-away gestures. However, there may be a price for the host to pay: there is an unremitting demand for carbohydrate to support the energy expended.

Trypanosome metabolism

The oxidation of carbohydrates by trypanosomes is dealt with elsewhere in this symposium by Dr Bowman (pp. 255-271). None of the metabolites along the several pathways available are recognizable as dangerous poisons; there is no evidence that trypanosomes produce toxins of any kind whatever. However, the carbohydrate turnover is massive and it has been suggested (Voorheis 1969) that animals that support a large population of trypanosomes may, as a result of the continuous demand for glucose, be in a condition resembling that in patients with diabetes. Moreover, *T. brucei* in the mammalian host can, on occasion, produce more pyruvate than the host's tissues can keep pace with.

TABLE 1

Pyruvate in blood and tissue fluid of a rabbit infected with *T. brucei*

Day of infection	Pyruvate (mg/100 ml)	
	Blood	*Tissue fluid*
0	0.82	1.11
6	0.9	1.27
9	0.82	1.15
13	1.31	1.4
16	3.36	1.64
19	1.7	1.4
21	1.81	1.89
23	2.3	1.97
27	4.47	2.59
28	3.12	3.04
29	3.86	3.04
30	5.91	4.93

The pyruvate concentrations in blood and tissue fluid of normal control rabbits remained at about 1 mg/100 ml throughout the experiment.

The peaks of concentration in the blood observed on the 16th, 27th and 30th days of infection corresponded with peaks of parasitaemia.

The metabolite accumulates in the blood, and Grant & Fulton (1957) and Coleman & von Brand (1957) found that, in mice, the amount of pyruvate was proportional to the number of trypanosomes present.

Our own work (Goodwin & Guy 1973) has been concerned with a study of the changes in blood and tissue fluid of infected rabbits and we have shown that, as the disease progresses, the pyruvate level in both fluids rises to about five times the normal value (Table 1). Tissue fluid contains about twice as much lactate as whole blood; during the course of the infection the level in both fluids rises to twice the original value. The high pyruvate concentration in tissue fluid seems to be associated with changes in the structure of the connective tissue. Tissue cages (plastic hair curlers) implanted subcutaneously in rabbits, become covered with a layer of new connective tissue composed mainly of fibroblasts, collagen fibres and blood vessels. The lining of such a curler in a normal rabbit is smooth, well organized and free from lipid. In an animal infected with *T. brucei*, the fibroblasts lining the cavity undergo a curious change, becoming laden with lipid droplets and gradually ceasing to produce collagen fibres (Fig. 1). They form a shaggy, rough surface to the new connective tissue and apparently float off into the tissue fluid (Goodwin *et al.* 1973). The normal metabolic activity of fibroblasts involves the production and storage of lipid

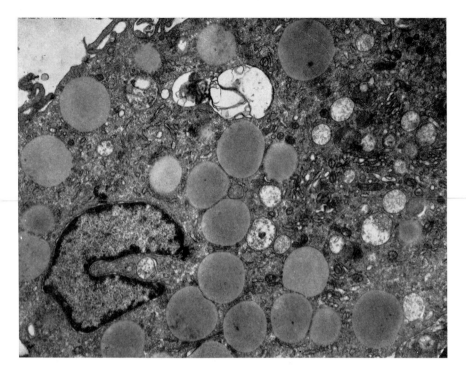

FIG. 1. A section passing through a cell lining the lumen of the tissue cage from a rabbit infected with *T.(T.) brucei*. Part of the Golgi zone is visible surrounded by vesicles containing diffuse material. The lipid droplets are a prominent feature of the cell. ($\times$ 10 135)

(Noble & Boucek 1955) but droplets rarely appear in the cytoplasm and if they do, are small, few and far between (Fernando & Movat 1963; Greenlee & Ross 1967). When exposed to concentrations of fatty acids in excess of their requirements, cultured fibroblasts collect lipid droplets in their cytoplasm (Geyer 1967; Mackenzie *et al.* 1967; Moskowitz 1967; Schneeberger *et al.* 1971). Persistently high concentrations of pyruvate, in the living animal, might provide a similar substrate for the accumulation of lipid in fibroblasts and, if so, this metabolite of the parasites could initiate the degenerative changes that take place in the connective tissues of infected rabbits. The fatty fibroblasts are quite clearly not doing their job. Skeletal and heart muscle also degenerate in infected animals and might also be affected by pyruvate accumulation, although heart muscle cells characteristically utilize pyruvate in the course of their normal activity. Experiments are in progress that should help to disentangle some of these possibilities.

Immunological reactions

The immune reactions of the host to trypanosome infections are a potent source of damage. Some years ago, at one of the annual seminars organized in London by the Trypanosomiasis Panel of the Overseas Development Administration, Professor R. R. A. Coombs pointed out the striking similarity between the events that lead to the death of rabbits infected with *T. brucei* and the syndrome described by Arthus (1903) as the 'generalized reaction' in rabbits sensitized to horse serum. The animal becomes oedematous and scabby around the face and the scrotum; the hair is rough, the ears flop and the muscles waste (Goodwin & Hook 1968). Antigen–antibody reactions are known to release potent pharmacologically active substances such as kinins, histamine, SRS-A (slow-reacting substance of anaphylaxis) and perhaps also 5-hydroxy-tryptamine and prostaglandins. The release of kinin certainly occurs during trypanosome infections of mice, rabbits, cattle and man (Goodwin & Richards 1960; Boreham 1968, 1970) and although the polypeptide is rapidly destroyed by plasma kininase, its effects could account for changes in vascular permeability leading to oedema, haemostasis, tissue anoxia and cardiovascular failure. Activation of the kinin system probably results from absorption of Hageman Factor onto the surface of antigen–antibody complexes (Boreham & Goodwin 1969). Boreham & Kimber (1970) have demonstrated the presence of aggregations of complex in the kidneys of infected rabbits—wherever these may originate, this is where one would expect to find them—and recent work in our own laboratories has shown that renal insufficiency is one of the main aspects of the pathology of *T. brucei* infections in rabbits (Goodwin & Guy 1973). There is progressive proteinuria; the protein in the urine resembles the normal serum proteins (Itazi & Enyaru 1973).

Boreham & Facer (1972) found fibrinoid deposits in the lung, indicating fibrinous exudation from the blood capillaries. More recently, Boreham & Facer (1973) showed that activation of plasminogen that occurred during the course of *T. brucei* infections in rabbits caused a measurable decrease in the plasminogen level in the plasma, and a fivefold increase in the level of fibrinogen degradation products. These substances are known to interfere with haemostatic processes.

The pathological process that takes place in the venules and capillaries can be observed using regenerative ear-chambers in infected rabbits. Although the first peak of temperature and parasitaemia occurs about three days after inoculation, the first signs of damage to the vessels appear on the 12th to 14th day of infection. The tissue spaces are crammed with mononuclear cells, large phagocytes stick to the vascular endothelium, collections of platelets and circulating leucocytes cause occlusions and the vessels disintegrate. At the same time, masses of trypanosomes can be seen in the connective tissue spaces and from time to time these are collected by phagocytic mononuclear cells and destroyed (Goodwin 1971; Losos & Ikede 1970). There is no apparent stimulation of the polymorphonuclear leucocytes.

Trypanosome infections cause the host to produce a great deal of immunoglobulin, particularly IgM, much of which is not specific to the antigens of the parasite and is useless in limiting the infection. Heterophile and autoantibodies also appear (Seed & Gam 1967), and Mackenzie et al. (1972, 1973) found that the levels of naturally occurring antibodies against homologous liver protein and fibrinogen, and against Wassermann antigen, were raised in rabbits and cattle infected with T. brucei, in cattle infected with T. congolense, and in human patients with sleeping sickness. Seed & Gam (1967) suggest that autoimmunity may be a factor in the pathology of trypanosome infections, but the rapidity and effectiveness with which health is restored when the parasite antigen is removed by chemotherapy suggests that it does not play a very important part. Although the concentration of protein in tissue fluid is lower than that in plasma and the capillary wall forms a barrier to proteins of high molecular weight, effective antibody titres are found in tissue fluid. In rabbits infected with T. brucei we showed, using the fluorescent antibody technique and blood films containing the trypanosomes as antigen, that titres about one-fifth of those in the serum appeared two days after the increase in the serum began (Goodwin & Guy 1973). The total globulin in the tissue fluid did not, at this stage of the infection, significantly increase; there was some evidence that the activity in tissue fluid at the time of the initial rise was due to IgG. Trypanosomes in the tissue spaces do not evade the humoral immune response.

As each antigenic trypanosome variant is suppressed by an antibody, another arises. The power to produce antibody wanes and the presence of the trypanosome interferes in some way with the ability of the host to respond to other antigens. This has been shown to occur in trypanosome-infected mice and rabbits challenged with sheep red cells (Goodwin 1970; Goodwin et al. 1972) and in rabbits injected with experimental allergic neuritis antigen (Allt et al. 1971). Also, Urquhart et al. (1972) have shown that rats with chronic trypanosomiasis are unable to mount a proper immune response to a primary infection with Nippostrongylus brasiliensis worms. Dr Brian Greenwood (unpublished) has recently shown that suppression of humoral and cell-mediated immunological responses also occurs in people infected with T. gambiense in an endemic focus of sleeping sickness in West Africa.

Murray et al. (1973) have recently studied the histopathological picture in rats infected with a strain of T. brucei that caused subacute disease; increased activity of phagocytic cells was observed throughout the infection. In the early stages, the lymph nodes and spleen were populated largely with lymphoblasts, dividing and differentiating into plasma cells, but later in the course of the disease these organs became steadily depleted of all immunological cell types. Similar observations were made on the lymphoid architecture of mice (Hudson & Byner 1973). It is unlikely that an animal in this condition would be able to produce antibodies to anything.

An attempt to explain the apparent paradox of heightened immunological activity accompanied by immunosuppression in trypanosomiasis has been made by Terry *et al.* (1973). They suggest that, by one means or another, trypanosome infections break the control link between thymus-dependent lymphocytes (T cells) and thymus-independent lymphocytes (B cells). In certain situations T cells appear to be able to prevent B cells from transforming into antibody-producing plasma cells (Allison 1971). Escape from control might allow B cells to proceed with the manufacture of IgM antibodies, some of which would be autoantibodies; other responses requiring cellular interactions would be suppressed. These ideas obviously need much experimental work to test them—but they mark the beginning of the elucidation of a fascinating immunological problem that could have effects in fields far removed from that of tropical parasitology.

Anaemia is also a characteristic sign of *T. brucei* infections; the cause is obscure. There is increased erythropoiesis, haemosiderin deposits accumulate and erythrophagocytosis occurs in the spleen. Murray *et al.* (1973) found that some rats underwent a major haemolytic crisis, with haemoglobinaemia and haemoglobinuria before they died. Herbert & Inglis (1973) suggest that erythrocytes may play a part in the immune response by adsorbing antigen on their surface; this may provide a clue to the cause of the anaemia. *T. congolense* and *T. vivax* infections also cause anaemia, which is very severe and is a frequent cause of death.

It is too soon to assess the part, if any, that may be played in pathogenesis by the amastigote phase of *T. brucei* described by Ormerod & Venkatesan (1971*a, b*).

PATHOLOGICAL EFFECTS OF T. CONGOLENSE AND T. VIVAX INFECTIONS

The basis of our knowledge of the pathogenesis of these important parasites of domestic stock was laid down during the first half of this century, largely by veterinarians working in East and West Africa. This work has been summarized by Hornby (1949) and by Fiennes (1970), both of whom made notable contributions of their own. More recently, the subject has been reviewed by Losos & Ikede (1972), who draw attention to the extent of our ignorance of the pathogenesis of these infections.

Unlike the trypanosomes of the *T. brucei* subgroup, *T. congolense* appears to be a parasite of the plasma; there is no evidence that it invades the tissues. This conclusion, reached by Hornby (1949) many years ago, has been confirmed by Losos *et al.* (1973), who made careful histological examinations of cattle infected experimentally with metacyclic *T. congolense* trypanosomes and slaughtered *in extremis* two to six months later. Large numbers of trypanosomes were found in the blood vessels of the brain, heart and skeletal muscles but the myocarditis, encephalitis, cellulitis and lymphadenitis commonly observed in *T. brucei* trypanosomiasis did not occur. The changes seen were anaemia, emaciation and polioencephalomalacia, probably caused by the accumulation of trypanosomes in the cerebral vessels. The uneven distribution of the parasites, which show a preference for swarming in the smaller blood vessels of selected organs, probably causes disturbances in the microcirculation, but Losos considers the main pathogenic factor to be anaemia. The cause of this, as with *T. brucei*, is unknown but is likely to be associated with immune reactions. Little work has so far been done to assess the effects of antigenic variation (Wilson & Cunningham 1972) and antigen–antibody reactions in *T. congolense* infections, but Fiennes (1950, 1970) suggested long ago that anaphylactic processes contribute to the lesions, and may bring about the serum dilution and hypoproteinaemia that he considers to be mainly responsible for the progressive decline of chronically infected animals.

The pathogenesis of *T. vivax* infections is equally obscure. Losos & Ikede (1972) think that the process differs in some respects from that caused by *T. congolense*; the organisms are distributed fairly evenly throughout the circulatory system, there are cyclical waves of heavy parasitaemia and the host often succumbs at the peak of a parasitaemic wave. In such animals there is evidence of massive terminal thrombosis in relatively large blood vessels. But the general progress of the chronic infection, with loss of weight and condition, anaemia and disturbance of the plasma proteins, indicates the involvement of immune reactions. As with *T. congolense*, little has yet been done to investigate this, although some useful observations have been made in experimental *T. vivax* infections in sheep by Clarkson & Awan (1969), and in cattle by Dar (1972).

Infections of different hosts with different species and strains of pathogenic trypanosomes quite clearly lead to pathological states of diverse nature and severity. But there is, surely, an underlying unity to the picture, based on the ability of the parasite to change its antigenic structure and to provoke the host's immunological defence mechanisms to repeated, often futile, activity. What happens to the host will depend on the length of time the process goes on, individual differences in the susceptibility of physiological systems, the habits of the trypanosome species or strain, and the influence of concurrent acute or chronic disease or stress. Death may occur from cardiovascular collapse, anaemia, myocardial or renal failure or acute thrombosis, or from an unrestrained secondary bacterial septicaemia or pneumonia; it depends on which system is most vulnerable and is the first to give way.

THE TREATMENT OF TRYPANOSOME INFECTIONS

A consideration of the pathogenesis of trypanosome infections gives an indication of what might be done to improve the treatment of infected patients. New medicines for the treatment of human trypanosomiasis are scarce; there has been no very great advance since the introduction by Friedheim of the melaminyl arsenical derivatives 25 years ago. The pharmaceutical industry does not find the difficult search for new drugs for a disease that affects a limited number of impoverished Africans an attractive financial proposition. But there is a need. And the trypanosomiases offer unique opportunities for unravelling basic principles of immunology and chemotherapy.

Secondary infection is a common cause of death in sleeping sickness; this is clearly linked with the immunosuppression that occurs during the later stages of the disease. In this connexion it may be recalled that Castellani was at first convinced that the cause of sleeping sickness was the coccus that he found in the brains of almost all fatal cases of the disease in Uganda at the turn of the century. When the ability of the host to manufacture antibody-producing cells has become impaired, antibiotic cover during treatment is clearly desirable. And this applies to all those diseases—leishmaniasis and malaria as well as trypanosomiasis—in which immunosuppression occurs.

A drug that would help to minimize the tissue damage caused by the presence of trypanosomes and hasten the repair processes would be a useful adjunct to treatment. Anti-inflammatory drugs, given with the purpose of damping down the catastrophic effects of successive allergic reactions, would be expected to benefit the patient. No real assessment has yet been made of the effects of giving corticosteroids or other antiphlogistic substances to sleeping sickness patients during treatment.

A drug that would 'freeze' or put the brake on the rate of antigenic variation might be a good medicine for trypanosomiasis; it would not necessarily be a trypanocide, and therefore new methods, different from the usual screening tests in infected mice, would be needed to detect useful activity of this kind.

Or there might exist a substance that would so affect the surface of the trypanosome that cells of the granulocytic series would take an interest in its presence and go into action to remove the parasite.

Pathology can often indicate directions, however fanciful, in which advances in therapy could be made.

References

ALLISON, A. C. (1971) Unresponsiveness to self antigens. *Lancet*, 2, 1401-1403

ALLT, G., EVANS, E. M. E., EVANS, D. H. L. & TARGETT, G. A. T. (1971) Effect of infection with trypanosomes on the development of experimental allergic neuritis in rabbits. *Nature (Lond.)* 233, 197-199

ARTHUS, M. (1903) Injections répétées de sérum de cheval chez le lapin. *C. R. Séances Soc. Biol. Fil.* 55, 817-820

BOREHAM, P. F. L. (1968) Immune reactions and kinin formation in chronic trypanosomiasis. *Br. J. Pharmacol. Chemother.* 32, 493-504

BOREHAM, P. F. L. (1970) Kinin release and the immune reaction in human trypanosomiasis caused by *Trypanosoma rhodesiense*. *Trans. R. Soc. Trop. Med. Hyg.* 64, 394-400

BOREHAM, P. F. L. & FACER, C. A. (1972) A histochemical investigation of fibrin deposits in the tissues of rabbits infected with *Trypanosoma brucei*. *Trans. R. Soc. Trop. Med. Hyg.* 66, 341

BOREHAM, P. F. L. & FACER, C. A. (1973) Fibrinogen degradation products in African trypanosomiasis. *Trans. R. Soc. Trop. Med. Hyg.* 67, 279

BOREHAM, P. F. L. & GOODWIN, L. G. (1969) The release of kinins as a result of an antigen-antibody reaction in trypanosomiasis. *Pharmacol. Res. Commun.* 1, 144-145

BOREHAM, P. F. L. & KIMBER, C. D. (1970) Immune complexes in trypanosomiasis of the rabbit. *Trans. R. Soc. Trop. Med. Hyg.* 64, 168-169

BOWMAN, I. B. R. (1974) This volume, pp. 255-271

CLARKSON, M. J. & AWAN, M. A. Q. (1969) The immune response of sheep to *Trypanosoma vivax*. *Ann. Trop. Med. Parasitol.* 63, 515-527

COLEMAN, R. M. & VON BRAND, T. (1957) Blood pyruvate levels of rats during hemoprotozoan infections. *J. Parasitol.* 43, 263-270

DAR, F. K. (1972) Antigenic variation of *Trypanosoma vivax* in cattle infected with strains from wild-caught tsetse flies. *Trop. Anim. Health Prod.* 4, 237-244

FERNANDO, N. V. P. & MOVAT, H. Z. (1963) Fibrillogenesis in regenerating tendon. *Lab. Invest*, 12, 214-229

FIENNES, R. N. T-W. (1950) The cattle trypanosomiases; some considerations of pathology and immunity. *Ann. Trop. Med. Parasitol.* 44, 42-54

FIENNES, R. N. T-W. (1970) Pathogenesis and pathology of animal trypanosomiases, in *The African Trypanosomiases* (Mulligan, H. W. & Potts, W. H., eds.), pp. 729-750, Allen & Unwin, London

GEYER, R. P. (1967) Uptake and retention of fatty acids by tissue culture cells, in *Lipid Metabolism in Tissue Culture Cells* (Rothblat, G. H. & Kritchevsky, D., eds.), pp. 33-47, Wistar Institute Press, Philadelphia

GOODWIN, L. G. (1970) The pathology of African trypanosomiasis. *Trans. R. Soc. Trop. Med. Hyg.* 64, 797-812

GOODWIN, L. G. (1971) Pathological effects of *Trypanosoma brucei* on small blood vessels in rabbit ear chambers. *Trans. R. Soc. Trop. Med. Hyg.* 65, 82-88

GOODWIN, L. G. & GUY, M. W. (1973) Tissue fluid in rabbits infected with *Trypanosoma (Trypanozoon) brucei*. *Parasitology* **66**, 499-513

GOODWIN, L. G. & HOOK, S. V. M. (1968) Vascular lesions in rabbits infected with *Trypanosoma (Trypanozoon) brucei*. *Br. J. Pharmacol. Chemother*. **32**, 505-513

GOODWIN, L. G. & RICHARDS, W. H. G. (1960) Pharmacologically active peptides in the blood and urine of animals infected with *Babesia rodhaini* and other pathogenic organisms. *Br. J. Pharmacol. Chemother*. **15**, 152-159

GOODWIN, L. G., GREEN, D. G., GUY, M. W. & VOLLER, A. (1972). Immunosuppression during trypanosomiasis. *Br. J. Exp. Pathol*. **53**, 40-43

GOODWIN, L. G., GUY, M. W. & BROOKER, B. E. (1973) Connective tissue changes in rabbits infected with *Trypanosoma (Trypanozoon) brucei*. *Parasitology* **67**, 115-122

GRANT, P. T. & FULTON, J. D. (1957) The catabolism of glucose by strains of *Trypanosoma rhodesiense*. *Biochem. J*. **66**, 242-250

GREENLEE, T. K. & ROSS, R. (1967) The development of the rat flexor digital tendon; a fine structure study. *J. Ultrastruct. Res*. **18**, 354-376

HERBERT, W. J. & INGLIS, M. D. (1973) Immunization of mice, against *T. brucei* infection by the administration of released antigen adsorbed to erythrocytes. *Trans. R. Soc. Trop. Med. Hyg*. **67**, 268

HORNBY, H. E. (1949) *Animal Trypanosomiasis in Eastern Africa*, H. M. Stationery Office, London

HUDSON, K. M. & BYNER, C. (1973) Changes in the lymphoid architecture of trypanosome infected mice. *Trans. R. Soc. Trop. Med. Hyg*., **67**, 265

ITAZI, O. K. A. & ENYARU, J. C. (1973) Nature of proteins excreted in the urine of rabbits infected with *T. brucei* subgroup organisms. *Trans. R. Soc. Trop. Med. Hyg*. **67**, 263

LOSOS, G. J. & IKEDE, B. O. (1970) Pathology of experimental trypanosomiasis in the albino rat, rabbit, goat and sheep—a preliminary report. *Canad. J. Comp. Med*. **34**, 209

LOSOS, G. J. & IKEDE, B. O. (1972) Review of pathology of the diseases in domestic and laboratory animals caused by *T. congolense, T. vivax, T. brucei, T. rhodesiense & T. gambiense*. *Vet. Pathol*. (suppl.) **9**

LOSOS, G. J., PARIS, J., WILSON, A. J. & DAR, F. K. (1973) Distribution of *Trypanosoma congolense* in tissues of cattle. *Trans. R. Soc. Trop. Med. Hyg*. **67**, 278

MACKENZIE, A. R., BOREHAM, P. F. L. & FACER, C. A. (1972). Non-trypanosome specific components of the elevated IgM levels in rabbit trypanosomiasis. *Trans. R. Soc. Trop. Med. Hyg*. **66**, 344

MACKENZIE, A. R., BOREHAM, P. F. L. & FACER, C. A. (1973) Autoantibodies in African trypanosomiasis. *Trans. R. Soc. Trop. Med. Hyg*. **67**, 268

MACKENZIE, C. G., MACKENZIE, J. B. & REISS, O. K. (1967) Regulation of cell lipid metabolism and accumulation. V: Quantitative and structural aspects of triglyceride accumulation caused by lipogenic substances, in *Lipid Metabolism in Tissue Culture Cells* (Rothblat, G. H. & Kritchevsky, D., eds.), pp. 63-83, Wistar Institute Press, Philadelphia

MOSKOWITZ, M. S. (1967) Fatty acid-induced steatosis in monolayer cell cultures, in *Lipid Metabolism in Tissue Culture Cells* (Rothblat, G. H. & Kritchevsky, D., eds.), pp. 49-62, Wistar Institute Press, Philadelphia

MURRAY, M., MURRAY, P. K., JENNINGS, F. W., FISHER, E. W. & URQUHART, G. M. (1973) The pathology of *Trypanosoma brucei* in the rat. *Trans. R. Soc. Trop. Med. Hyg*. **67**, 276

NOBLE, N. L. & BOUCEK, R. V. (1955) Lipids of the serum and connective tissue of the rat and rabbit. *Circ. Res*. **3**, 344-350

ORMEROD, W. E. (1970) Pathogenesis and pathology of trypanosomiasis in man, in *The African Trypanosomiases* (Mulligan, H. W. & Potts, W. H., eds.), pp. 587-601, Allen & Unwin, London

ORMEROD, W. E. & VENKATESAN, S. (1971*a*) The occult visceral phase of mammalian trypanosomes with special reference to the life cycle of *Trypanosoma (Trypanozoon) brucei*. *Trans. R. Soc. Trop. Med. Hyg*. **65**, 722-735

ORMEROD, W. E. & VENKATESAN, S. (1971*b*) An amastigote phase of the sleeping sickness trypanosome. *Trans. R. Soc. Trop. Med. Hyg.* **65**, 736-741

SCHNEEBERGER, E. E., LYNCH, R. D. & GEYER, R. P. (1971) Formation and disappearance of triglyceride droplets in strain L fibroblasts. *Exp. Cell Res.* **69**, 193-206

SEED, J. R. & GAM, A. A. (1967) The presence of antibody to a normal rabbit liver antigen in rabbits infected with *Trypanosoma gambiense. J. Parasitol.* **53**, 946-950

SLATER, M. (1946) In *Peter Grimes and Other Poems*, p. 35, John Lane, London

TERRY, R. J., FREEMAN, J., HUDSON, K. M. & LONGSTAFFE, J. A. (1973) Immunoglobin M production and immunosuppression in trypanosomiasis: a linking hypothesis. *Trans. R. Soc. Trop. Med. Hyg.* **67**, 263

URQUHART, G. M., MURRAY, M. & JENNINGS, F. W. (1972) The immune response to helminth infection in trypanosome-infected animals. *Trans. R. Soc. Trop. Med. Hyg.* **66**, 342

VOORHEIS, H. P. (1969) The effect of *T. brucei* (S-42) on host carbohydrate metabolism: liver production and peripheral tissue utilization of glucose. *Trans. R. Soc. Trop. Med. Hyg.* **63**, 122-123

WILSON, A. J. & CUNNINGHAM, M. P. (1972) Immunological aspects of bovine trypanosomiasis. I: Immune response of cattle to infection with *Trypanosoma congolense* and the antigenic variation of the infecting organisims. *Exp. Parasitol.* **32**, 165-173

Discussion

Newton: Seed (1969) has described the preparation of a protein fraction from homogenates of trypanosomes which he claims will produce increased vascular permeability and other changes that you have described in your paper, Dr Goodwin. Does this fraction release kinins or does it act directly on blood vessels?

Goodwin: I think it acts by releasing kinin.

Bowman: Pyruvate could possibly have some effect. In the chronic infection in the rabbit it was about 10 mg/l, rising to 60 mg/l. How did you sample the blood? Grant & Fulton (1957) showed a massive increase in pyruvate in the plasma of infected rats, but they waited perhaps a minute after drawing the blood before deproteinizing it. There are so many trypanosomes busily churning out pyruvate that Coleman & von Brand (1957) thought Grant & Fulton's values were artifactually high, so they withdrew infected blood directly into a syringe containing cold trichloroacetic acid. Of course trypanosome metabolism stopped immediately. Were the parasitaemia levels in your rabbits high?

Goodwin: No. But the pyruvate in the tissue fluid increased steadily as the infection progressed. The fluid is very easy to withdraw and to deal with immediately. I don't think the trypanosomes artifactually increased the pyruvate in tissue fluid after withdrawal.

Njogu: Alanine, which is obtained from pyruvate by transamination, is also increased in rabbits infected by *T. brucei.* It looks as if the system is trying to remove pyruvate but can't manage it.

Bowman: Given these vast increases in concentration, would you consider that those rabbits have an acidosis? Did you measure the alkali reserve in the terminal stages of the infection? Could the toxic effect of pyruvate just be due to an upset in acid-base regulation?

Goodwin: The alkali reserve goes down and there are changes in electrolyte balance, but only towards the end. The pyruvate increases from the beginning.

Bowman: Did you notice any changes in the structure of bone, for example, which might have maintained the alkali reserve?

Goodwin: We have not examined the mineral content of bone, but there are no gross changes. The impressive changes are the destruction of connective tissues and muscle.

de Raadt: In the very last stages of the disease, signs of acidosis are seen in man too. Some French workers (Bertrand *et al.* 1968; Dutertre & Labusquière 1966) who used cortisone clinically found that damage to the heart decreased, according to their ECG findings. Robertson (1963) and myself (unpublished) have tried giving cortisone to patients with sleeping sickness but we didn't use such high doses as Bertrand and co-workers did. The great difficulty, of course, is that one hesitates to apply the results from laboratory animals directly to the treatment strategy in humans. This is especially so because the most typical pathological lesion in human trypanosomiasis, meningoencephalitis, is very difficult to reproduce in the same constant way in animals. The basic pathological mechanisms may well be similar in animals and in man, but the question remains, why are so few cerebral lesions or perivascular infiltrations seen in rabbits?

Goodwin: There is perivascular cuffing with mononuclear cells in all tissues, including the brain, of infected rabbits. I agree that there is no good animal model for the encephalitis of human trypanosomiasis and it is probably time somebody tried to find one. Even monkeys don't always show much encephalitis, although some of Peruzzi's (1928) had brain lesions. Maybe the sphaeromastigotes found by Dr W. E. Ormerod (Ormerod & Venkatesan 1971) in the meningeal vessels will give us a lead as to what is going on.

Baker: Chimpanzees are a good model.

Goodwin: Yes, but they are very expensive and are a rare and protected species.

de Raadt: Dogs might be good but they are not so easy to handle. Of 20 monkeys which we have used for experimental infections in *T. rhodesiense* recently, only one developed a typical encephalitis. It is strange that the same strain produces encephalitis in an absolutely haphazard way in individual animals of the same species.

Goodwin: Doesn't this add weight to my suggestion that there is a general underlying situation? What eventually happens depends on which organ of a particular species or a particular individual gives way first.

Baker: Neitz & McCully (1971) and McCully & Neitz (1971) have made a detailed study of *T. brucei* in horses with an encephalitic picture similar to that in humans.

Goodwin: There are, of course, several ways in which brain damage can occur. In *T. congolense* infections in cattle, Losos *et al.* (1973) have observed polioencephalitis, a degeneration caused by blockage of blood vessels with trypanosomes. This is probably different from the mechanism in human sleeping sickness.

de Raadt: Have you looked for IgM agglutinating antibodies in the hair curlers [see p. 110]?

Goodwin: Not yet.

Njogu: We have found that the amount of protein in the urine is much increased in *T. brucei*-infected rabbits. In relation to what you said about antigen–antibody complexes, I assume you mean that the kidneys are damaged?

Goodwin: Both the glomeruli and the tubules suffer. They begin to leak during the third week of infection and we see increasing proteinuria. The serum proteins come through.

Newton: Did you actually detect the presence of the immune complexes and were they present in the glomeruli?

Goodwin: Boreham & Kimber (1970) detected complexes in the renal arterioles and venules; we found them in the glomeruli also. The glomeruli showed lesions in ordinary histological sections.

Peters: How general is the marked decrease in mitochondria in muscle in the infected animal? And do you think there might be a fundamental lesion behind all these changes? It has been suggested that in malaria a toxic material sets the vicious circle going through mitochondrial damage (Maegraith & Fletcher 1972).

Goodwin: Muscle cells lose most of their mitochondria when the trypanosomes have been at them: the damage is always patchy. There are 'nests' of trypanosomes in some places and none in others. No one has yet detected a specific toxin from trypanosomes.

Bowman: The fat in fibroblasts may accumulate because it is not being further oxidized, due to mitochondrial incompetence and eventually mitochondrial degeneration. I am not terribly happy about the vast pool of pyruvate feeding in to build up the lipids.

Goodwin: Nor am I.

Peters: What happens to the liver in this infection?

Goodwin: It is surprisingly resistant to damage. Enormous numbers of macrophages stick in the sinusoids and if we inject Indian ink into a rabbit infected with *T. brucei*, the liver goes black with particles taken up by the mononuclear phagocytic cells. The liver cells themselves look reasonably normal until the end of the infection, when they show signs of fatty degeneration. The liver is not entirely unscathed (Lumsden *et al.* 1972).

de Raadt: Three out of 100 of our patients had jaundice, which we couldn't explain, and M. Gelfand (personal communication) saw higher incidences in Rhodesia. Whether this has anything to do with the anti-liver antibodies found by Mackenzie *et al.* (1972) or with the different pathology in man than in animals, I don't know.

Bray: If the antigen–antibody complex gives a sort of glomerular nephritis, does that suggest to you that this might also occur at the blood–brain barrier and might be the chief way in which trypanosomes can leak into the central nervous system due to damage at that site? Has the *T. brucei* subgroup any special ability in this regard, since you find it largely in tissue spaces whereas you find *T. congolense* and *T. vivax* largely in blood?

Goodwin: *T. brucei* trypanosomes can probably get through the 'blood–brain barrier' very easily, slipping in between endothelial cells. They can also get out into the tissue when a vessel which has been stopped-up with leucocytes and platelets—or trypanosomes—starts to disintegrate. A trypanosome in a disintegrating cerebral vessel would be in the brain straight away.

Baker: If so, why don't they get in much quicker in, say, *T. gambiense* infection, when it seems to take them a long time to get into the central nervous system?

de Raadt: We found trypanosomes in the cerebral tissues of a mouse which had been inoculated intraperitoneally the previous day with *T. rhodesiense*. With regard to direct inoculation into the cerebrospinal fluid, in another experiment we inoculated a large dose of trypanosomes into the suboccipital space of a rabbit and were unable to find them in the central nervous system three days later. In other words, the pathological changes in the cerebrospinal fluid are necessary to maintain the trypanosomes in the fluid.

Bray: I am not necessarily surprised that you do not find the trypanosomes. Did you, for instance, get a rise in cell numbers or of protein in the central nervous system three weeks later?

de Raadt: No, the trypanosomes disappeared. My interpretation is that in hosts susceptible to brain lesions in trypanosomiasis, the brain has first to be damaged to provide the necessary conditions for the parasites to maintain themselves in the cerebrospinal fluid—the liquid has to be enriched, as it were. The penetration itself does not seem to be the problem.

Baker: Didn't Regendanz (1932) inoculate directly into the cerebrospinal fluid of baboons and produce infections of the brain? It is the only way one can infect a baboon.

Martinez-Silva: Infection of newborn mice with *T. cruzi* by the intracerebral route gives excellent results. Inoculation of a few parasites (1 to 10) of a virulent strain results 20 days later in a harvest of 1×10^7 parasites per gram of brain.

Newton: When you kindly sent us samples of tissue fluids withdrawn from implanted hair curlers they seemed to contain a variable amount of blood, Dr Goodwin. Do you think this has affected your analyses?

Goodwin: It affects the electrolytes; potassium leaks out of the erythrocytes. It is difficult to avoid getting some blood if samples are taken frequently because the needle has to pass through an exceedingly vascular tissue. A piece of silicone rubber tubing round the middle of the hair curler dissuades the tissue from growing over it on the inside and helps us to get a nice clear sample.

Lumsden: In the natural situation most animals are infected with all three species at once. Could a significant infection with *T. brucei* underlie the terminal parasitaemia with *T. vivax*, say? In man parasites are not easily found in the terminal situation, yet there are obvious lesions.

Goodwin: An inapparent infection with *T. brucei* might interfere with the immune response to other antigens. And the other antigen could well be another trypanosome.

Bray: But *T. gambiense* sleeping sickness is a very complicated situation, with general depression of the patient's health and consequently poor nutrition. Nutrition has a profound effect on the immune responses of the host and on other processes. In that situation, how do you work out which was acting on what?

Njogu: Cattle at our field station at Lugala, as I mentioned earlier, start with *T. brucei* and eventually *T. congolense* predominates.

References

BERTRAND, E., RIVE, J., BOUDIN, L., BARABE, P. & AYE, M. (1968) Le rôle des corticoïdes dans le traitement de la trypanosomiase humaine africaine. *Bull. Soc. Pathol. Exot.* **61**, 617-625

BOREHAM, P. F. L. & KIMBER, C. D. (1970) Immune complexes in trypanosomiasis of the rabbit. *Trans. R. Soc. Trop. Med. Hyg.* **64**, 168-169

COLEMAN, R. M. & VON BRAND, T. (1957) Blood pyruvate levels of rats during hemoprotozoan infections. *J. Parasitol.* **43**, 263-270

DUTERTRE, J. & LABUSQUIÈRE, O. (1966) Le traitement de la trypanosomiase humaine africaine. *Méd. Trop.* **26**, 342-356

GRANT, P. T. & FULTON, J. D. (1957) The catabolism of glucose by strains of *Trypanosoma rhodesiense*. *Biochem. J.* **66**, 242-250

LOSOS, G. J., PARIS, J., WILSON, A. J. & DAR, F. K. (1973) Distribution of *Trypanosoma congolense* in tissues of cattle. *Trans. R. Soc. Trop. Med. Hyg.* **67**, 278

LUMSDEN, R. D., MARCIACQ, Y. & SEED, J. R. (1972) *Trypanosoma gambiense* cytopathologic changes in guinea pig hepatocytes. *Exp. Parasitol.* **32**, 369-389

MACKENZIE, A. R., BOREHAM, P. F. L. & FACER, C. A. (1972) Non-trypanosome specific components of the elevated IgM levels in rabbit trypanosomiasis. *Trans. R. Soc. Trop. Med. Hyg.* **66**, 344-345

MCCULLY. R.M. & NEITZ, W. M. (1971) Clinicopathological study on experimental *Trypanosoma brucei* infections in horses. 2: Histopathological findings in the nervous system and other organs of treated and untreated horses reacting to nagana. *Onderstepoort J. Vet. Res.* **38**, 141-175

MAEGRAITH, B. & FLETCHER, A. (1972) The pathogenesis of mammalian malaria. *Adv. Parasitol.* **10**, 49-75

NEITZ, W. O. & MCCULLY, R. M. (1971) Clinicopathological study on experimental *Trypanosoma brucei* infections in horses. 1: Development of clinically recognisable nervous symptoms in nagana-infected horses treated with subcurative doses of Antrypol and Berenil. *Onderstepoort J. Vet. Res.* **38**, 127-139

ORMEROD, W. E. & VENKATESAN, S. (1971) The occult visceral phase of mammalian trypanosomes with special reference to the life cycle of *Trypanosoma (Trypanozoon) brucei. Trans. R. Soc. Trop. Med. Hyg.* **65**, 722-735

PERUZZI, M. R. I. (1928) Pathologico-anatomical and serological observations on trypanosomiases, in *Final Report, League of Nations International Commission on Human Trypanosomiasis*, **3**, 245-328, League of Nations, Geneva

REGENDANZ, P. (1932) Die experimentelle Erzeugung von Schlafkrankheit beim naturlich immunen Pavian durch Infektion des Liquor cerebrospinalis. *Arch. Schiffs- & TropenHyg.* **36**, 409-425

ROBERTSON, D. M. M. (1963) The treatment of sleeping sickness (mainly due to *T. rhodesiense*) with Melarsoprol. *Trans. R. Soc. Trop. Med. Hyg.* **57**, 122-133

SEED, J. R. (1969). *Trypanosoma gambiense* and *T. lewisi:* increased vascular permeability and skin lesions in rabbits. *Exp. Parasitol.* **26**, 214-223

Pathogenic mechanisms in Chagas' cardiomyopathy

ALFONSO ANSELMI and FEDERICO MOLEIRO

Laboratory of Experimental Cardiology, Institute of Tropical Medicine, Caracas, and Department of Cardiology, University Hospital, Central University of Caracas

Abstract The fundamental properties of cardiac tissue are correlated with the structural changes in the heart and the clinical picture in Chagas' disease. The electrophysiological changes are analysed in relation to the arrhythmias and the disturbances in impulse conduction that occur independently of heart size and configuration. The clinical manifestations of heart enlargement are analysed in relation to cardiac dynamics.

The infection produced by *Trypanosoma cruzi* is one of the most widespread endemics affecting the rural inhabitants of southern America. It extends from the southern United States to the Argentine Republic, the number of persons exposed to the infection being estimated by the World Health Organization in 1960 as 35 million, according to the distribution of the vector.

WHO (1960) reported that epidemiological studies based on the complement fixation test for *T. cruzi*, together with electrocardiographic studies in several countries, indicated that seven million people living in endemic areas had Chagas' infection, and 20% of these showed ECG alterations compatible with myocardial lesions.

In man, American trypanosomiasis initially affects the histiocyte reticular system, and later its most frequent site is the heart, where it produces either acute myocarditis or chronic cardiomyopathy, according to the stage the disease has reached. The clinical picture in these two phases depends on the type of histological alterations caused by the lesions in the cardiac muscle, and on the changes in heart function caused by the penetration and development of *T. cruzi* in the vertebrate host.

PATHOLOGY

Acute phase

The histopathological picture in acute Chagas' myocarditis (Table 1) has three basic elements: (*a*) the infiltration of mononuclear cells into the interstitial space; (*b*) variable degenerative processes in the myocardial fibres; and (*c*) the development of leishmanial cysts. The inflammatory infiltrate varies in extent and intensity, depending on the immunoallergic reaction of the individual and regardless of the total number of parasites present. The inflammation may be mild and localized in any area of the muscular mass of the heart, or conversely it may be very dense and extensive, affecting practically the whole myocardium.

The morphology of the heart in the acute phase of Chagas' cardiomyopathy depends on the extent and density of the inflammatory infiltrate. Hearts with mild inflammation in small areas of the muscular mass do not show morphological alterations, and the ventricular walls have normal consistency and tone. If the cellular infiltrate is very dense and extensive the shape of the heart is modified: the interventricular notch disappears and the ventricular walls become flaccid. In cases of the latter type, the pathologist sees organs of normal size and weight even though, for reasons to be analysed later, radiological study may have shown hearts of increased size and with variable enlargement of the different cavities.

Chronic phase

Histologically, the chronic phase of Chagas' cardiomyopathy is characterized by the presence (Table 1) of (*a*) fibrous tissue, (*b*) degenerating myocardial fibres and (*c*) infiltrates of mononuclear cells.

The destruction of the cardiac fibres and the fibroblastic proliferation are characteristic of this phase of the cardiomyopathy. Several theories have been advanced to explain the mechanism by which myocardial fibres are destroyed:

The mechanical theory, relating the chronic phase to the invasion of the cardiac fibres by the parasite and to the destruction of the muscle fibres through the rupture of the leishmanial cysts (Chagas 1909).

The toxic theory, according to which the fibres are destroyed by toxic metabolic products of the parasite, or by substances released when the parasitized cells rupture or when the parasitic bodies disintegrate (Vianna 1911). The

TABLE 1

The histopathological picture of Chagas' disease

Acute phase	(a)	Infiltration of mononuclear cells (lymphocytes, histiocytes, plasmacytes)
	(b)	Myocardial fibres with degenerative processes
	(c)	Cysts of leishmanial forms of T. cruzi
Chronic phase	(a)	Presence of fibrous tissue
	(b)	Myocardial fibres with degenerative processes
	(c)	Infiltration of mononuclear cells

toxic theory became more important when Mayer & Rocha Lima (1914), working on infected animals, found that the degeneration phenomena bore no relation to the presence of the parasite in the immediate tissues.

The allergic theory. By 1940 Mazza & Jörg had found that the number of aggressor organisms and the responses were not related, and they suggested that an allergic factor was responsible. Cossio (1943) also found that the number of parasites and the intensity of the inflammatory process were not related, and Jaffe (1943) observed that, if the cardiac lesions were caused by toxins produced by the parasites, the cases with the most serious lesions should be those with the larger numbers of parasites.

According to Jaffe (1943), toxic metabolic substances produced in the parasitized fibres give rise to specific antibodies against the myocardial fibres and so cause the lesions. According to this hypothesis, the lesions in the tissue should be diffuse but in fact chronic Chagas' cardiomyopathy is the result of a *focal inflammatory process* that evolves towards fibrosis (Laranja *et al.* 1956).

Andrade (1958) considered that the inflammatory lesions of the cardiac tissue were produced by immunoallergic mechanisms.

The vascular theory. Laranja *et al.* (1951) attributed the ischaemic phenomena to a reduction of the blood supply to the myocardial tissue, this reduction being due to the lesions originating in the small branches of the coronary arteries. Nevertheless, this kind of lesion is the exception during the acute phase of the disease, and Rosenbaum & Moia (1953) concluded that Chagas' disease did not endanger the arterial coronary tree during the chronic phase.

The neurogenic theory. Köberle (1956) related the cardiomyopathy to the direct action of the parasite on the cardiac adrenergic ganglia. However, in experimental studies, Andrade (1958) and Dominguez & Suárez (1963) reproduced the cardiomyopathy without finding alterations in the autonomic nervous system of the heart.

The anoxic theory related the destruction of fibres to a disturbance in oxygen diffusion due to the increase in the interstitial space caused by the inflammatory infiltrate (Anselmi *et al.* 1966). This would lead to fibroblastic proliferation, whose mechanism of production has been analysed by Sanabria & Aristimuño (1971) in experimental myocarditis.

Fibrosis varies in extent and distribution, taking the appearance of leaves, bands or striae. The fibrotic foci may be small, scattered throughout the myocardium and few in number, or conversely they may be very dense, forming large plates of fibrotic tissue which thin the ventricular wall. These fibrous tissue plates are separated from one another by normal cardiac muscular tissue. Among the fibrotic foci, muscle fibres may be isolated or grouped in irregularly distributed bundles. The muscle fibres in the fibrotic areas generally show degenerative changes of variable extent and severity, ranging from vacuolation of the cytoplasm to atrophy or total lysis of the cell.

The shape, size and appearance of the heart in chronic Chagas' cardio-myopathy are related to the intensity of the fibrotic process. If the fibrotic foci are scattered, forming small nuclei, and few in number, the morphology of the heart is not altered. Conversely, when the fibroblastic proliferation is very dense and extensive the size of the heart increases, since the replacement of contractile by fibrous tissue elongates the muscle fibres. This, together with the presence of fibrotic plates, reduced the thickness of the ventricular walls and of the muscular mass of the ventricular septum. The cardiac chambers are seen to be dilated, and the trabeculae are accentuated. Intramural thrombi, mainly at the apex of the left ventricle and the right atrial appendage, are frequent (Anselmi *et al.* 1965). The formation of these thrombi is conditioned by the roughness of the endocardium due to subendocardial fibrosis, and by the delayed circulation resulting from the dilatation of the chambers and the diminished contractility of the wall at that level.

Thinning of the ventricular wall by large plates of fibrous tissue produces a foliaceous texture which allows transillumination and is the starting point for the formation of aneurysms. For reasons not yet satisfactorily explained, these aneurysms are usually found at the apex of the left ventricle and the posterior area of the mitral valve.

Post-mortem injection of the coronary arteries has shown that the system is normal (Suárez 1967). The shape of the heart is rounded because dilatation of the ventricular chambers results in the disappearance of the interventricular notch. The fibrous tissue gives the heart a rosy colour, which becomes paler as the quantity of fibrous tissue increases.

PHYSIOPATHOLOGY

(a) Alterations in heart function

Experimental studies have shown that the fundamental properties of the heart are profoundly altered by the acute inflammatory changes in the myocardium resulting from T. cruzi infection and by the sequelae of these changes (the chronic phase).

The contractile force of the myocardial fibres decreases in both the acute and chronic phases of the cardiomyopathy. In the acute inflammatory process, the distensibility of the muscle fibres is altered by the increased interstitial space produced by the inflammatory infiltrate, and some loss of contractility results (Cross et al. 1961). Damage to the muscle fibre itself is another factor that reduces contractility (Salisbury et al. 1960).

The speed of propagation of the impulse is reduced in the atrial and ventricular muscular mass, both when there is an inflammatory reaction and when fibroblastic proliferation occurs.

Experimentally, in dogs with dense and extensive inflammation of the auricles, the speed of propagation of the impulse was considerably reduced, going as low as 50 mm/s, whereas normal values range between 0.5 and 1 m/s. In the ventricular muscular mass of dogs with acute inflammation of the myocardium, the speed of propagation was 120 mm/s in the right ventricle and 80 mm/s in the left (Moleiro et al. 1970), the normal values for ventricular propagation being 400 mm/s. This reduction at the free ventricular walls explains, through the mechanism of focal 'blocks' (Cabrera et al. 1961), the positive, wide and slurred appearance of electrocardiographic records obtained from the precordial leads in patients with severe Chagas' myocarditis (Anselmi et al. 1971).

The speed of propagation is likewise diminished in chronic Chagas' cardiomyopathy, figures of 90 mm/s being recorded at sites having connective tissue proliferation and degenerated and atrophic myocardial fibres (Anselmi et al. 1965).

The excitability of cardiac tissue undergoes important changes in Chagas' cardiomyopathy (Moleiro et al. 1970). When there are inflammatory infiltrates in the atrial and ventricular muscular masses, the excitability of the cardiac tissues is altered. It should be pointed out that when the myocardium showed profound histological changes the cardiac tissues became inexcitable. This phenomenon was more frequently observed in dogs undergoing repeated super-infections and with a long period of evolution of the disease. In these cases

multifocal extrasystoles and paroxysmal tachycardia did not follow high frequency stimulation.

The *functional refractory period* (FRP) of the cardiac tissues showed important
changes (Anselmi *et al.* 1965; Moleiro *et al.* 1970), depending on the extent of
the histological alterations produced by *T. cruzi*. As a rule, during the first
days of the infection, when the inflammatory reaction was very dense and
extensive, the FRP was greatly prolonged: 200–258 ms in the atrial muscle,
250–311 ms in the ventricle, and 289–335 ms in the auriculoventricular (AV)
conduction system. Animals killed after three months with the infection
showed shorter than normal FRP values in the atrium and ventricle. In these
cases histopathological study showed changes corresponding to the chronic
phase of cardiomyopathy.

Experimentally it has been proved that the *disturbances in the AV conduction
system* depend on the location of the inflammatory infiltrate (Anselmi *et al.*
1967). When this is at the bundle of His, the propagation of the impulse is
obstructed, increasing the AV conduction time. The FRP of the cells of this
tissue does not influence the AV conduction time. This type of lesion is recognized by the fact that the ventricles follow the high atrial frequencies, with the
P-R interval remaining at the same length. Conversely, when the inflammatory
infiltrate settles on the AV node, the conduction disturbance is caused mainly
through alteration of the FRP; the slow propagation speed of the impulse in
this instance has little influence. Prolongation of the FRP increases AV
conduction time at low atrial frequencies, and blocks the impulses completely
when the atrial frequency is increased.

(b) Dynamic alterations of the heart

The dynamic and morphological alterations in the heart during the acute
phase of cardiomyopathy are conditioned fundamentally by the type of
changes taking place in the cardiac tissues and depend on the intensity of the
immunological reaction (Table 2). When the inflammatory reaction is scanty
and localized in small isolated foci, the dynamics of the heart are not altered.

Conversely, if the immunological reaction is very intense, the fibres are
separated from one another by the cellular infiltrate and by oedema fluid. In
this situation the distensibility of the cardiac fibre diminishes; this becomes
apparent when the amount of oedema fluid attains 4 to 5% of the original
weight of the heart (Cross *et al.* 1961). Also, the myocardial fibres themselves
are damaged and become less distensible (Salisbury *et al.* 1960). This in turn
results in reduced contractility (Johnson 1945), which manifests itself as a

TABLE 2

Correlation between histopathological, functional and structural, and dynamic changes in the heart in Chagas' cardiomyopathy

Histopathological picture	Functional and structural changes in the myocardial fibres		Dynamic changes
Infiltration of mononuclear cells	(a) Functional changes	Reduced distensibility of myocardial fibres	Reduced systolic force
		Diminished contractility of fibres	Reduced systolic volume
Interstitial oedema			Increased end-diastolic pressure
			Decreased aorto-coronary sinus gradient
Myocardial fibres with degenerative processes	(b) Structural changes	Enlarged interstitial spaces	Decreased amplitude of heart beats
		Decreased resistance of wall	Reversible dilatation of cardiac chambers
Presence of fibrous tissue	(a) Mechanisms of cardiac reserve	Elongated muscular fibres (Starling's law)	Irreversible dilatation of cardiac chambers
	(b) Structural changes	Decreased resistance of the wall	Reduced systolic force
Myocardial fibres with degenerative processes	(a) Functional changes	Reduced distensibility of myocardial fibres	Reduced systolic volume
		Diminished contractility of fibres	Increased end-diastolic pressure
Infiltration of mononuclear cells	(b) Structural changes	Enlarged interstitial spaces	Decreased aorto-coronary sinus gradient
		Decreased resistance of wall	Decreased amplitude of heart beats

decrease in the systolic contraction force of the heart, a reduction of the stroke volume, and an increase in the intracavity end-diastolic pressure. The free ventricular walls, whose resistance is diminished by the increased interstitial space, the cellular infiltrate and the oedema, yield to the increased intracavitary pressure, causing the cavity to expand and the heart to increase in size.

The systolic contraction force and the stroke volume, together with the peripheral resistance, control the blood pressure. The decrease in the first two factors influences the regulation of the systemic pressure or the pulmonary pressure, or both. The reduction in contractility and the diminished resistance of the walls are factors tending to reduce the amplitude of the heart beats. On the other hand, the reduced stroke volume and the increased ventricular end-diastolic pressure cause the aorto-coronary sinus gradient to decrease, so lessening the coronary flow. The displacement of the aortic and pulmonary valves, and of the atrioventricular valves, is diminished through a reduction of the aorto-ventricular gradient.

As the inflammation of the tissue subsides, the distensibility of the fibre improves through the reduction in the interstitial space; the contractility of the fibre, and consequently of the cardiac muscle, improves. The stroke volume increases, the end-diastolic pressure within the cardiac cavities diminishes, and the resistance of the free ventricular walls increases slowly, as the oedema and interstitial infiltrate are reduced.

The dynamic alterations undergone by the cardiac muscle during the chronic phase of Chagas' cardiomyopathy can be related to the intensity of the destruction of the myocardial fibres (see Table 2).

When the amount of muscular tissue destroyed is small, the functional reserve of the healthy fibres is sufficient to maintain the dynamics of the heart. If the amount of contractile tissue destroyed is appreciable efficient cardiac function can still be maintained, since Starling's law applies (Starling 1918).

These adaptive mechanisms (Rosenblueth et al. 1959a, b) cause the heart to maintain its circulatory dynamics, keeping an efficient contractile force and a normal amplitude of cardiac pulsations, except where areas of fibrosis are confluent and form extensive thinned areas. As more contractile tissue is destroyed, the muscle fibre elongates until it reaches a dilatation limit at which the contractile force of the fibre begins to decrease (Doy 1921). The systolic contraction force then becomes less, the stroke volume is reduced, and some blood remains within the ventricular cavity, thus increasing the end stroke volume. The increased intraventricular end-diastolic pressure and the reduced aortic pressure cause the aorto-coronary sinus gradient to diminish and the displacement of the aortic, pulmonary and atrioventricular valves to become less.

CLINICAL ASPECTS

Acute form

The clinical picture of acute Chagas' myocarditis depends on the dynamic changes resulting from histological alterations and on the changes in the fundamental properties of the heart. The clinical manifestations during this phase are therefore very varied.

When the inflammatory reaction of the myocardium to the presence of *T. cruzi* is mild, the clinical manifestations depend on the localization of the mononuclear infiltrate. Thus, if the inflammatory infiltrate is scanty, the heart maintains its normal functioning and the tissue changes can be detected only by the electrocardiogram. The increased interstitial space produced by oedema and cellular infiltration causes a disturbance in oxygen diffusion (Anselmi *et al.* 1965) and negative T waves or positive deviations of the ST-T segment can be observed in the leads oriented towards the affected zones.

Scanty and not very extensive inflammatory infiltrations of the AV conduction system endanger propagation of the supraventricular impulse and produce AV blocks of all kinds, from first-degree block to complete block, including the Stokes-Adams syndrome. It is important to note that in the incomplete blocks the localization of the cellular infiltrate in the bundle of His permits the ventricle to follow the high atrial rates, while localization of the infiltrate in the AV node blocks the supraventricular impulses when the atrial rate increases (Anselmi *et al.* 1967). This allows one to make an approximate prognosis of the further evolution of the disease.

Dense and extensive inflammatory infiltrations severely endanger the distensibility of the myocardial fibre and jeopardize the dynamics of the heart.

The diminution of the systolic contraction force and the reduction of the stroke volume bring about arterial hypotension and the rapid and filiform pulse frequently observed at this stage of the disease.

The intensity of the second sound is decreased; this is caused by the reduction in the displacement of the atrioventricular, aortic and pulmonary valves. Functional murmurs occur as a result of valvular incompetence produced by the dilatation of the valvular rings. In this form of the disease, precordial pain, similar to that of angina pectoris, is frequent. The pain is of an oppressive type, radiating to the neck and left arm, but it differs from that of angina in not being relieved by nitroglycerin or by rest, since it is due not to an imbalance between demand and supply but to a reduction in the pressure gradient between the aorta and the coronary sinus. The symptoms and signs of right, left, or bilateral cardiac failure occur in accordance with the distribution and severity of the inflammatory lesions. In experimental animals, if the inflammation is intense but confined to certain areas of the free ventricular walls, the functional alterations to the fibres and the structural changes in the tissue are limited to the level of the affected zone, giving rise to aneurysms (Anselmi *et al.* 1971). Parietal aneurysms of the acute phase have not yet been reported in man.

The decreased speed of propagation of the impulse in the atrial muscular mass depolarizes this tissue slowly, thus prolonging the duration of atrial activation. The P wave of the electrocardiogram widens and the PR segment shortens as the duration of atrial activation increases.

The reduction in the propagation speed of the impulse and the shortening of the FRP are the basic elements that can lead to the appearance of circus movement, causing atrial fibrillation and flutter.

The reduction of the excitability threshold and the shortening of the FRP favour the appearance of supraventricular and ventricular tachycardia.

In the acute phase of the disease, death can occur as a consequence of the dynamic or functional alterations of the fibres. Cardiac failure, either bilateral or with predominance of one of the cavities, is the most frequent form of death. AV conduction disturbances with the occurrence of the Stokes-Adams syndrome and sudden death are other less frequent forms.

With the passing of the acute stage of the disease, the dynamics of the heart improve and the cardiac shadow decreases in size. When the cellular infiltration disappears, or is reduced to small isolated foci, the shape, size and kinetics become normal.

Chronic form

If the quantity of muscular tissue destroyed by the inflammatory process is small, the healthy fibres are sufficient to maintain the dynamics of the heart, which keeps its normal shape and size. Nevertheless, the myocardial fibres surrounded by small plates of fibrous tissue alter their fundamental properties, and ectopic beats may be produced as a result of the increased excitability and the reduced FRP. Unifocal or multifocal ventricular extrasystoles may occur, with episodes of paroxysmal ventricular tachycardia, and this may be the only manifestation of the disease. Lesions of the atrioventricular conduction system may produce bradycardia and the Stokes-Adams syndrome.

The presence of fibrous plates in the subendocardium may produce mural thrombi, which, when detached, cause embolism in various organs. Hemiplegia and acute pulmonary embolism are not uncommon.

Death in the chronic phase of the disease may be caused by arrhythmias, such as paroxysmal tachycardias, ventricular fibrillation or flutter disturbances in the AV conduction system, followed by cardiac failure or by embolism.

PROGNOSIS

The foregoing analysis of the pathogenic mechanisms of Chagas' myocardiopathy is sufficient to demonstrate the difficulty of establishing a prognosis for the disease. A classification based on the size of the heart, correlated with the evolution of the disease and the prognosis, has been sought, but this simplified concept, applicable in other fields of cardiovascular pathology, is unacceptable for Chagas' cardiomyopathy. Laranja et al. (1951) have shown that neither sudden death nor subjective manifestations of the disease necessarily bear any relation to the degree of cardiomegaly. It is difficult to predict, in the light of present knowledge, when a circus movement may begin, whether or not this will lead to ventricular fibrillation or flutter, when intractable ventricular paroxysmal tachycardia may appear, or at what time an AV block may be accentuated to produce a fatal Stokes-Adams attack.

Likewise, criteria that base the prognosis on an accentuation of the deviation of the electrical axis of the heart towards the left, are oversimplified and unacceptable. In most such patients, deviation of the electrical axis towards the left is due to a block of the anterior subdivision of the left branch of the bundle of His (Rosenbaum et al. 1968) and no prognostic value can be assigned to this.

References

ANDRADE, Z. A. (1958) Anatomía patológica da doença de Chagas. Rev. Goiana Med. 4 (2) 103-119

ANSELMI, A., PIFANO, F., SUÁREZ, J. A., DOMÍNGUEZ, A., DÍAZ VÁZQUEZ, A. & ANSELMI, G. (1965) Experimental Schizotrypanum cruzi myocarditis. Am. Heart J. 70, 638-656

ANSELMI, A., PIFANO, F., SUÁREZ, J. A. & GURDIEL, O. (1966) Myocardiopathy in Chagas disease: comparative study of pathologic findings in chronic human and experimental Chagas myocarditis. Am. Heart J. 72, 469-481

ANSELMI, A., GURDIEL, O., SUÁREZ, J. A. & ANSELMI, G. (1967) Disturbances in the AV conduction system in Chagas myocarditis in the dog. Circ. Res. 20, 56-64

ANSELMI, A., MOLEIRO, F., SUÁREZ, R., SUÁREZ, J. A. & RUESTA, V. (1971) Ventricular aneurysms in acute experimental Chagas' myocardiopathy. Chest 59, 654-658

CABRERA, E., HERNÁNDEZ, Y., GIORDANO, M. & SIMÓN, J. (1961) Bloqueo intrainfarto, in Cardiologia, p. 169, Editorial Interamericana, Mexico

CHAGAS, C. (1909) Nova trypanosomiase humana. Mem. Inst. Oswaldo Cruz Rio de J. 1, 159-218

COSSIO, F. (1943) Estado actual de nuestros conocimientos sobre la miocarditis chagásica. Rev. Med. Tucumán. 7, 11-21

CROSS, C. E., RIEBEN, P. A. & SALISBURY, P. F. (1961) Influence of coronary perfusion and myocardial edema on pressure-volume diagram of left ventricle. *Am. J. Physiol.* **201**, 102-108

DOMINGUEZ, A. & SUÁREZ, J. A. (1963) Untersuchungen über das intrakardiale vegetative Nervensystem bei myocarditis chagasica. *Z. Tropenmed. Parasitol.* **14**, 81-85

DOY, Y. (1921) Studies on muscular contraction. II: Relation between the maximal work and the tension developed in muscle twitch, and the effects of temperature and extension. *J. Physiol. (Lond.)* **54**, 335-341

JAFFE, R. (1943) Consideraciones sobre la patogenia de la miocarditis. *Rev. Sanid. Asist. Soc. (Caracas)*, **8**, 85-93

JOHNSON, J. R. (1945) Factors controlling intramyocardial pressure. *Fed. Proc.* **4**, 37-38

KÖBERLE, V. F. (1956) Patogenese dos Megas. *Rev. Goiana Med.* **2** (2), 101-110

LARANJA, F. S., DIAS, E., DUARTE, E. & PELLEGRINO, J. (1951) Observacões clinicas e epidemiologicas sobre a molestia de Chagas no Oeste de Minas Gerais. *Hospital (Rio de J.)* **40**, 137-192

LARANJA, F. S., DIAS, E., NOBREGA, G. & MIRANDA, A. (1956) Chagas' disease: a clinical, epidemiologic and pathologic study. *Circulation* **14**, 1035-1060

MAYER, M. & ROCHA LIMA, H. (1914) Zum Verhalten von Schizotrypanum cruzi in Warmblütern und Arthropoden. *Arch. Schiffs- & Tropenhyg.* **18**, 101-136

MAZZA, S. & JORG, M. E. (1940) Períodos anatomoclínicos de la enfermedad de Chagas. *Prensa Med. Argent.* **27**, 2361-2363

MOLEIRO, F., ANSELMI, A., SUÁREZ, R., SUÁREZ, J. A. & DRAYER, A. (1970) Effect of Peruvosid (Cd412) on excitability and functional refractory period of atrial and ventricular tissues in cardiomyopathy caused by *Trypanosoma cruzi*. *Br. Heart J.* **32**, 189-194

ROSENBAUM, M. B. & MOIA, B. (1953) Miocarditis crónica chagásica y enfermedades asociadas, in *I Conf. Nac. Enfermedad de Chagas*, Buenos Aires, pp. 95-103

ROSENBAUM, M. B., ELIZARI, M. V. & LAZZARI, J. O. (1968) *Los Hemibloqueos*, Editorial Paidos, Buenos Aires

ROSENBLUETH, A., ALANIS, J. & RUBIO, R. (1959a) Some properties of the mammalian ventricular muscle. *Arch. Int. Physiol. Biochem.* **67**, 276-293

ROSENBLUETH, A., ALANIS, J., LÓPEZ, E. & RUBIO, R. (1959b) The adaptation of ventricular muscle to different circulatory conditions. *Arch. Int. Physiol. Biochem.* **67**, 358-373

SALISBURY, P. F., CROSS, C. E. & RIEBEN, P. A. (1960) Distensibility and water content of heart muscle before and after injury. *Circ. Res.* **8**, 788-793

SANABRIA, A. & ARISTIMUÑO, J. (1971) Nuevos estudios acerca de las lesiones ultraestructurales en la miocarditis chagásica aguda en el ratón. *Acta Cient. Venez.* **22**, 182-193

STARLING, E. H. (1918) *The Linacre Lecture on the Law of the Heart*, Longman, Green, London & New York

SUÁREZ, J. A. (1967) Coronariografía post-mortem en miocardiopatía chagásica. *Gac. Med. Caracas* **75**, 57-93

VIANNA, G. (1911) Contribuiçao para o estudo da Anatomía Patológica da 'Molestia de Carlos Chagas' (Esquizotrypanozis humana ou tireoidite parasitaria). *Mem. Inst. Oswaldo Cruz Rio de J.* **3**, 276-294

WORLD HEALTH ORGANIZATION (1960) Chagas' disease. *Wld Hlth Org. Tech. Rep. Ser.*, 202

Pathogenesis of Chagas' disease

F. KÖBERLE

Department of Pathology, Faculty of Medicine, University of São Paulo, Ribeirão Preto

Abstract In addition to the well-known Chagas' disease with its acute and chronic phases, Chagas' syndromes are distinguished as sequelae of Chagas' disease. These (also called late manifestations) develop as a result of the destruction of nerve cells in the peripheral or central nervous systems or both, during the acute phase. So these late manifestations caused by a numerical reduction of nerve cells are essentially neuropathies. This provides a different orientation for the treatment of this widespread disease since these nervous system lesions are not reversible—Chagas' disease is not a problem for curative medicine but a challenge for preventive medicine.

When Carlos Chagas reported the disease he had discovered to the National Academy of Medicine in Rio de Janeiro he referred to it several times as a 'new world in pathology' (Chagas 1911). However, American trypanosomiasis passes after an acute septicaemic phase to a chronic one with a very low parasitaemia and few parasitic pseudocysts in the body tissue; accordingly inflammatory foci after the rupture of these pseudocysts are rarely seen. This classic concept of Chagas' disease, shown in Fig. 1, is nothing more than the well-

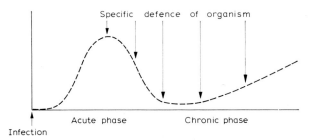

FIG. 1. The classic concept of Chagas' disease. Dotted line represents parasitaemia and parasitism.

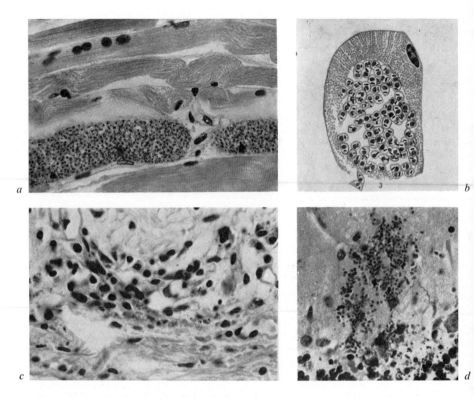

FIG. 2. Parasitism and ganglion cell damage.

(a) Parasitized striated muscle fibres in the human oesophagus.
(b) Rupture of a parasitized striated muscle fibre; only two leishmania forms are transformed into trypanosomes (Vianna 1911).
(c) Leishmania forms in the myenteric plexus of a human oesophagus in the acute disease; complete destruction of ganglion cells.
(d) Destruction of Purkinje cells after dissemination of leishmania forms in the cerebellum of a rat; acute disease.

known course of any infectious disease. There is nothing new in it to justify Chagas' assertion that this was a 'new world in pathology'.

Let us revise this concept, analysing the series of changes that occur after a parasitized cell has ruptured in the human host. Obviously there is no alteration while the parasitic pseudocyst remains intact (Fig. 2a). After transformation of the first intracellular leishmania form into a mature trypanosome, this latter form leaves the cell actively (Fig. 2b), penetrates the bloodstream and maintains the infection in the body. All the other leishmania forms not yet transformed into trypanosomes (and therefore not viable outside the host cell) die and disintegrate, causing the local lesions. This mechanism was

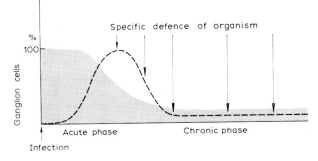

FIG. 3. Present concept of Chagas' disease.

demonstrated by Vianna (1911) in the first published report on the pathological anatomy of American trypanosomiasis and has been confirmed by all later investigators. The first reactions in the vicinity of a ruptured pseudocyst are degeneration, necrosis or lysis of the surrounding cells. All types of cells can suffer in this way but nerve cells are especially sensitive and vulnerable, as Vianna also observed. These very early lesions are immediately followed by much more impressive inflammatory reactions, which is why they went unnoticed or underestimated by later investigators. The ganglion cell lesion in the peripheral and central nervous system is shown in Fig. 2c, d.

We have studied these lesions of the central and peripheral nervous system during acute Chagas' disease in hundreds of inoculated animals and in five human cases. The reduction in the number of ganglion cells in the chronic phase was quantified by counting some millions of ganglion cells in several hundred human cases and in animals with natural or experimental infection. These quantitative studies of the nervous system in Chagas' disease led us to a new concept of the pathogenesis of American trypanosomiasis (Fig. 3). In addition to the well-known Chagas' disease with its acute and chronic phases, we distinguished so-called 'Chagas' syndromes' which result from the destruction of ganglion cells in distinct parts of the human body. These lesions are therefore *neuropathies* of the central or peripheral nervous system, or both, and they really constitute a 'new world in pathology', even today as new as in Chagas' time.

Let us take a quick and superficial look at this new world, or rather at a small part of it. I shall deal solely with the changes which have generally been called 'idiopathic hypertrophies and dilatations' in the hollow muscular organs, including the heart. In our material from more than 1700 autopsies of cases of American trypanosomiasis we found cardiopathy in 90%, megacolon in 20%, megaoesophagus in 18%, bronchiectasis in 7%, and other megaformations in 5%.

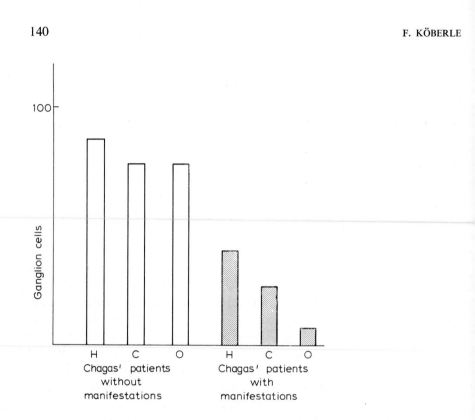

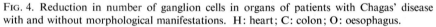

F<small>IG</small>. 4. Reduction in number of ganglion cells in organs of patients with Chagas' disease with and without morphological manifestations. H: heart; C: colon; O: oesophagus.

If the reduction in number of ganglion cells in these organs really causes this curious type of 'idiopathic' dilatation, it is essential to know how many ganglion cells there are in normal hollow organs. In normal organs (material from Vienna), we found the following total numbers of ganglion cells:

$$
\left.\begin{array}{lr}
\text{Oesophagus} & 2 \\
\text{Stomach} & 20 \\
\text{Small intestine} & 200 \\
\text{Large intestine} & 120 \\
\end{array}\right\} \times 10^5
$$

Total number of ganglion cells in the myenteric plexus of the digestive tract $\quad\quad 342 \quad \times 10^5$

Total number of ganglion cells in the intracardiac plexus

$$0.3 \quad \times 10^5$$

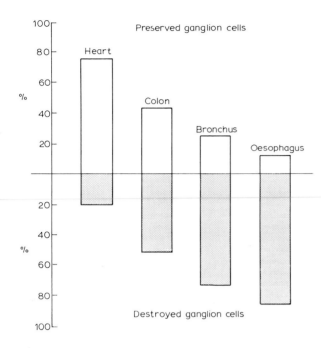

F<small>IG</small>. 5. Limits of tolerance of denervation.

We then compared these average values of the ganglion cell population in normal organs with the number of ganglion cells in the heart, colon and oeso-phagus from patients with chronic Chagas' disease with and without megalic manifestations (Fig. 4). A reduction in the number of ganglion cells is clearly seen in all chagasic organs, but the denervation in the organs with hypertrophy and dilatation (cardiomegaly, megacolon and megaoesophagus) is several times higher than in the chagasic organs without these morphological mani-festations. This difference is especially evident in the oesophagus. Apparently the sensitivity to denervation is different for each organ, being very high for the heart and very low for the oesophagus. For that reason we established the limits of tolerance to denervation in the heart, the colon, the bronchi and the oesophagus (Fig. 5). It is perfectly understandable that the heart is the most sensitive and the oesophagus the most tolerant organ. Whereas the heart is working day and night, the oesophagus has to work only intermittently, the law of gravity helps it during swallowing, and a large part of its musculature is striated, which means that it does not suffer from the destruction of the ganglion cells that occurs in the myenteric plexus. As the oesophagus is a relatively simple organ and its tolerance to denervation is very high, we selected it for a

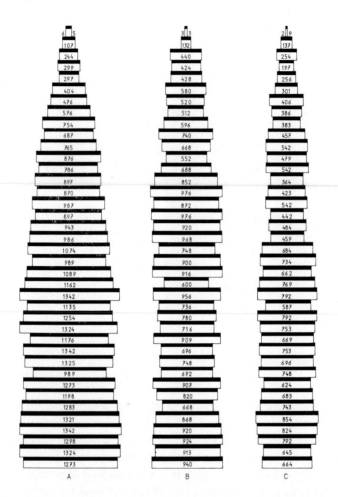

FIG. 6. Numbers of ganglion cells in rings of 1 mm thickness in the myenteric plexus of the human oesophagus; Above: cricoid cartilage level; below: cardia. From men aged (A) 20 years, (B) 60 years and (C) 75 years.

short demonstration of the essential pathogenic mechanisms in Chagas' syndromes.

Quantitative studies at 40 levels of three normal oesophagi show that ganglion cells in the myenteric plexus appear just below the level of the cricoid cartilage (Fig. 6). The numbers increase slowly up to the middle portion and then remain fairly uniform as far as the cardia. Fig. 6 shows that (1) the number of ganglion cells at different levels of the lower half of the oesophagus stays about the same, (2) this number decreases with age; (3) this decrease appears

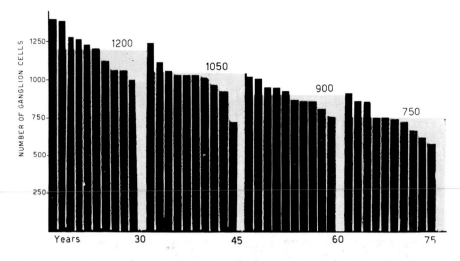

FIG. 7. Physiological denervation of the human oesophagus with increase in age.

to be uniform over the whole organ, and (4) for quantitative investigations on a large scale it seems to be sufficient to count the ganglion cells at only one level in the lower half of the organ.

The physiological decrease in the number of ganglion cells with age is demonstrated (Fig. 7) in 40 normal oesophagi from patients in Vienna who did not have Chagas' disease. This physiological denervation is the cause of the well-known difficulty in swallowing—presbyoesophagus—experienced by old people. We also investigated in the same way 40 oesophagi from patients with chronic Chagas' disease but without morphological alterations of this organ. As we had already learned that the nerve cells decrease in all chagasic organs, we expected a much steeper decrease with age than in the normal cases, but exactly the opposite happened (Fig. 8): more ganglion cells were found in oesophagi from older patients with Chagas' disease than from younger cases. The only possible interpretation of this apparently paradoxical result is that the chagasic patient dies sooner the more pronounced the destruction of his ganglion cells had been. Although nearly all of these patients died from a cardiopathy, the oesophagus was a very good indicator of the damage to their ganglion cells in general.

The more or less marked changes seen in parallel with the more or less accentuated denervation of the oesophagus are shown in Fig. 9. The first alteration in consequence of the disturbed peristalsis is dilatation of the organ. This dilatation may appear on X-ray examination but not at autopsy (rigor mortis) or in a surgical specimen. The initial dilatation is only temporary and is soon

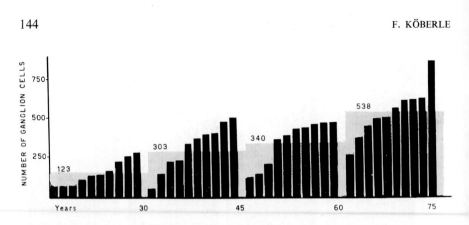

F<small>IG</small>. 8. 'Increase' in number of ganglion cells with increased age in chagasic oesophagus without morphological alterations.

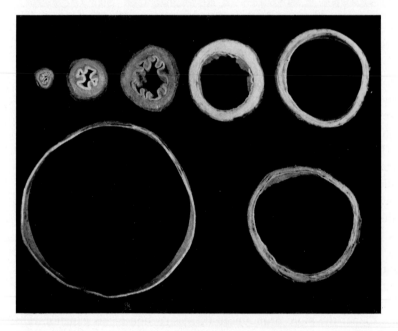

F<small>IG</small>. 9. Evolution of Chagas' oesophagopathy from a normal organ passing through hypertrophy and dilatation to megaoesophagus (approx. $^1/_3$ normal size).

compensated for by hypertrophy of the musculature, principally of the inner circular layer. Through a vicious cycle of dilatation and hypertrophy this muscle layer may increase by up to 25 times the normal thickness. But cases with such intense hypertrophy are very rare, because insufficient irrigation of the megaoesophagus soon leads to atrophy of the muscle and atony of the wall, with tremendous dilatation and elongation of the organ (megadolicho-oeso-phagus).

The same pathogenic mechanism leads to identical alterations in all the other muscular hollow organs during the final stage of megaformation. The essential lesion is a more or less intense denervation of the organ, with the immediate consequence that there are functional changes; time and overloading are the two main factors which produce the later morphological alterations which culminate in the impressive megaformations.

Whereas the oesophagus is the best paradigm with which to explain the pathogenesis of Chagas' syndromes in an easy and understandable way, the heart seems to be the most difficult and inadequate model. This seems strange, because a possible chagasic aetiology for South American megaoesophagus has been steadily denied, whereas the same aetiology for the different forms of a heart disease (myocarditis idiopathica, obscura, tropica, venezuelana, giganto-cellular etc.) that is very common in South America has been put forward by many authors and accepted by a few.

Cardiopathy is the most frequent and most dangerous of all Chagas' syndromes, with very distinctive clinical and electrocardiographic manifestations. The morphology of the chronic Chagas' heart is even more peculiar and shows some features completely unknown outside the American continent. We consider it to be a neurogenic heart disease, a neurocardiopathy caused by poor regulation of the nervous control of the activity of the heart. It seems obvious that every disturbance of cardiac function caused by changes in the autonomic nervous system must inevitably lead to morphological alterations in the organ. It also seems understandable that—because of the inherent automatism of the heart—such morphological alterations will not appear immediately but only after some time and in accordance with more or less severe overloading of the denervated organ. This is exactly what happens in Chagas' cardiopathy, yet only a few investigators accept that this characteristic heart disease is neurogenic in origin. It is not agreeable but it is in no way fatal if the chagasic oesophagus stops working for some minutes in consequence of a spasm or a palsy. The same event in cardiac activity leads to sudden and unexpected death, which in fact occurs in 60–70% of patients with Chagas' disease.

Because sudden death is extremely frequent and may occur at any stage of chagasic heart disease, the heart in Chagas' disease can vary in size from normal to huge (cardiomegaly) (Fig. 10). In addition to hypertrophy of the heart muscle and dilatation of the cavities, we find in more than 50% of cases a lesion that is not only characteristic but pathognomonic—an apical aneurysm. It is more frequent at the apex of the left ventricle, less frequent in both ven-

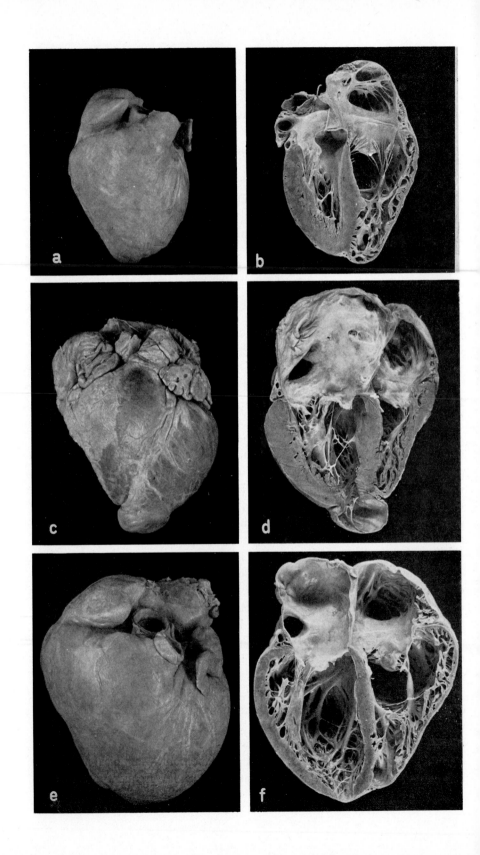

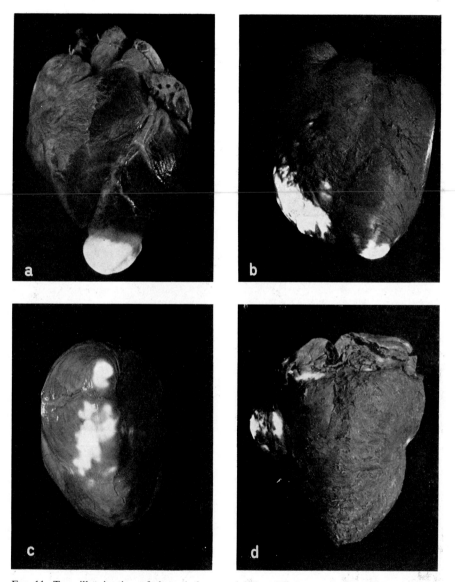

Fig. 11. Transillumination of chagasic hearts, showing different types of aneurysms.

tricles and rare at the apex of the right ventricle only. Very occasionally an aneurysm in the submitral part of the posterior wall of the left ventricle can be seen. The presence of an apical aneurysm often gives the heart the appearance

←

Fig. 10. Chagas' cardiopathy; heart weights 215 g, 420 g and 680 g ($^3/_8$ normal size).

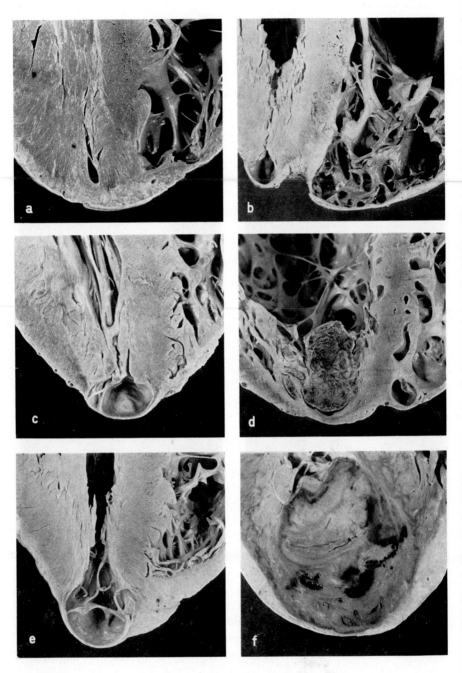

FIG. 12. Apical aneurysms with (right) and without (left) thrombosis (approx. $^5/_8$ size).

of a 'cor bifidum'. But even without an aneurysm the heart may show this peculiar shape, suggesting that the two ventricles have separated because of asynchronous activity. Transillumination of the heart shows the extreme thinness of the ventricular wall, which in these areas consists of endocardium and epicardium only (Fig. 11).

For a good demonstration of the peculiar morphological alterations we inject the hearts with formalin and fix them in the same solution (10%) for 24 hours. Then the organ is divided by a frontal cut into anterior and posterior halves (Fig. 12). Hypertrophy, dilatation, mural thrombosis and especially the pathognomonic aneurysms—even if they are very small—are clearly seen. As in the other hollow muscular organs, dilatation is always much more pronounced than hypertrophy of the heart muscle.

Those histological findings in chagasic hearts whose interpretation and significance led to so much controversy need not be discussed here. As an example of the futility of such discussion, I shall mention the categorical declaration by Doerr (1967) that Chagas' heart disease is a 'chronic parasitic myocarditis', although he found no parasites in the hearts!

Counts of ganglion cells in the intracardiac plexus reveal a striking decrease and sometimes a complete absence of parasympathetic nerve cells (Köberle 1957, 1959; Reis 1966; Alcântara 1970). Counts of the stellate ganglion showed a similar but smaller decrease in the number of sympathetic ganglion cells (Alcântara 1970). The average denervation of the heart was 55% and of the stellate ganglion 35%.

The verification of this denervation is difficult and tiresome. Therefore many pathologists simply deny the fact or its importance instead of investigating how much there is. But we now have a very easy method for demonstrating denervation of the cardiac valves (Ferreira & Rossi 1972). This method, using osmium impregnation of the valvular nervous network, is very convincing (Fig. 13) but unfortunately it works only in relatively fresh material (two to three hours *post mortem*), a condition very rare in our material.

The demonstration of the destruction of parasympathetic and sympathetic ganglion cells of the heart and the destruction of nerve fibres in the cardiac valves helps to provide evidence that Chagas' cardiopathy arises through a neurogenic mechanism. Previously no absolutely convincing proof of such a hypothesis existed. Because of the marked destruction of parasympathetic ganglion cells we assumed that the sympathetic influence on the heart predominated. The clinical symptomatology speaks in favour of this. Oliveira (1969) therefore injected isoproterenol (isoprenaline: 20 to 340 mg/kg subcutaneously) into rats and with only one application produced cardiac lesions exactly resembling those in Chagas' cardiopathy in man (Fig. 14). We do not know

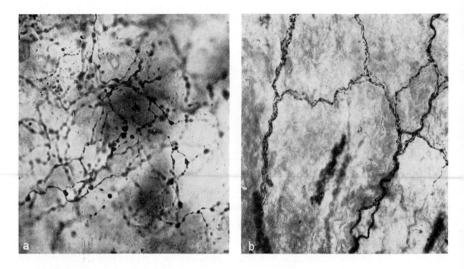

FIG. 13. Innervation of a normal tricuspid valve (left) and destruction of nerve fibres in the tricuspid valve of Chagas' cardiopathy (right).

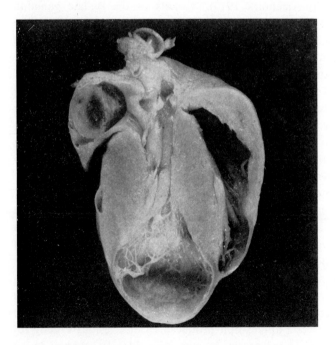

FIG. 14. Catecholamine-induced cardiopathy in rat.

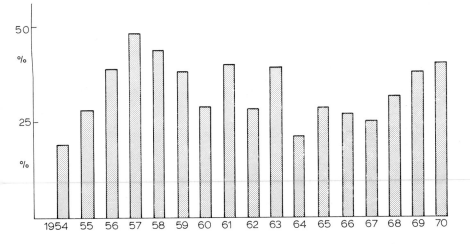

FIG. 15. Incidence of Chagas' disease as the cause of death in autopsy material (adults only) in Ribeirão Preto, Brazil.

whether our interpretation of sympathetic predominance is correct, because the amount of catecholamines in the hearts of chronic chagasic rats is not increased (J. S. M. Oliveira, 1972, personal communication). However these investigations have not been done in stress situations but at rest only. Another possible explanation is that the sympathetically denervated heart muscle is hypersensitive to catecholamines. As the cardiac valves mainly show destruction of sympathetic nerve fibres, this theory gains some credibility. It is more than likely that catecholamines play an important or decisive role in the pathogenesis of human Chagas' cardiopathy, since chagasic patients are extremely sensitive to sympathomimetic drugs (Brasil 1951).

In spite of all our efforts and all our knowledge of Chagas' cardiopathy we are still very far from a complete understanding of this terrible heart disease. Just as unsatisfactory is our knowledge of the mechanism and time of nerve cell destruction, two questions of fundamental importance for successfully combating the most frequent and terrible plague on the American continent.

My last illustration shows the extraordinarily high incidence of chronic Chagas' disease in our autopsy material, in which Chagas' disease is the cause of death of one-third of all adult cases (Fig. 15). This is by no means a local exaggeration, for many regions of Brazil and other countries show an even higher incidence. I can end my paper in no better way than by repeating the prophetic words of Carlos Chagas, who considered 'his disease' the most important and severe medico-social problem in Latin America.

152 F. KÖBERLE

References

ALCÂNTARA, F. G. (1970) Desnervação dos ganglios cardiacos e cervicotoracicos na molestia de Chagas. *Rev. Goiana Med.* **16**, 159-177

BRASIL, A. (1951) Estudo do sistema nervoso autonomo de coração na cardiopatia chagásica crônica. *Rev. Assoc. Med. Minas Gerais* **2**, 67-77

CHAGAS, C. (1911) Nova entidade mórbida do homen. *An. Acad. Med. Rio de J.* **76**, 45-84

DOERR, W. (1967) Entzündliche Erkrankungen des Myokard. *Verh. Dtsch. Ges. Pathol.* **51**, 67-99

FERREIRA, A. & ROSSI, M. (1972) Über die Denervierung des Herzens bei der Chagaskrankheit. *Beitr. Pathol.* **145**, 213-220

KÖBERLE, F. (1957) Die chronische Chagaskardiopathie. *Virchows Arch. Pathol. Anat. Physiol. Klin. Med.* **330**, 267-295

KÖBERLE, F. (1959) Cardiopathia parasympathicopriva. *Münch. Med. Wochenschr.* **101**, 1308-1310

OLIVEIRA, J. S. M. (1969) Cardiopatia chagásica experimental. *Rev. Goiana Med.* **15**, 77-133

REIS, E. L. (1966) Contribuição ao estudo dos ganglios cardiacos em chagásicos crônicos. *Hospital (Rio de J.)* **70**, 1421-1433

VIANNA, G. (1911) Contribuições para o estudo da anatomia patologica da 'molestia de Carlos Chagas'. *Mem. Inst. Oswaldo Cruz Rio de J.* **3**, 276-294

Discussion

Sanabria: In ultrastructural studies on chronic Chagas' myocarditis in the mouse, in spite of the parasitaemia present at the moment of death, we found no parasites within the muscle fibres. On the other hand, some muscle fibres had oedema under the sarcolemma and among the myofibrils, as well as vacuoles of different sizes. The mitochondria appeared to be swollen, with complete disorganization of the cristae and some inclusions. The mitochondrial membranes were separated by large spaces, and the external membrane extended into these spaces. Presynaptic buttons of the intramyocardial nerve endings also showed altered mitochondria. In the interstices, as well as within some muscle fibres, large bundles of collagen fibres and fibroblasts with intense secretory activity were observed (Sanabria & Aristimuño 1972).

Köberle: Acute Chagas' myocarditis in man is caused by parasites (leishmania forms) after their disintegration in the vicinity of ruptured pseudocysts. The so-called 'chronic Chagas' myocarditis' has nothing to do with parasites, which are hardly ever found in the hearts of chronically infected patients. Inflammatory changes appear after focal or massive lysis of heart muscle cells. Lysis is due to metabolic changes that occur because the muscle cells are denervated and become hypersensitive to catecholamines.

Maekelt: Three fundamental problems in the pathogenesis of Chagas' disease are the aetiology of chronic cardiomyopathy, the factors responsible for its evolution, and the factors responsible for damage to the heart.

The chagasic origin of chronic cardiomyopathy in Latin America can in most cases be confirmed only by serodiagnostic procedures. In many cases, because of a very low parasitaemia, it is not possible to confirm the presence of *T. cruzi* in the blood. Thus, a correlation between the presence of *T. cruzi* and its specific antibodies and the chronic cardiomyopathy can be established only by statistical methods.

We found that in Venezuela chronic cardiomyopathy is always much more frequent in individuals with specific *T. cruzi* antibodies. Statistical evaluation of 1286 hospitalized patients showed that a clinical diagnosis of chronic myocarditis was ten times more frequent in patients with *T. cruzi* antibodies (78 out of 402 cases: 19.4%) than in those with a negative complement fixation test (18/884: 2.0%). Statistical evaluation of 381 autopsies showed that the histopathological diagnosis of chronic cardiomyopathy was twelve times more frequent (62/78: 79.4%) in those with *T. cruzi* antibodies in the blood than in those with a negative complement fixation test (20 out of 303 cases: 6.6%) (Maekelt 1966). Also, in material from a non-selected rural population, electrocardiographic (ECG) changes were three times more frequent in *T. cruzi* antibody carriers (874/4262: 20.5%) than in individuals without trypanosomal infection (406/5738: 7.0%) (Maekelt 1970).

Our epidemiological survey of 10 000 people from different rural zones of Venezuela demonstrated that only 22.7% of 4525 *T. cruzi* antibody carriers (with or without positive xenodiagnosis) had ECG changes compatible with Chagas' disease (Maekelt 1970). We don't know why *T. cruzi* infection may lead to severe heart damage in one individual and to none in another. We may find *T. cruzi* (by xenodiagnosis) in the blood of individuals without any ECG changes.

Statistical evaluation of the results of our epidemiological survey showed that in individuals with *T. cruzi* antibodies the percentage of ECG changes depended mainly on the presence of *T. cruzi* in the blood. Of 3716 individuals with *T. cruzi* antibodies, but without positive xenodiagnosis, only 452 (12.3%) showed ECG changes. Of 546 individuals with *T. cruzi* antibodies who also had *T. cruzi* in the blood (positive xenodiagnosis), 422 (77.3%) showed ECG changes (Maekelt 1971).

From these results it seems that the presence of *T. cruzi* in blood and tissue may be an important factor in the pathogenesis of chronic heart disease. This finding does not favour theories which exclude the parasitic factor in the pathogenesis of chronic Chagas' cardiomyopathy.

Köberle: We are not able to exclude completely the 'parasitic factor' in the pathogenesis of chronic Chagas' disease, but we are convinced that it is not an important one.

For people living and working in an area of tremendous infestation there are two main problems. One is the mechanism of destruction of ganglion cells, which is not yet known; the other is the period of time over which this destruction occurs. We have sufficient proof that this destruction occurs mainly or exclusively in the acute phase of the disease and therefore we are convinced that the destiny of the patient with Chagas' disease is determined in the acute phase. This conclusion is of fundamental importance. If a child has severe poliomyelitis with paralysis of the right leg one can treat him for his whole life and he will still have a paralysed right leg. In the same way a child with severe degeneration of the oesophagus during acute Chagas' disease in the first year of his life will get an enlarged oesophagus in the course of time, with or without treatment.

We studied the alterations of peristalsis and the intensity of denervation in different segments of rat gut (Frederigue 1972). In the duodenum the functional manifestations were the same one month, six months and one year after acute Chagas' disease. According to this study the extent of denervation of the gut (75%) in these three different groups was also the same.

In a two year-old girl we examined, 99% of ganglion cells in the oesophagus had been destroyed, 95% in the small intestine and 95% in the colon. She had had acute Chagas' disease eight months earlier, after which she could neither swallow nor defaecate. Defaecation could be obtained with the help of enemas but dysphagia had to be treated three times by oesophagomyotomy. After the last operation the child died of mediastinitis. The autopsy revealed a megaoesophagus and a megacolon. In this case destruction of ganglion cells obviously occurred in the acute phase of Chagas' disease. We have other similar cases.

Maekelt: Megaoesophagus is rarely seen in Chagas' disease in Venezuela. Most of our cases with chronic cardiomyopathy have apparently never had an acute clinical phase of Chagas' disease—the phase in which you said that a tremendous number of ganglion cells had to be destroyed to explain the later development of chronic heart damage.

Köberle: Simple country people always answer according to the question one puts to them. Therefore it is very difficult to obtain an accurate history of their diseases in general, especially those they had in childhood. We must also consider the possibility of a congenital infection, not remembered by the patient.

Goodwin: In the rat experiments, you gave a catecholamine and the muscle disappeared. Does the lack of nervous control around the heart lead to an aneurysm because of the rise in blood pressure produced by the catecholamine?

Köberle: We do not know yet. In 80 rats with chronic Chagas' disease which may or may not affect the heart, the concentration of catecholamines in the heart muscle was not increased (J. S. M. Oliveira, personal communication). But these examinations have not been done on animals under stress, and it is well known that stress may increase the amount of catecholamines more than 100 times. We know that the hearts of patients with chronic Chagas' disease are very sensitive to catecholamines and this hypersensitivity could explain the heart muscle lesions.

Goodwin: Your patients produce endogenous adrenaline to which they must be sensitive and which could produce aneurysms in their hearts through the increased blood pressure. Do beta-blocking drugs help those patients?

Köberle: I have no personal experience but in haemodynamic studies clinical investigators in our medical school (D. S. Amorim, personal communication) have given propranolol to chagasic patients without cardiopathy. Beta-blocking drugs must not be given to a patient with manifest Chagas' cardiopathy because they would kill him, apparently by completely blocking sympathetic action on the heart muscle.

Pulido: In the University Hospital, Caracas, a group interested in the physiological responses of these patients as shown in renal clearance tests is testing beta-blocking drugs. The results are not published yet but the patients certainly improve (H. Acquatella, personal communication). Are the catecholamine concentrations diminished in the rat hearts you studied, Professor Köberle?

Köberle: No.

Pulido: What about the response with atropine and similar drugs?

Köberle: Some Chagas' cases respond and some do not. There is no exact concordance between the presence or intensity of chronic Chagas' cardiopathy and the denervation (verified by functional methods) of the heart (D. S. Amorim, personal communication). There is denervation of both the parasympathetic and the sympathetic systems of the heart (usually 55% parasympathetic and 35% sympathetic denervation). The situation of the heart is much more difficult and complex than that of the oesophagus. We are now beginning to study the hearts of patients with chronic Chagas' disease in collaboration with the clinical investigators. But there are many difficulties, one of the greatest being that patients who die have usually not been clinically and haemodynamically studied, while patients who have had an extensive functional examination do not die.

Pulido: There has been no real investigation of the incidence of megaoesophagus or megacolon in Chagas' disease in Venezuela, as you indicated, but can you explain the difference between the Brazilian findings and ours?

Köberle: I don't know why there are differences in pathology in different countries. In Paraguay, Argentine, Chile and Bolivia there are thousands of cases with megacolon and only a few cases of megaoesophagus. In Brazil we have thousands with megaoesophagus and more or less the same number of megacolons. In Venezuela you have very few cases of either megaoesophagus or megacolon.

Pulido: Could variations in the antigenic composition of the trypanosomes be the basis for this difference?

Köberle: It is very difficult to know. Chagas' cardiopathy is characterized by alterations in shape and in the conduction of stimuli, and all over South America the heart symptomatology is the same. The manifestations in the digestive tract are quite different.

Newton: Has anybody made a really detailed and careful comparison of the pathogenicity and symptoms produced by strains from different geographical areas?

Köberle: Andrade *et al.* (1970) studied three strains and verified a different tropism. We are working exclusively with the Y strain and cannot confirm these results. The variation in tropism of our Y strain was discouraging. When we wanted to study the encephalic lesions in a large group of rats, all the parasites were in the viscera or in the striated muscle. When we planned a systematic study of visceral lesions, all metastases were found in the central nervous system, and so on.

Pulido: That is why I asked about antigenic composition. Gonçalves & Yamaha (1969) claim that the polysaccharide and protein compositions are different in two different strains.

Newton: If one is comparing the protein and carbohydrate composition of different strains it is vital that the organisms should be grown under precisely the same conditions and examined at the same stage of growth. Without knowing whether this was done in the work of Gonçalves & Yamaha, I think it is difficult to assess the significance of reports of differences in polysaccharide and protein composition.

Sanabria: Thromboembolism often occurs in Chagas' disease and the embolus frequently reaches the kidney. Determinations of lactate dehydrogenase and alkaline phosphatase levels in urine have proved helpful in the diagnosis of renal infarction in patients with Chagas' disease and advanced heart failure. In four series of necropsies by other workers, renal infarcts were reported in 27% (74 out of 274) of patients dying from Chagas' disease. In our study (Sanabria *et al.* 1970) half the patients had increased levels of enzymes in urine and renal infarcts were found in three out of four cases at autopsy. We suggest that the incidence of renal infarction in Chagas' disease may be even higher than that previously reported.

Peters: John Edgcomb and Carl Johnson, who have studied the pathology of Chagas' disease in Panama in depth, have told me that they see a lot of typical acute cardiopathy of the type Professor Köberle described, but they do not see megasyndromes at all. Dr Walter Petana, who has been studying fresh isolates of *T. cruzi* in a 'standard mouse' from various parts of South America from British Honduras down to Rio de Janeiro, has good evidence (personal communication) that there are distinctive trypanosome strains with clearly defined tropisms for cardiac muscle, nervous tissue and so on. We really do not know whether there is just one organism or a complex of organisms.

Goodwin: It is probably a complex of organisms. Presumably, if a large number of parasites collect in a certain place, they will produce a certain effect on the tissues near to them. Therefore, they must either release or remove something for a local action to be produced. Surely experiments could be done to help us to understand this. Have you any idea what these parasites do to the cells near to them, Professor Köberle?

Köberle: We have some ideas but no definite proof of the mechanism of ganglion cell destruction. Studies of human and experimental material allow us to exclude several mechanisms proposed as being responsible for the nerve cell damage: parasitism of the ganglion cell, parasitism of the Schwann cells and inflammatory infiltration. We think that the ganglion cell destruction is closely connected with the rupture of the parasitic pseudocysts because it appears immediately after this rupture but before the inflammatory reaction begins. Mayer & Rocha Lima (1912) long ago saw a liquid inside the pseudocysts before their rupture, when the transformation of leishmania forms into trypanosomes begins. This fluid, liberated after the cell rupture, could be responsible for the nerve cell damage. We are more inclined to consider that destruction is caused by disintegration of the leishmania forms which are not viable outside the host cells. Meyer *et al.* (1958) showed a small vesicle at the posterior end of the trypanosomes which obviously contains a membranolytic substance (enzyme) necessary for the penetration of the parasites into the host cells. If the leishmania forms also contain this enzyme or its precursor, it may when liberated damage the membranes of the surrounding cells and so destroy them. The ganglion cells appear to be very sensitive or susceptible to the postulated substance. So it is not a neurotoxin but rather a cytotoxin or cytolysin, which can damage every cell in the organism.

Bray: Dr R. J. W. Rees at the National Institute of Medical Research in London has been examining the effect of lysosomes on *Mycobacterium* inside cells in tissue culture. Briefly, if the parasite is dead or is one which cannot establish itself in the cell system the lysosomes converge on the phagosome containing the parasite and eventually surround and destroy the parasite. If the parasite is successful as with *M. leprae* in a macrophage the cell's lysosomes completely ignore the parasite. Now Dr Sanabria has published very interesting electron micrographs (Sanabria 1971) which show a Kuppfer cell having engulfed a trypomastigote of *T. cruzi* and the trypomastigote is surrounded by what Dr Sanabria believes to be a lysosome. In other photomicrographs, however, he shows amastigotes of *T. cruzi* in Kuppfer cells where no lysosomes are to be seen in the vicinity. Thus there appears to be some evidence for a similar lysosomal activity in *T. cruzi* infection as with mycobacteria. A point to remember is that muscle cells have no lysosomes, I believe.

References

ANDRADE, S. G., CARVALHO, M. L. & FIGUEIRA, R. M. (1970) Caracterização morfobiologica e histopatologica de diferentes cêpas de *Trypanosoma cruzi*. *Gaz. Med. Bahia* **70**, 32-42

FREDERIGUE, U., JR. (1972) Correlação entre alterações functionaes e destruição neuronal no duodeno isolado de ratos chagasicos. Thesis, Faculty of Medicine, Ribeirão Preto

GONÇALVES, J. M. & YAMAHA, T. (1969) Immunochemical polysaccharide from *Trypanosoma cruzi*. *J. Trop. Med. Hyg.* **72**, 39-44.

MAEKELT, G. A. (1966) La evaluación longitudinal de las campañas contra la enfermedad de Chagas por procedimientos parasitológicos e inmunológicos. *Rev. Venez. Sanid. Asist. Soc.* **31**, 163-181

MAEKELT, G. A. (1970) Seroepidemiology of Chagas' disease. *J. Parasitol.* **56**, 557

MAEKELT, G. A. (1971) Die Serodiagnose der Trypanosomiasen, insbesondere der Chagaskrankheit, in *Kongressbericht über die II Tagung der Österreichischen Gesellschaft für Tropenmedizin und der IV Tagung der Deutschen Tropenmedizinischen Gesellschaft e.V. 1969 vom 21 bis 23 April in Salzburg und in Bad Reichenhall* (Flamm, H. & Mohr, W., eds.), pp. 111-121, Hansisches Verlagskontor H. Scheffler, Lübeck

MAYER, M. & ROCHA LIMA, H. (1912) Zur Entwicklung von *Schizotrypanum cruzi* in Säugetieren. *Arch. Schiffs.- & Tropenhyg.* **17**, 376-380

MEYER, H., OLIVEIRA MUSACCHIO, M. DE & ANDRADE MENDONÇA, I. DE (1958) Electron microscopic study of *Trypanosoma cruzi* in thin sections of infected tissue cultures and of blood-agar forms. *Parasitology*, **48**, 1-8

SANABRIA, A. (1971) Ultrastructure of *Trypanosoma cruzi* in mouse liver. *Exp. Parasitol.* **30**, 187-198

SANABRIA, A. & ARISTIMUÑO, J. (1972) Estudio ultramicroscopico de la miocarditis chagasica cronica en el raton. *Acta Cient. Venez.* **23**, 66-74

SANABRIA, A., ACQUATELLA, H., PULIDO, P. A. & SUÁREZ, J. A. (1970) Diagnóstico del infarto renal en la enfermedad de Chagas por las enzimas urinarias deshidrogenasa láctica y fosfatasa alcalina. *Acta Med. Venez.* Jan./Feb., pp. 7-14

Cutaneous leishmaniasis

The clinical and immunopathological spectrum in South America

J. CONVIT and M. E. PINARDI

Instituto Nacional de Dermatologia, Caracas

Abstract The correlation between the clinical, histopathological and immunological aspects of American cutaneous leishmaniasis suggests that the various clinical forms of this disease in South America may be conditioned mainly by the various types of response of the human host towards the leishmanial parasite.

Cutaneous leishmaniasis is a public health problem in all the South American countries where it has been described. Its importance varies according to the country. The only South American country where it has not been seen so far is Chile.

When its multiple forms are considered, especially in relation to the predominance of skin or mucocutaneous lesions, the general impression is that the cutaneous type is more common in the countries to the north, while the mucocutaneous form is seen more frequently in the south, especially in Brazil, Argentina and Paraguay. When we compare the ratio between the cutaneous and mucocutaneous forms, we see that each country has areas where the mucocutaneous form is predominant, and that there are other areas where the percentage is much lower, or where such cases are not seen. The pattern in Venezuela is of this kind: the mucocutaneous form is important in the southern region, while the central region presents no cases of this type.

Another interesting epidemiological finding in Venezuela is that, although there are areas where patients with the mucocutaneous form are not normally seen, when the numbers of cases in these areas increase during serious epidemic outbreaks, mucocutaneous lesions begin to appear among the population.

The characteristics of the disease in South America are quite different from those in Central America and Mexico, where mucous involvement is very seldom seen. The picture varies from Panama, where some cases appear, to Mexico, where they seem to be rare.

Cutaneous leishmaniasis becomes a public health problem when the human population is affected, especially when previously uninfected individuals come to forest areas to work in agricultural or industrial expansion projects. Nevertheless, man is only an accidental host and as a general rule he is the end of the transmission chain, not playing any role in the maintenance of the parasite in nature. This chain starts as a zoonosis of various wild and domestic animals, from which transmission takes place when man appears on the ecological scene. In spite of the large amount of research which has been done, there are still areas where the wild or domestic reservoir has not been determined.

Although man is only an accidental host constituting the end of the transmission chain, the appearance in endemic areas of a clinical form of the disease which has been called diffuse cutaneous leishmaniasis (Convit *et al.* 1972) suggests that the human hosts could act as reservoirs for transmission, since the skin lesions contain an enormous population of parasites.

Cutaneous leishmaniasis has been described according to the most diverse criteria. Initially it was classified according to the clinical and dermatological aspects and given names such as cromomicoid, piodermoid, lupoid, etc. Later, on the basis of the clinical aspects in relation to the parasitological aspects, it was classified (Pessôa 1961) as having two forms, one with invasion of nasal mucous tissue and one with cutaneous lesions only.

The cases with invasion of nasal mucous tissue are subdivided into forms produced by *Leishmania braziliensis*, where the mucous involvement can affect up to 80% of the patients, and those produced by *L. braziliensis guyanensis*, which affects the mucous tissue in about 5% of cases.

The forms where the lesions are strictly cutaneous include the benign form, in which there is only one lesion, produced by *L. braziliensis peruviana*, and the malignant form, with diffuse involvement due to *L. braziliensis pifanoi*.

More recently, cutaneous leishmaniasis in the New World has been considered to be divided into two complexes: the *L. mexicana* complex and the *L. braziliensis* complex (Lainson & Shaw 1972).

The *L. mexicana* complex is characterized by a fast-growing parasite, which multiplies abundantly in NNN culture medium and produces, in the hamster, tuberous lesions which are very rich in amastigotes; sometimes these lesions show metastatic spread to the extremities.

The *L. braziliensis* complex is characterized by a slow-growing parasite, which multiplies poorly in NNN medium and produces limited lesions in the hamster, with few parasites and a tendency to regress.

We consider that the characteristics of cutaneous leishmaniasis within a community follow patterns similar to those of other chronic granulomatous diseases such as leprosy and deep mycosis. In these diseases, the immune

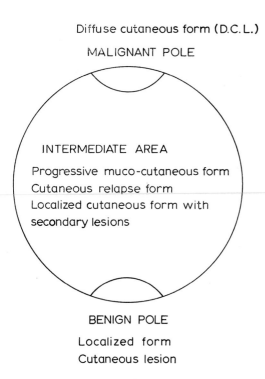

Diffuse cutaneous form (D.C.L.)

MALIGNANT POLE

INTERMEDIATE AREA

Progressive muco-cutaneous form
Cutaneous relapse form
Localized cutaneous form with
secondary lesions

BENIGN POLE

Localized form
Cutaneous lesion

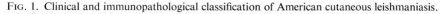

Fig. 1. Clinical and immunopathological classification of American cutaneous leishmaniasis.

pattern of a community reflects the various ways that individuals within the community respond to the infecting agent. In the deep mycoses and especially in leprosy the response can range from total immunity, without development of the disease, through the benign tuberculoid form and the borderline intermediate form to the other extreme, the malignant lepromatous form. The type of response seems to be conditioned by genetic factors.

In American cutaneous leishmaniasis, the immunological responses of the human host could well explain the clinico-pathological polymorphism of this disease. Correlation of the clinical, histopathological and immunological factors provides a further basis for this proposition.

In relation to the clinical aspects, Fig. 1 shows a classification in which we propose two polar forms of American cutaneous leishmaniasis. The malignant pole is represented by diffuse cutaneous leishmaniasis, characterized by massive invasion of the skin and mucous tissue of the nasopharynx, as well as certain lymph nodes. The lesions have large numbers of parasites and the response to the Montenegro test is negative. There is little or no improvement with

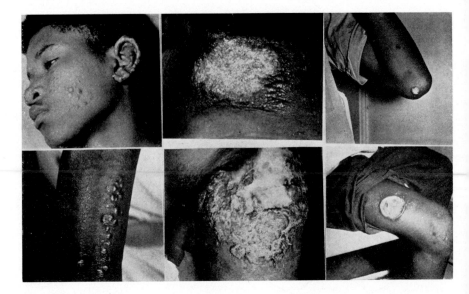

Fig. 2. Left, diffuse leishmaniasis lesions; centre, cutaneous relapse lesions; right, typical localized cutaneous lesions.

treatment. Parasites taken from skin lesions of these patients and inoculated into normal human volunteers, or into patients with lepromatous leprosy, give localized cutaneous lesions which disappear without leaving any sequelae (Convit *et al.* 1972). We therefore conclude that this form of the disease is due to an immunological defect in the host and not to a special strain of the parasite.

At the other pole there is the localized form of the disease, with few parasites, a positive Montenegro test and a clear tendency towards complete involution after treatment.

In the intermediate zone are those forms which show cutaneous or mucous relapses, or cases with cutaneous lesions appearing at a distance from the primary lesion. These clinical forms usually give a positive Montenegro test and have parasites in varying numbers in the lesions. They frequently respond more slowly to treatment than the benign localized forms. Figs. 2–4 show the clinical characteristics of the polar and intermediate forms.

The correlation between the clinical and histopathological appearances has some interesting aspects. For this study, we selected patients who had had their disease for several months, so that the immunopathological character-istics would be well established. We were also careful to study leishmanial granulomas which had not been secondarily modified by complicating factors

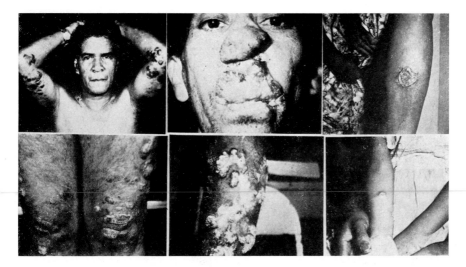

Fig. 3. Left, diffuse leishmaniasis lesions; centre top, mucutaneous form; centre bottom cutaneous relapse; right, localized cutaneous form.

such as ulcerations or secondary infection of the lesion. This requirement was easy to fulfil in diffuse cutaneous leishmaniasis where the lesions generally do not ulcerate. In the ulcerated forms of the disease it was necessary to take the biopsies from the outer edge of the border of the lesion.

Histopathological examination showed a clear difference between the polar forms. Diffuse cutaneous leishmaniasis shows a granuloma formed almost exclusively by macrophages filled with parasites; in localized forms we often saw epithelioid or tuberculoid nodules, surrounded by a thick infiltration of lymphoid cells. In the intermediate forms we found granulomas formed by macrophages, giant cells, and lymphoid and plasma cells, irregularly grouped. In some instances, we saw epithelioid nodules with few lymphocytes and peripheral plasmocytes. Fig. 5 shows the clinico-pathological correlation in these cases.

Histological analysis of these structures suggests that in the malignant forms (diffuse forms) an immunological alteration affects the cellular composition of the granuloma, with no lymphocytic infiltration. Therefore, we have a purely macrophagic granuloma, perhaps because of the absence of the clone of lymphocytes which corresponds to the leishmania antigen. At the benign pole, the granuloma shows good balance between lymphocytes and macrophages. In the intermediate zone, the cellular balance is altered and the granuloma is formed mainly by macrophages, with some lymphocytes.

This clinico-pathological correlation supports the proposition that in leish-

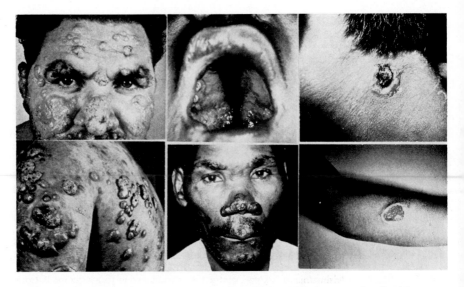

FIG. 4. Left, diffuse form; centre, mucocutaneous form; right, cutaneous localized form.

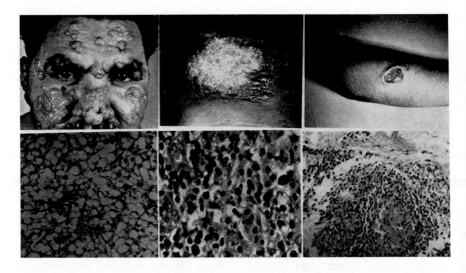

FIG. 5. Left, pure macrophagic granuloma, diffuse lesion; centre, granuloma formed mainly by macrophages with few lymphocytes, cutaneous relapse lesion; right, granuloma formed by epithelioid cells surrounded by thick infiltration of lymphocytes, localized cutaneous form. Microphotographs, haematoxylin-eosin stain, × 40, × 40, × 16.

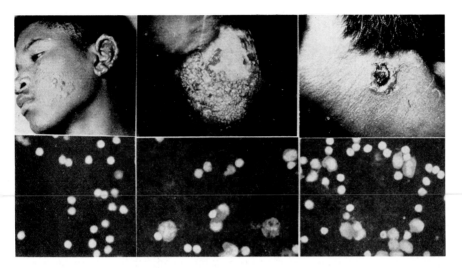

FIG. 6. Left, diffuse case, no blast formation; centre, cutaneous relapse, and right, localized cutaneous form, both showing blast formation.

manial infection the immunological response of the host conditions the defensive processes through which the organism either destroys the parasite, as in the benign cutaneous forms, or lets it proliferate *ad infinitum*, as in diffuse cases or allows it to survive for several years, after which it produces a metastatic lesion, either cutaneous or mucocutaneous.

We also did studies with delayed hypersensitivity tests *in vitro* and *in vivo*, with the Montenegro test, and by stimulating cultured lymphocytes with specific antigen. These tests also showed a clear difference between the malignant pole, where the diffuse cases showed a negative Montenegro test and no blast formation, and the benign pole, where the cases had a positive Montenegro test and a high percentage of blast formation when their lymphocytes were challenged with a leptomonad antigen. Cases in the intermediate zone showed blast formation and a positive Montenegro test.

Fig. 6 shows blast formation in the various forms of leishmaniasis we studied. The preparation is stained with acridine orange and was observed and photographed under ultraviolet light.

These findings lead us to think that the clinical polymorphism of American cutaneous leishmaniasis is due fundamentally to the response of the host, and that the characteristics of the infecting strain of *Leishmania* can only secondarily influence the type of lesion that appears.

References

CONVIT, J., PINARDI, M. E. & RONDÓN, A. J. (1972) Diffuse cutaneous leishmaniasis: a disease due to an immunological defect of the host. *Trans. R. Soc. Trop. Med. Hyg.* **66**, 603-610

LAINSON, R. & SHAW, J. J. (1972) Leishmaniasis of the New World: taxonomic problems. *Br. Med. Bull.* **28**, 44-48

PESSÔA, S. B. (1961) Classificação das leishmanioses e das especies do genero *Leishmania*. *Arq. Hig. Saude Publica (São Paulo)* **26**, 41-50

Discussion

Peters: This question of the different clinical forms is going to remain confused until we really know which organism we are dealing with. Lainson & Shaw (1972) have characterized as 'fast-growing' those strains causing the rather simple type of cutaneous lesion. Certainly the organisms from their cases with diffuse leishmaniasis appear to be identical to these, as is the case in Ethiopia to which Dr Bray referred (p. 102). The classical espundia type of lesion is producing a 'slow-growing' strain. I am sure we are dealing with different organisms as well as with a difference in the host response.

Convit: When we studied an endemic zone in eastern Venezuela we found, living in the same house, a girl with the localized form and her sister with the diffuse cutaneous form. It is difficult for me to explain this as due to two different strains of the parasite. My explanation is that it is the same strain but there are different host responses.

Peters: This is exactly what we are saying is possible.

Bray: Certainly in Ethiopia we think the same parasite causes both conditions but the situation in Amazonia is slightly different. Every organism isolated by Lainson & Shaw (1972) from patients with diffuse cutaneous leishmaniasis has been a fast-growing *L. mexicana* type, whereas all of those from espundia and most of those from single-lesion cutaneous leishmaniasis in Amazonia are the slow-growing *L. braziliensis* type. I don't think, however, that our minds should boggle at two sisters having two different organisms, because the reservoir host for the two organisms can be the same. The sandflies transmitting them may be different but they may coexist, and this is almost certainly the case in Amazonia. However, we simply don't know this about Venezuela. I am quite sure that this taxonomic system of Lainson & Shaw (1972) does not apply yet to Panama or to Costa Rica, where we don't have sufficient information to go on.

Newton: A single fly may well carry more than one strain or species of leishmania.

Bray: I doubt it but in any case I don't think this is any real objection. Some of our work on diffuse cutaneous leishmaniasis and normal cutaneous leishmaniasis in Ethiopia, relating to a number of the correlates of cell-mediated immunity, bear out Dr Convit's results, that is that the 'diffusa' patients are immunologically incompetent in relation to *Leishmania* (see below).

Baker: If two sisters can have two different organisms then surely one sister can have two different organisms at the same time, which would confuse the issue even further.

Lumsden: It seems to me inevitable that there are going to be differences among the organisms and differences in the reactivities of the hosts. We know there are differences in virulence among the organisms. I think one cannot polarize this and say that one or other is more important. We have to stabilize one end of the thing before we can do anything about the other. If we untangle the organisms then we can start untangling host responses.

Zeledón: Two histopathological pictures were presented by Dr Convit. In the tuberculoid type of granuloma, epithelioid cells predominated, while in the other type histiocytes were the most common. This is exactly what we see in hamsters inoculated with *L. braziliensis* and *L. mexicana*, respectively. Guimarães (1951) isolated a strain of *Leishmania* which produced a lesion very much like the *L. mexicana* type in hamsters. He called the tumour in the hamster a histiocytoma, on histological grounds.

Bray: We are using four tests for correlates of cell-mediated immunity in leishmaniasis: the lymphocyte transformation test, the leucocyte migration test (inhibition of leucocyte migration in the presence of antigen), and two tests on lymphocyte activation products, in which the lymphocytes are put in with antigens for a certain time and the supernatants are then tested for either mitogenic activity on normal lymphocytes or for their activity in inhibiting macrophage migration. We have now done this for active cutaneous leishmaniasis, cured cutaneous leishmaniasis, diffuse cutaneous leishmaniasis, cured diffuse cutaneous leishmaniasis, and kala azar in Ethiopia (where unfortunately the cutaneous strains seem to be not nearly as strongly immunogenic as those from the Middle East) and in some patients from the Middle East. In active cutaneous leishmaniasis while the infection is going on the lymphocytes are not transformed, though they are transformed by phytohaemagglutinin. The same is true in diffuse cutaneous leishmaniasis whether cured or not and in kala azar, except that some patients with kala azar fail to respond to phytohaemagglutinin. In cured cutaneous leishmaniasis we get good lymphocyte transformation in response to antigen. In case enhancing antibody interferes with the test in kala azar, we wash the lymphocytes and test them and also test washed lymphocytes reconstituted with the serum: we get absolutely no difference whatsoever throughout. It is as if in kala azar the lymphocytes have never been sensitized at all.

In leucocyte migration we see considerable inhibition of the movement of the leucocytes in healed cutaneous leishmaniasis but none in active cutaneous leishmaniasis, diffuse cutaneous leishmaniasis whether cured or not, or kala azar. When we looked for a mitogenic factor, we saw very little activity in the controls. In healed cutaneous leishmaniasis, there was considerable activity but nothing much in kala azar or diffuse cutaneous leishmaniasis, whether cured or not. So in diffuse cutaneous leishmaniasis there was no lymphocyte activation product containing a mitogenic factor. Exactly the same happened when we looked at the inhibition of macrophage migration. With phytohaemagglutinin there is enormous inhibition. In healed cutaneous leishmaniasis, there is considerable inhibition; with kala azar there is no inhibition, and in diffuse cutaneous leishmaniasis, whether cured or not, there was no inhibition except in one possible case. I think Dr Convit will agree that this is more or less the same as he has been getting. Finally, in two patients with something approaching leishmaniasis recidivans, activity in all tests was recorded.

Zeledón: Have you tried to transfer lymphocytes from an immune person to a person with the diffuse type of leishmaniasis?

Bray: Dr A. D. M. Bryceson (1970) attempted something of the sort, without success. One doesn't really expect success in this unless one can match recipient and donor, because the recipient is going to destroy the donated lymphocytes in any case, if the HL-A antigens are not the same. Instead one extracts 'transfer factor' (Lawrence & Landy 1969) and uses this, which we have done. 'Transfer factor' has been apparently successful in diffuse dermatomycoses and generalized variola. It has had a slight success in converting borderline lepromatous leprosy to borderline tuberculoid leprosy. We have tried it only once and had absolutely no success. That is, we freeze-thawed known active lymphocytes from recovered patients, then dialysed the mixture and inoculated the dialysate into a patient with diffuse cutaneous leishmaniasis. At the 'lepromatous leprosy' end of the spectrum, which is where we assume diffuse cutaneous leishmaniasis is, I don't think there is any hope in any case of resuscitating a person's lymphocytes with something like transfer factor because I don't think the relevant clone of lymphocytes any longer exists. One would have to transfuse whole lymphocytes which would live, in order to get a result. This is not possible without an enormous HL-A matching programme.

References

BRYCESON, A. D. M. (1970) Diffuse cutaneous leishmaniasis in Ethiopia. III: Immunological studies. *Trans. R. Soc. Trop. Med. Hyg.* **64**, 380-393

GUIMARÃES, F. N. (1951) Leishmaniose experimental. IV: Reprodução em hamsters *(Cricetus auratus)* de uma leishmaniose cutanea nodulotumoral oriunda de Amazonia (histiocitoma leishmaniótico). *Hospital (Rio de J.)* **40**, 665-676

LAINSON, R. & SHAW, J. J. (1972) Leishmaniasis of the New World: taxonomic problems. *Br. Med. Bull.* **28**, 44-48

LAWRENCE, H. S. & LANDY, M. (1969) *Mediators of Cellular Immunity*, pp. 143-245, Academic Press, New York

The ultrastructure
of pathogenic flagellates

KEITH VICKERMAN

Department of Zoology, University of Glasgow, Scotland

Abstract   Changes occur in the kinetoplast–mitochondrion and in surface structure as trypanosomatid flagellates pass through their life cycles. There is progressive elaboration of the single mitochondrion in the transition from multiplicative to non-multiplicative forms in the mammal and on to early vector (or culture) stages. This increase in structural complexity is paralleled by the development of new respiratory pathways and changes in ability to utilize respiratory substrates. The mitochondrion of dyskinetoplastic flagellates lacks the ability to complete these changes.

The surface coat present on metacyclic and bloodstream stages of salivarian trypanosomes may be a secretion which contains the variant antigens, the ability to replace its antigenic surface layer enabling the trypanosome to avoid the host's defences.

Lysosomes detected in trypanosomes may have a role in organelle turnover and in the control of secretion as well as in parasite feeding. Lysosomal enzymes secreted into the flagellar pocket may damage host cells.

Intracellular stages differ in their relationship with the host cell. In phagocytic host cells the parasite lies in a vacuole but *Trypanosoma cruzi* in muscle and nerve lies free in the cytoplasm; parasite lysosomal enzymes may invoke more damage in the latter case.

The ability of flagellates to attach to vector surfaces is associated with the development of special flagellar junctional complexes of the hemidesmosome/desmosome type.

Supporting microtubules are present beneath the plasma membrane and in the dividing nucleus where they form a primitive mitotic spindle apparatus. Acting in consort with the mitochondrial changes, the growth and regression of surface microtubules may be responsible for trypanosome morphogenesis.

In this short review I shall try to show that the electron microscope is not only revealing a wealth of ultrastructural detail in trypanosomes and leishmanias but is also helping to answer the question 'Why do these flagellates assume so many different forms in the course of a single life cycle?' We are at last beginning to see the adaptive significance of minute changes in the flagellate's anatomy in relation to the gross changes visible at the light microscope level and to the accompanying physiological changes which are to be discussed in greater detail by other contributors to this symposium.

THE SALIENT FEATURES OF TRYPANOSOMATID FINE STRUCTURE

Most of our knowledge of the fine structure of trypanosomes and leishmanias comes from the study of sectioned material by electron microscopy. Electron micrographs reveal a certain constancy of basic structure in these flagellates. This is depicted in Fig. 1 and can be summarized as follows.

The nucleus (Figs. 3, 7, 11) is typically eukaryote with its two-membrane envelope (punctured by pores), prominent endosome and peripheral chromatin. The outer nuclear membrane is continuous with ribosome-studded (granular) endoplasmic reticulum. The ground cytoplasm of the flagellates (Fig. 2 etc.) is packed with ribosomes; sparse distribution of ribosomes indicates suboptimal fixation. The entire flagellate is bounded by a unit plasma membrane. Beneath the plasma membrane of the body lies a palisade of longitudinally arranged microtubules linked to one another by fine lateral bridges (Fig. 4). These microtubules are believed to support the external body form. The flagellum arises from a basal body which lies in the floor of a flask-shaped surface intucking —the flagellar pocket (Figs. 2, 8). A second (aflagellate) basal body (Fig. 2) lies close to the first, and both have classical centriolar construction. In addition to the usual axoneme ('9 + 2') structure in the flagellum shaft, however, trypanosomatids have a paraxial rod of paracrystalline structure (Figs. 3, 4, 12, 13).

Close to the flagellar basal bodies lies the kinetoplast (Figs. 2, 5, 6). What we identify by light microscopy as the kinetoplast is seen by electron microscopy as a fibrous nucleoid of overall discoid shape, and numerous studies (reviewed by Simpson 1972) have shown that this nucleoid is composed of circular and linear DNA molecules. The nucleoid is housed in a capsular expansion of the mitochondrial apparatus or chondriome. In all kinetoplastid flagellates the chondriome appears to be a single mitochondrion which may be highly branched (Figs. 2, 4, 5, 7) and which most commonly forms an interconnected series of double-membrane-bound canals lying beneath the pellicle. These canals as well as the kinetoplast capsule often have typical mitochondrial cristae arising from their inner membrane (Figs. 2, 5, 7). The kinetoplast nucleoid is connected to the inner mitochondrial membrane by a loose felt of filaments (Fig. 6).

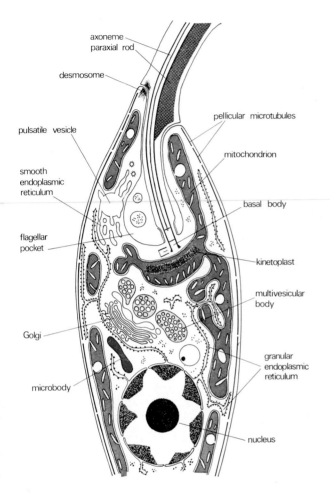

axoneme
paraxial rod
desmosome
pellicular microtubules
pulsatile vesicle
mitochondrion
smooth
endoplasmic
reticulum
basal body
flagellar
pocket
kinetoplast
multivesicular
body
Golgi
granular
endoplasmic
reticulum
microbody
nucleus

FIG. 1. Diagram of longitudinal section of a trypanosomatid flagellate, *Leishmania mexicana*, promastigote form, showing location and relationships of principal structures observed by electron microscopy (the posterior third of the flagellate is not shown).

The kinetoplast has long been known to have genetic continuity. During division the kinetoplast divides before the nucleus. In fact, kinetoplast division reflects a splitting of the entire mitochondrion into two daughter organelles.

The granular endoplasmic reticulum is frequently found plunging into cytoplasmic invaginations of the mitochondrion (Figs. 2, 4) and in some trypanosomatids (Fig. 10) complex labyrinths of mitochondrion and endoplasmic reticulum may be formed.

In the vicinity of the flagellar pocket are several smooth-membraned sacs

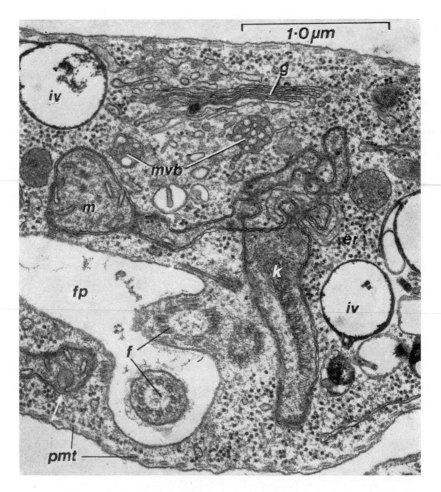

Fig. 2*. Electron micrograph of longitudinal section through kinetoplast region of *Leish-mania mexicana*, culture promastigote early division stage. Shows kinetoplast profiles of mitochondrial network (crista arrowed) with granular endoplasmic reticulum dissecting the mitochondrion, flagellum bases in flagellar pocket, Golgi apparatus, ribosomes in cytoplasmic matrix, pellicular microtubules, microbodies and inclusion vacuoles of unknown significance but possibly containing polyphosphate (see p. 195) × 40 000.

* The electron micrographs illustrating this article are of sectioned material fixed in phosphate-buffered glutaraldehyde and postfixed in osmium tetroxide, similarly buffered, except for Figs. 8-10 which are of material fixed in veronal acetate buffered osmium tetroxide only. Embedding was in Araldite resin and the sections were stained with uranyl acetate and lead citrate.

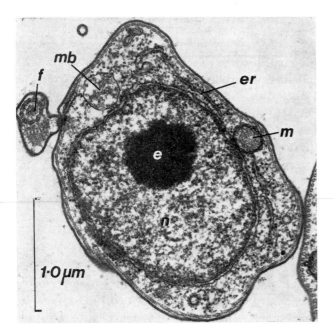

FIG. 3. Transverse section of *Trypanosoma brucei* intermediate bloodstream form in region of nucleus. Note profile of single mitochondrial canal. × 30 000.

and tubes; the most recognizable conformation is the Golgi apparatus (Figs. 2, 7, 11) whose proximal face is subtended by a branch of the granular endoplasmic reticulum. At the distal end of the pile of Golgi saccules lie smooth vesicles and multivesicular bodies (Fig. 2). A pulsatile (contractile) vacuole, present in leishmanias, empties from this region into the flagellar pocket (Fig. 1).

Abbreviations used in labelling:

ax	– axoneme of flagellum	*kr*	– remnant of kinetoplast
bb	– basal body of flagellum	*m*	– mitochondrion
dbf	– desmosome between body and flagellum	*mb*	– microbody-like organelle
		mvb	– multi-vesicular body
dff	– desmosome between adjacent flagella	*n*	– nucleus
e	– endosome (nucleolus)	*np*	– nuclear pore
er	– granular endoplasmic reticulum	*pl*	– plasma membrane
f	– flagellum	*pmt*	– pellicular microtubules
fp	– flagellar pocket	*pr*	– paraxial rod of flagellum
g	– Golgi apparatus	*sr*	– smooth endoplasmic reticulum
iv	– inclusion vacuole	*ss*	– secretion storage vacuole of *sr*
k	– kinetoplast nucleoid		

In some trypanosomes at least, the pellicular microtubules near the opening of the flagellar pocket may be deflected inwards to form a cytopharynx through which colloidal proteins are ingested into food vacuoles where digestion takes place. Single membrane-bound organelles have been designated lysosomes and peroxisomes (microbodies, Figs. 2–7, 11) by various authors, and although such structures are undoubtedly present, the cytochemical evidence supporting identification is conflicting and difficult to assess.

As yet no striking ultrastructural differences have been discerned between pathogenic and non-pathogenic species of these flagellates.

CYCLICAL CHANGES IN THE KINETOPLAST–MITOCHONDRION

My early comparison of the fine structure of bloodstream and culture forms of *Trypanosoma brucei* (Vickerman 1962) showed that the most striking difference was in the appearance of the mitochondrion. Synthesizing these observations with the contemporary work of Ryley (1962) on the respiratory metabolism of the same strains, I concluded that the physiological and morphological changes in cyclical development of trypanosomes might prove intelligible in terms of adaptive mitochondrial proliferation and regression. Subsequent work on these trypanosomes has amplified the correlation between mitochondrial structure and respiratory economy (reviewed by Vickerman 1971; Brown *et al.* 1973; Newton *et al.* 1973).

In the slender multiplicative bloodstream forms of *Trypanosoma brucei* the mitochondrion is reduced to a single peripheral canal (Fig. 3) which extends the length of the trypanosome on either side of the kinetoplast capsule. Cristae are sparse or absent. These trypanosomes break down glucose to pyruvate which they cannot degrade further, and oxidize their $NADH_2$ via a glycerophosphate oxidase cycle which is cyanide-insensitive (see Bowman, this symposium). Progression to the stumpy form is marked by swelling of the mitochondrial canal which develops tubular cristae. Stumpy forms can oxidize 2-oxoglutarate and, at a low rate, proline, with some decarboxylation, suggesting some mitochondrial participation in metabolism, but succinate is not respired.

In some stumpy forms, especially those derived from hosts immunosuppressed by irradiation, the simple mitochondrial canal shows localized intrusions of the cytoplasm and especially the endoplasmic reticulum (Fig. 4). When bloodstream trypanosomes are put into culture this dissection of the mitochondrion is carried further (Figs. 5–7), and within 24 h the chondriome becomes a reticulum with noticeable amplification of the post-kinetoplastic

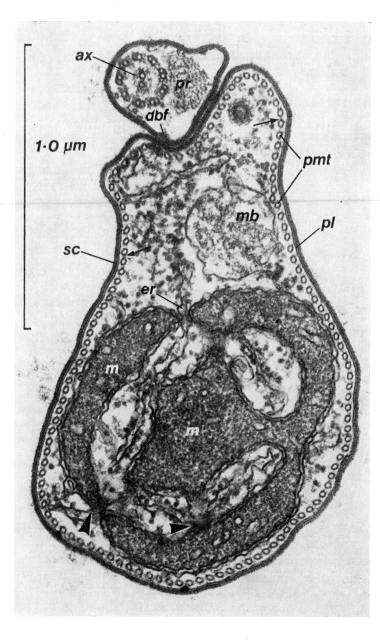

FIG. 4. Transverse section of *T. brucei* stumpy bloodstream form showing incipient dissection of mitochondrion by endoplasmic reticulum. The latter may supply the outer membrane of the former; possible continuities are indicated by arrowheads. Arrows indicate bridges between pellicular microtubules. × 75 000.

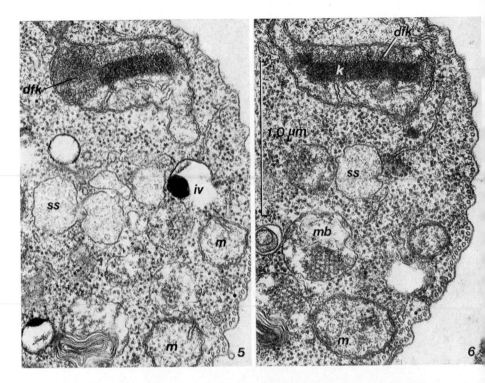

FIGS. 5 & 6. Non-consecutive serial sections of kinetoplast region of *T. brucei* after 24 h in primary culture. Apart from the prominent band of dense anisotropic fibrils, the kinetoplast shows associated diffuse fibrils (dfk) connecting the dense nucleoid to the kinetoplast capsule (mitochondrial membrane). Note paracrystalline structures in microbodies and absence of surface coat on plasma membrane. The regressing secretory reticulum is represented by isolated saccules. × 40 000.

portion as the kinetoplast becomes further removed from the posterior end of the body. The tubular cristae of the stumpy forms become replaced by plate-like cristae but these are small and sparse (Figs. 5, 6). These ultrastructural changes are accompanied by a marked increase in oxidative capacities, especially of proline, and by the acquisition of succinoxidase activity. After two days in the monophasic blood broth medium used in our laboratory (Brown *et al.* 1973), morphological transformation to the culture form is completed but all oxidase activities are still cyanide-insensitive. Morphologically these trypanosomes correspond to the early developmental stages found in the vector gut after a similar period. The longer thinner flagellates which characterize the later stages of infection in the ectoperitrophic space and proventriculus (cardia) of the fly gut have maximum mitochondrial reticulation and a greater number

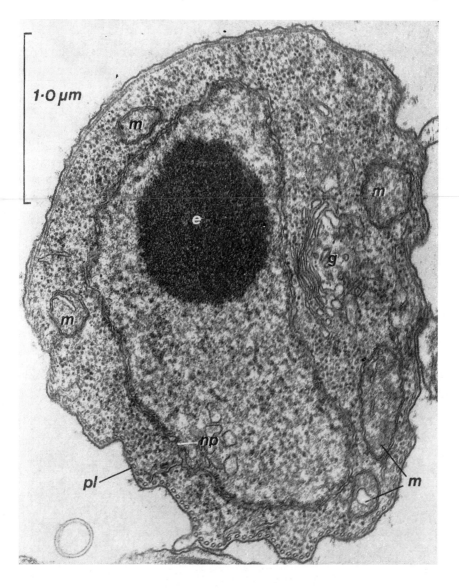

FIG. 7. Transverse section of nuclear region of *T. brucei* after 36 h in primary culture showing Golgi apparatus and several profiles of mitochondrial network (cf. Fig. 3). × 45 000.

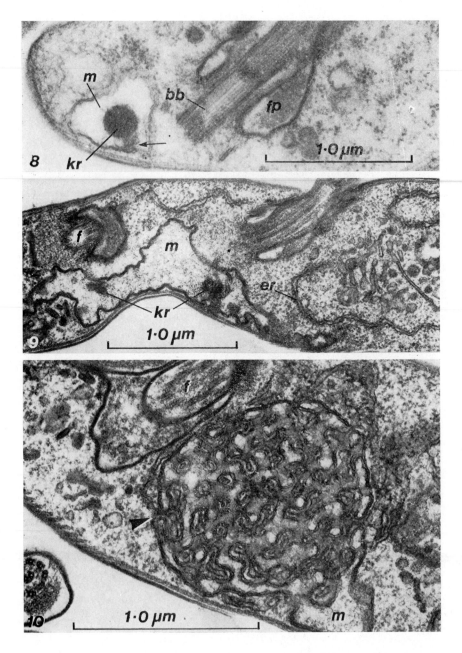

FIGS. 8-10. Longitudinal sections of flagellum base region of the dyskinetoplastic trypanosome *T. evansi equinum.*
                                                                                                    →

of large plate-like cristae than the culture forms. We have not yet conducted *in vitro* studies on respiration of the proventricular forms, but Balber & Ward (1972) have shown cytochemically that diaminobenzidine oxidation by the mitochondrion of these forms is cyanide-sensitive.

The proventricular forms probably represent the peak of mitochondrial development in the *T. brucei* life cycle, for electron micrographs of the fly salivary gland stages show regression of the mitochondrial reticulation and reversion to tubular cristae. In the metacyclic trypanosome the single mito-chondrial canal of the bloodstream forms is present. We know nothing of the respiration of these stages, however. In *T. congolense* and *T. vivax* all the blood forms have tubular cristae and all the vector forms have plate-like cristae (Fig. 12) but the overall pattern of the mitochondrial changes is as in *T. brucei*.

The significance of tubular *versus* plate-like cristae remains to be explored, but in our correlated physiological/ultrastructural studies on *T. brucei* (Brown *et al.* 1973) the acquisition of plate-like cristae paralleled the development of succinoxidase and cytochrome *c* reductase activities though not necessarily cytochrome oxidase activity (cyanide sensitivity).

The leishmanias show simpler mitochondrial cycles than the salivarian trypanosomes (Rudzinska *et al.* 1964; Creemers & Jadin 1967; reviewed by Simpson 1972). The transition from intracellular amastigote to culture promastigote is accompanied by an increase in the number of mitochondrial profiles per section of flagellate, but cristae are plate-like (Fig. 2) and res-piration is cyanide-sensitive in both forms of the parasite. From the frag-mentary evidence available, *T. cruzi* likewise shows plate-like cristae and probably cyanide-sensitive respiration at all stages in the life cycle. Although Brack (1968) was dubious about a mitochondrial cycle in *T. cruzi* comparable to that of *T. brucei*, the electron microscope studies of Sanabria (1966) and Maria *et al.* (1972) suggest progressive mitochondrial development in the sequence from intracellular amastigote to bloodstream trypomastigote to vector epimastigote.

A remarkable feature of the mitochondrial cycle of *T. cruzi*, however, is the

---

←

FIG. 8. Showing kinetoplast remnant—a dense mass which replaces the fibrillar nucleoid of the intact kinetoplast (cf. Figs. 5 & 6). The kinetoplast remnant retains a diffuse fibrillar connection (arrowed) with the mitochondrial envelope. This connection appears to be missing from non-viable dyskinetoplastic forms. × 40 000.

FIG. 9. Dividing trypanosome showing that kinetoplast remnant is replicated along with mitochondrion at division. × 35 000.

FIG. 10. Section showing localized dissection of mitochondrion (cf. Fig. 4) by cytoplasmic channels containing endoplasmic reticulum. Arrowhead indicates ingress of one channel. × 50 000.

amplification of the kinetoplast nucleoid in metacyclic and bloodstream trypo-mastigotes (Brack 1968; Meyer 1968). Instead of the characteristic double-layered row of fibrils found in other stages, the trypomastigote kinetoplast has three or four such rows arranged in tiers. Presumably such kinetoplasts are polyenergid, the monoenergid condition returning in the ensuing division phase.

In dyskinetoplastic trypanosomatids the fibrous nucleoid is reduced to a compact mass of dense material (Fig. 8). This mass still shows fibrillar attach-ment to the mitochondrial envelope in the viable dyskinetoplastic species of *Trypanozoon* and appears to be replicated along with the crista-less mito-chondrial envelope (Fig. 9).

By analogy with other mitochondrial systems, the kinetoplast genome is thought to be concerned with the synthesis of inner mitochondrial membrane components, while the outer mitochondrial membrane may be derived from the endoplasmic reticulum—its proteins the products of nuclear genes. Evidence that in trypanosomatids the endoplasmic reticulum feeds membrane into the mitochondrial envelope cannot as yet be described as conclusive (Fig. 4). Mitochondrion–endoplasmic reticulum complexes are usually found in the vector stages or, in *T. brucei*, in stumpy forms which are 'preadapting' to life in the vector. The presence of such a complex in dyskinetoplastic *T. evansi* (Fig. 10), however, shows that an intact kinetoplast is unnecessary for this early stage in mitochondrial proliferation.

SURFACE CHANGES

An interesting feature of the bloodstream forms of all the salivarian trypano-somes is the presence of a compact coat, 12–15 nm thick overlying the entire plasma membrane (reviewed by Vickerman 1969b, 1971, 1972). This coat (Fig. 4) is discarded within 24 h of entering the culture tube (Figs. 5–7) or vector, but in *T. brucei* and *T. congolense* the coat is subsequently regained when the epimastigote trypanosomes transform into metacyclic forms. The coat is present in freeze-etched trypanosomes (Seed *et al.* 1972) and so is not a fixation artifact. It can be removed by proteolytic enzymes (Vickerman 1969b; Wright & Hales 1970) and contains a carbohydrate layer next to the under-lying plasma membrane (Wright & Hales 1970).

The surface coat appears to be an adaptation to bloodstream living and I have argued (Vickerman 1969b) that it contains the variant antigens demon-strated by agglutination reactions for bloodstream trypanosomes. The evidence for this is (1) loss of variant antigen character is correlated with loss of the coat,

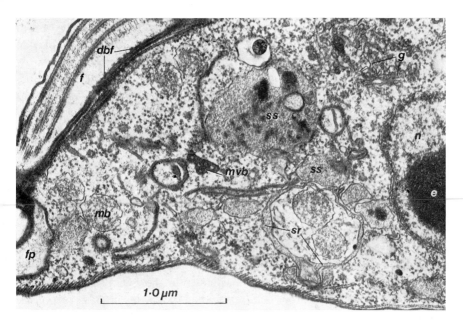

Fig. 11. Longitudinal section of stumpy bloodstream *T. brucei* to show smooth-membraned secretory reticulum systems close to the Golgi apparatus in the region between flagellar pocket and nucleus. The distended sacs of secretion contain regions of differing electron density suggesting heterogeneity of composition. × 35 000.

(2) the metacyclic trypanosomes carry the same surface antigen as the first bloodstream population and both possess a coat, (3) both variant antigens and surface coat appear to be glycoproteins, (4) ferritin-conjugated antibody to a specific variant will bind only to the surface of homologous trypanosomes whose coat is intact and not to homologous trypanosomes from which the coat has been removed or to the coat of heterologous trypanosomes (Vickerman & Luckins 1969), (5) a compact coat has not been reported from the stercorarian trypanosomes which do not have the capacity for antigenic variation (see de Raadt, this symposium).

A further characteristic of the surface of salivarian trypanosomes is its mobility: the surface membrane of these flagellates can be seen streaming from body and flagellum by light microscopy (Wright *et al.* 1970). These streamers carry the surface coat and their shedding into drawn blood probably accounts for the 'exoantigen' found in infected serum (reviewed by Allsopp *et al.* 1971).

If trypanosomes have the ability to shed coated membrane, they must also have an efficient means of replacing it. I have suggested that the Golgi apparatus and associated smooth membrane systems of the bloodstream forms are concerned with the production of coated membrane—just as they are in *Amoeba* (Stockem 1969): there are several well substantiated examples of flagellates producing surface glycoprotein complexes in this way (reviewed by Vickerman 1969*a*). The smooth reticulum of membranous sacs and tubes between the Golgi apparatus and flagellar pocket is locally dilated with what appears to be a secretion (Fig. 11). This secretory reticulum regresses (Figs. 5, 6) as the flagellate loses the surface coat in culture (Brown *et al.* 1973).

Another possible interpretation of the surface coat is that it represents adsorbed host serum protein, but the presence of the coat in the metacyclic trypanosome argues against this. There is good evidence, however, that *T. vivax* binds host serum protein to its surface (Desowitz 1970). This trypanosome has a surface coat in its bloodstream phase and the coat is lost (Figs. 12, 13) when the trypanosome anchors itself to the tsetse proboscis wall to become epimastigote (Vickerman 1973). Paradoxically, after what has been said, the epimastigote retains the secretory reticulum of the bloodstream form. Moreover, electron micrographs of trypomastigotes in the hypopharynx show a scarcely discernible filamentous coat rather than the thick coat of *T. congolense* in this location. These trypomastigotes may be preinfective forms rather than true metacyclic ones, but if they are metacyclic forms a study of the origin of the surface coat in *T. vivax* should provide an illuminating comparison with *T. brucei*.

The bloodstream (but not culture) stages of stercorarian trypanosomes have an uneven filamentous coat (Vickerman 1969*b*; Maria *et al.* 1972) whose significance has not yet been debated.

NUTRITION AND THE ROLE OF LYSOSOMES

Many of the free-living kinetoplastid flagellates are known to ingest bacteria by way of a cytostome and cytopharynx (Brooker 1971b). A similar cytopharynx is prominent in the electron micrographs of the trypanosomes of poikilotherms (Steinert & Novikoff 1960; Preston 1969), the cytostome lying close to the opening of the flagellar pocket. Preston demonstrated uptake of exogenous ferritin via the cytopharynx, and formation of pinosomes from the distal end of this structure. The ferritin-containing pinosomes were found to fuse with acid phosphatase-containing vesicles, i.e. primary lysosomes, digestion presumably taking place in the resulting secondary lysosomes (multivesicular bodies). The Gomori reaction used to demonstrate phosphatase also showed enzyme activity in the Golgi apparatus which is commonly regarded as the generator of primary lysosomes.

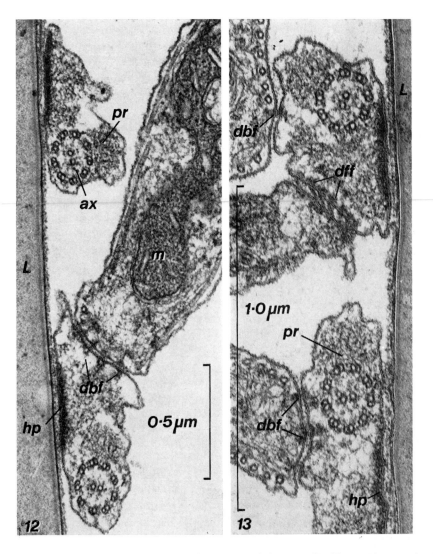

Figs. 12 & 13. Transverse sections of proboscis of the tsetse fly *Glossina fuscipes* showing regions of attachment of *Trypanosoma vivax* epimastigotes to the labrum (L). Note junctional complexes of the macula adherens (desmosome) type between trypanosome body and flagellum and between flagella of adjacent trypanosomes. A prominent zonular hemidesmosome plaque (*hp*) occurs along the flagellar membrane where it is attached to the labrum. × 60 000 and × 86 000.

The existence of a differentiated cytopharynx in the trypanosomes of mammals is not so obvious. No traces of such a structure have been found in the salivarian trypanosomes and it is doubtful that the leishmanias possess one. *T. cruzi* has a cytostome in the amastigote tissue and epimastigote culture forms (Milder & Deane 1969; Sanabria 1970). Nevertheless pinocytosis of colloids has been claimed for both salivarian trypanosomes and leishmanias (reviewed by Jadin 1971), caveolae in the flagellar pocket providing the portal of entry. Acid phosphatase activity has been located in the nearby cytoplasm and in the flagellar pocket itself (reviewed by Jadin 1971). Although these lysosomal vesicles and secreted enzymes have been ascribed a role in digestion of nutrients (heterophagy), it is equally possible that the lysosomes play a part in autophagy (digestion of damaged or unwanted cell structure) or in crinophagy (the control of secretion release by digestion). Fragments of ejected cytoplasm are frequently found in the flagellar pocket and may be digested there. The possibility of secretion into the pocket has been raised for salivarian trypanosomes and may be more widespread. Do leishmanias, for example, secrete a mitogen that stimulates their host cell to divide? The fact that hydrolases are discharged to the exterior by these flagellates is of obvious potential significance in pathogenesis.

ATTACHMENT MECHANISMS

Many trypanosomatids have a phase of development in the vector where they are attached to one another or to host tissues, e.g. the lining of salivary glands or gut. This stage is usually a multiplicative epimastigote in the trypanosomes and is essential for reinfection of the vertebrate host as its eventual products are metacyclic trypanosomes. The firmness of attachment of the trypanosomes in this vital period is obviously an important adaptation as in most cases muscular contraction or movement of the lumen contents must tend to expel the parasite.

Recent electron microscope studies suggest that the trypanosomatid flagellum is unique among cilia and flagella in its ability to form junctional complexes of the desmosome or hemidesmosome type with other flagellates or with the substratum to which the flagellates are clinging. A trypomastigote's flagellum is linked to its body by a single row of macular desmosomes (Fig. 3) basically similar in structure, and presumably in function, to the desmosomes which bind epithelial cells to one another (Vickerman 1969*b*).

Similar macular desmosomes bind the emerging leishmania flagellum to the wall of its flagellar pocket (Fig. 1).

Electron micrographs of sectioned clusters of *T. vivax* epimastigotes (Figs. 12, 13) in the proboscis of *Glossina fuscipes* (Vickerman 1973) show that bands of macular desmosomes can also occur between the flagella of adjacent flagellates, and the cohesion of flagellates in clusters may depend on similar mechanisms in other trypanosomatids. In the *T. vivax* epimastigote clusters some of the flagella are attached directly to the wall of the fly's proboscis and the junctional complex found here is comparable to that which secures epithelial cells to their underlying basal lamina, i.e. a hemidesmosome, but this hemidesmosome is zonular (strip-like) rather than macular (spot-like), extending for several microns along the flagellum wherever it adheres to the host. Paralleling this hemidesmosome in the host-attached flagellum, the number of rows of macular desmosomes binding flagellum to body may be increased from one to as many as six. This localized increase in support for the flagellum–body junction has only been observed in the epimastigote and this stage appears to be designed specifically for attachment to host surfaces in the salivarian trypanosomes.

Experimental studies on the attachment of the trypanosomatid *Crithidia fasciculata* to various substrates (Brooker 1971*a*) suggest that flagellum hemidesmosome formation is not specific for the gut lining of the host. Whether such lack of specificity characterizes the attachment of pathogenic trypanosomatids is not known.

PENETRATION OF HOST CELLS

Information about the mode of entry of intracellular flagellates into their host cells is scanty. The leishmania promastigote appears to be phagocytosed by the macrophage into a membrane-lined vacuole. This shrinks during the parasite's transformation to the amastigote, which appears to be surrounded by two membranes (Rudzinska *et al.* 1964), the outer one of host origin. Intracellular *T. cruzi* amastigotes, however, lack this outer membrane and lie free in the host cell cytoplasm of muscle or nerve (R. E. Howells, unpublished). Presumably the infecting trypomastigote actively bores through the host cell membrane (compare certain coccidian parasites: see Vickerman 1971). If the breach that it creates in doing so remains unhealed, the resulting leakage of cell components may well be a factor in cardiac tissue destruction.

NUCLEAR DIVISION AND THE LIFE CYCLE

In dividing trypanosomatids the electron microscope has disclosed the presence of an intranuclear bundle of microtubules which envelop the persistent endosome as the nucleus elongates. Presumably growth of the microtubule bundle pushes the poles of the nuclear envelope apart, causing the nucleus to constrict and divide into two. Whether the chromosomes are attached to the nuclear envelope (as in dinoflagellates) or to the microtubules of this spindle apparatus (as in classical mitosis) remains unsettled (reviewed by Vickerman & Preston 1970), but the obvious difference between nuclear division of trypanosomes and that of mammalian cells may be amenable to exploitation in chemotherapy.

The assembly and dissembly of pellicular microtubules, and the formation of bridges between microtubules so that they act as scaffolding, are probably most important in morphogenesis of the different stages in the trypanosome life cycle as well as in nuclear division. Thus vinblastine (an inhibitor of microtubule assembly) will prevent the *in vitro* morphological transformation of *T. brucei* to culture forms, though it does not prevent the mitochondrion from undergoing its characteristic ultrastructural changes (K. Vickerman, unpublished). Mitochondrial proliferation alone, then, does not appear to provide the mechanical driving force for morphogenesis, as I previously thought. If stumpy forms are inoculated into biphasic medium with proline replacing glucose in the overlay, morphogenesis of the culture form is delayed for three or four days and in the meantime mitochondrial development stops in the persistent stumpy forms, as shown by their ultrastructure and the absence of succinoxidase activity (D. A. Evans & K. Vickerman, unpublished). These arrested stumpy forms, however, accumulate microtubules beneath those of the pellicle in the region of the flagellar pocket. An interpretation of this result is that, in the absence of mitochondrial changes, microtubules can be assembled but cannot fulfil their architectural role in morphogenesis, possibly through failure of bridge formation *inter alia*. The acquisition of the ability to oxidize succinate may step up production of guanosine triphosphate and this substance is known to limit microtubule-dependent morphogenesis (Tilney 1971).

Our corpus of knowledge about the control of microtubule behaviour by the environment, both extracellular and intracellular, is growing daily. From this knowledge we may expect a substantial contribution to our understanding of how gross morphological changes in the trypanosome relate to the ultrastructural adaptations that I have described, and so we may achieve a better understanding of the life cycles of the pathogenic flagellates.

ACKNOWLEDGEMENTS

The author wishes to thank the Wellcome Trust, the Royal Society and the Nuffield Foundation for financial support. A grant from UK Foreign and Commonwealth Office Overseas Development Administration is also gratefully acknowledged.

References

ALLSOPP, B. A., NJOGU, A. R. & HUMPHRYES, K. C. (1971) Nature and location of *Trypanosoma brucei* subgroup exoantigen and its relationship to 4s antigen. *Exp. Parasitol.* **29**, 271-284

BALBER, A. E. & WARD, R. A. (1972) Diaminobenzidine staining of the mitochondrion of *Trypanosoma brucei*. *J. Parasitol.* **59**, 1004-1005

BOWMAN, I. B. R. (1974) This symposium, pp. 255-271

BRACK, C. (1968) Elektronenmikroskopische Untersuchungen zum Lebenszyklus von *Trypanosoma cruzi. Acta Trop.* **25**, 289-356

BROOKER, B. E. (1971a) Flagellar adhesion of *Crithidia fasciculata* to millipore filters. *Protoplasma* **72**, 19-25

BROOKER, B. E. (1971b) Fine structure of *Bodo saltans* and *Bodo caudatus* (Zoomastigophorea: Protozoa) and their affinities with the Trypanosomatidae. *Bull. Br. Mus. (Nat. Hist.) Entomol.* **22**, 90-102

BROWN, R. C., EVANS, D. A. & VICKERMAN, K. (1973) Changes in oxidative metabolism and ultrastructure accompanying differentiation of the mitochondrion in *Trypanosoma brucei*. *Int. J. Parasitol.* **3**, 691-704

CREEMERS, J. & JADIN, J. M. (1967) Etude de l'ultrastructure et de la biologie de *Leishmania mexicana* Biagi 1953. I. Les modifications qui surviennent lors de la transformation leishmania-leptomonas. *Bull. Soc. Pathol. Exot.* **60**, 53-58

DESOWITZ, R. S. (1970) African trypanosomes, in *Immunity to Parasitic Animals* (Jackson, G. J., Herman, R. & Singer, I., eds.), Appleton-Century-Crofts, New York

JADIN, J. M. (1971) Cytologie et cytophysiologie des Trypanosomidae. *Acta Zool. Pathol. Antverpiensia* **53**, 5-168

MARIA, T. A., TAFURI, W. & BRENER, Z. (1972) The fine structure of different bloodstream forms of *Trypanosoma cruzi. Ann. Trop. Med. Parasitol.* **66**, 423-431

MEYER, H. (1968) The fine structure of the flagellum and kinetoplast–chondriome of *Trypanosoma (Schizotrypanum) cruzi* in tissue culture. *J. Protozool.* **15**, 614-621

MILDER, R. & DEANE, M. P. (1969) The cytostome of *Trypanosoma cruzi* and *T. conorhini*. *J. Protozool.* **16**, 730-737

NEWTON, B. A., CROSS, G. A. M. & BAKER, J. R. (1973) Differentiation in Trypanosomatidae. *Symp. Soc. Gen. Microbiol.* **23**, 339-373

PRESTON, T. M. (1969) The form and function of the cytostome–cytopharynx of the culture forms of the elasmobranch haemoflagellate *Trypanosoma raiae* Laveran & Mesnil. *J. Protozool.* **16**, 320-333

RAAD, P. DE (1974) This symposium, pp. 197-224

RUDZINSKA, M. A., D'ALESANDRO, P. A. & TRAGER, W. (1964) The fine structure of *Leishmania donovani* and the role of the kinetoplast in the leishmania–leptomonad transformation. *J. Protozool.* **11**, 166-191

RYLEY, J. F. (1962) Studies on the metabolism of the protozoa. 9: Comparative metabolism of bloodstream and culture forms of *Trypanosoma rhodesiense. Biochem. J.* **85**, 211-223

SANABRIA, A. (1966) Ultrastructure of *Trypanosoma cruzi* in the rectum of *Rhodnius prolixus*. *Exp. Parasitol.* **19**, 276-299

SANABRIA, A. (1970) Nuevos estudios acerca de la ultraestructura del *Trypanosoma cruzi* en el miocardio del raton. *Acta Cient. Venez.* **21**, 107-118

SEED, T. M., GNAU, J. M., KREIER, J. P. & PFISTER, R. M. (1972) *Trypanosoma congolense:* fine structure study by the carbon replica and freeze-etch technique. *Exp. Parasitol.* **31**, 399-406

SIMPSON, L. (1972) The kinetoplast of haemoflagellates. *Int. Rev. Cytol.* **32**, 139-207

STEINERT, M. & NOVIKOFF, A. B. (1960) The existence of a cytostome and the occurrence of pinocytosis in the trypanosome, *Trypanosoma mega. J. Biophys. Biochem. Cytol.* **8**, 563-569

STOCKEM, W. (1969) Pinocytose und Bewegung von Amöben. III: Die Funktion des Golgi-apparates von *Amoeba proteus* und *Chaos chaos*. *Histochemie* **18**, 217-240

TILNEY, L. (1971) Origin and continuity of microtubules, in *Origin and Continuity of Cell Organelles* (Reinert, J. & Ursprung, H., eds.), pp. 222-260, Springer, Berlin

VICKERMAN, K. (1962) The mechanism of cyclical development in trypanosomes of the *Trypanosoma brucei* sub-group: an hypothesis based on ultrastructural observations. *Trans. R. Soc. Trop. Med. Hyg.* **56**, 487-495

VICKERMAN, K. (1969a) The fine structure of *Trypanosoma congolense* in its bloodstream phase. *J. Protozool.* **16**, 54-69

VICKERMAN, K. (1969b) On the surface coat and flagellar adhesion in trypanosomes. *J. Cell Sci.* **5**, 163-194

VICKERMAN, K. (1971) Morphological and physiological considerations of extracellular blood protozoa, in *Ecology and Physiology of Parasites* (Fallis, A. M., ed.), pp. 58-59, Toronto University Press, Toronto

VICKERMAN, K. (1972) The host-parasite interface of parasitic protozoa. *Symp. Br. Soc. Parasitol.* **10**, 71-91

VICKERMAN, K. (1973) The mode of attachment of *Trypanosoma vivax* in the proboscis of the tsetse fly *Glossina fuscipes*. *J. Protozool.* **20**, 394-404.

VICKERMAN, K. & LUCKINS, A. G. (1969) Localization of variable antigens in the surface coat of *Trypanosoma brucei* using ferritin-conjugated antibody. *Nature (Lond.)* **224**, 1125-1126

VICKERMAN, K. & PRESTON, T. M. (1970) Spindle microtubules in the dividing nuclei of trypanosomes. *J. Cell Sci.* **6**, 365-383

WRIGHT, K. A. & HALES, H. (1970) Cytochemistry of the pellicle of *Trypanosoma (Trypanozoon) brucei*. *J. Parasitol.* **56**, 671-683

WRIGHT, K. A., LUMSDEN, W. H. R. & HALES, H. (1970) The formation of filopodium-like processes by *Trypanosoma (Trypanozoon) brucei*. *J. Cell Sci.* **6**, 285-297

Discussion

Newton: With regard to your reference to kinetoplast DNA, Dr Vickerman, if all this DNA is in the form of identical 'minicircles' it can be calculated that there would be sufficient genetic information for only three or four small proteins. However, there is an increasing amount of evidence that some kinetoplast DNA is in the form of long linear molecules (Laurent & Steinert 1970), although we don't yet know what proportion of the total is in this form.

Martinez-Silva: Dr Vickerman, you said that *T. cruzi* is surrounded by the cell membrane. We have photographed the penetration of parasites into beef primary fibroblasts cultured in a perfusion chamber and we observed a vacuole in which epimastigotes were actively moving. Very often they divided inside the vacuole, producing two similar forms. The vacuole, however, is not a unique mechanism of epimastigotes, since we have also observed trypomastigotes.

Vickerman: I should extend my statement from macrophages to cover mesenchymal cells in general.

Sanabria: I have not seen a vacuolar membrane surrounding the parasites housed inside the macrophages.

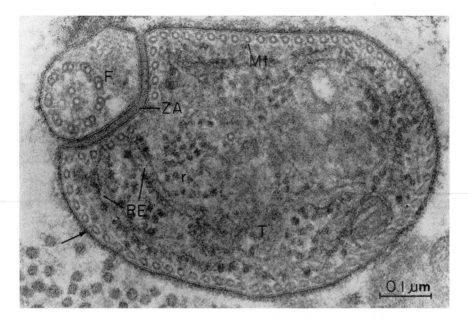

FIG. 1 (Sanabria). Trypomastigote, showing its asymmetrical cell membrane covered by a fuzzy layer (arrow). The microtubules (Mt) of the periplast appear in a row underlining the cell membranes. The flagellum (F) is bound to the parasite body (T) by the attachment zone (ZA) between both membranes. The cytoplasm contains abundant ribosomes (r) free or attached to the endoplasmic reticulum cisterns (RE). (From Sanabria & Aristimuño 1970.)

Trager: When trypanosomes are in the process of entering a nerve or muscle cell could a membrane be present which is later lost?

Martinez-Silva: I have pictures made from cells (beef primary fibroblasts kept in a perfusion chamber) inoculated with *T. cruzi*, from the moment of penetration by the parasite up to the moment in which the cell was disrupted. At the magnification used ($\times$ 1600) it is not possible to see membranes, but whether they are there or not should be determined by electron microscopy. Trypomastigotes are very fast in penetrating the cell and vacuoles are only exceptionally observed, while epimastigotes are slow and vacuoles are frequently produced.

Trager: This matter of the membranes around intracellular parasites of course is of great interest. Parasites seem to be able to do things in various ways. For example in erythrocytes we have malaria parasites with their own membranes and somebody else's membrane around them, while microsporidia have only their own membrane. Amastigotes of *Leishmania donovani* have two membranes and the amastigote forms of *T. cruzi*, at least in muscle cells,

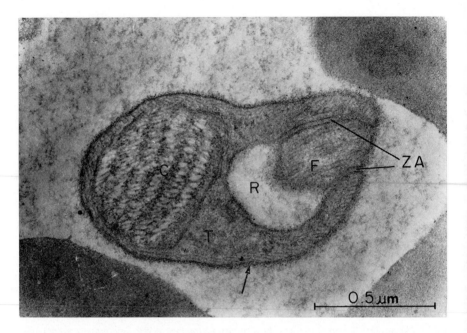

Fig. 2 (Sanabria). Bloodstream trypomastigote (T) showing: the kinetoplast (C) formed by three spirals piled up (one on another), the reservoir (R) and the flagellum (F) with the attachment zone (ZA). The parasite's membrane appears to be covered by a fuzzy layer (arrow). (From Sanabria & Aristimuño 1970).

apparently have only one membrane. Even for coccidia I don't feel the matter is yet settled. In Jones's work (Jones & Hirsch 1972) toxoplasma entering a non-phagocytic cell like the fibroblast seem not to puncture the membrane, but rather to be engulfed essentially by a phagocytic process which perhaps is induced by some enzymes at the tip of the parasite. So it can go either way.

Sanabria: I have been unable to see *T. cruzi* passing through the membrane in my electron microscope studies in different tissues. Figs. 1–5 (Sanabria) show bloodstream forms of *T. cruzi.*

Zeledón: Have you worked with the so-called stumpy and slender blood forms of *T. cruzi* in relation to their mitochondria?

Sanabria: In general, the mitochondria in bloodstream forms are less developed than in the other forms.

de Raadt: Dr Vickerman, you spoke about the trypanosome taking up a new coat. This, in my opinion, is always very difficult, because if it occurred in the bloodstream, I would expect a more gradual shift of antigenic variation than we see—that is, for instance, 10^5 trypanosomes/ml blood going down to virtually

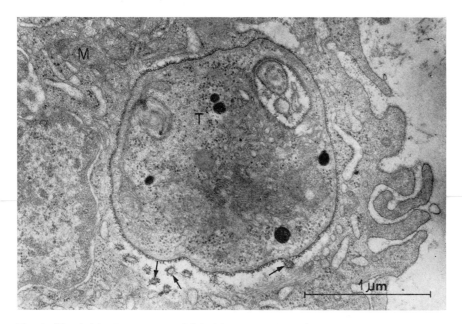

Fig. 3. (Sanabria). Trypanosome (T) inside a macrophage (M). The fuzzy layer appears detached in certain regions and forms rounded profiles (arrows). (From Sanabria & Aristimuño 1972.)

nothing, with an interval of several days before parasitaemia occurs again. If this were a process regulated by the cells themselves, one would expect the populations to change in a more gradual way, with a more even replacement of one variant population by the other. If one assumes that the formation of a new coat takes place in the tissues, that would be a solution, of course, but it seems unlikely to me that this could occur in the bloodstream. It does not exclude the cell from regulating the whole process. But I cannot imagine two new trypanosomes with a different coat emerging from a dividing cell, nor that renewal of the coat of one individual trypanosome would be the whole mechanism of variation, because of the dynamics of the process.

Njogu: We have been following a more chemical approach to the study of the surface of the trypanosome. We have identified a complex of eight glycoproteins which we have shown to be antigenic. We label live trypanosomes with ^{125}I using the enzyme lactoperoxidase, which is supposed to label only the surface of the cell. Of the eight proteins, only two so far seem to get labelled and so we assume that these are the ones on the surface. Maybe when we get this going properly we will test some of the variants and see whether their surfaces contain different groups of proteins from among the eight in the com-

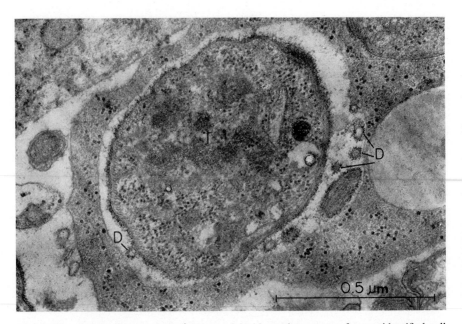

Fig. 4 (Sanabria). Trypanosome (T) housed inside a phagosome of an unidentified cell. Rounded profiles bound by a fuzzy contour (D) are seen in the clear zone around the parasite. These profiles correspond to detachment of the fuzzy layer of the parasite. (From Sanabria & Aristimuño 1969.)

plex. We are also trying to find out how these eight proteins are set up on the surface of the trypanosome, using papain to digest the ones on the top. Our results are not yet complete.

Bowman: It seems a very wasteful process for the trypanosome to manufacture a lot of protein for export or to make a surface coat of protein, for example. While some surface coat protein will be made, could Desowitz's (1969) idea also be involved, that is that some of the plasma proteins will then bind on the surface coat protein and so act as a cement? I am very alarmed at the shortage of energy produced during metabolism in a trypanosome, especially by the bloodstream forms. There just doesn't seem to be enough ATP for all that is going on in the trypanosome during its generation time. We can't simply pull out of the sky a lot of other proteins and say that plenty of energy for protein biosynthesis will appear for this somehow. I would like to apply a law of limitation!

Vickerman: Maybe the trypanosome can recoup some of this energy when it transforms from a stumpy form to a midgut form. The secretion that I mentioned, if it is a surface coat material, seems to be digested at this time, and

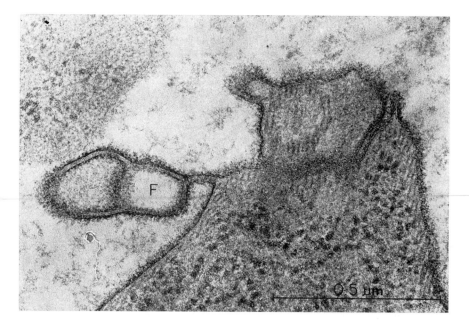

Fig. 5 (Sanabria). Part of a trypomastigote showing at the tip a cross-section of the flagellum and near it a 'filopodium' (F).

then the products of its breakdown may be responsible for induction of the switch-over to using amino acids as respiratory substrates.

Bowman: Yes, but on paper energy deficiency seems to be a problem not for the culture or the midgut form but for the bloodstream form, which goes to the trouble of making a coat protein. It can't recoup that energy.

Newton: We know very little about the nature of endogenous energy reserves in trypanosomes. We have heard that *T. cruzi* can exist for long periods of time (maybe months) in stored blood, in conditions where synthesis and respiration are probably minimal but the cells must be using some energy—where do they get it from? Many flagellates contain polymetaphosphates which contain a large number of high energy bonds. Are similar substances present in trypanosomes?

Bowman: One would then have to postulate that polyphosphates are being synthesized during the life cycle in the insect, where energy provision and energy trapping metabolism are at a maximum. Then the polyphosphates are used, but that wouldn't last very long in the bloodstream forms, would it?

Newton: I don't think we have enough information to answer that. My point was that it seems to be extremely difficult, if not impossible, to exhaust the endogenous reserves of many trypanosomatid flagellates by, for example, incubating them in a buffered salt solution, as can readily be done with bacteria.

Bowman: I don't have much problem with endogenous metabolism in salivarian trypanosomes, but I certainly agree with you that in *T. cruzi* there is the serious problem of background endogenous metabolism. Professor Zeledón has also had this problem of poor stimulation of amino-acid-supported oxygen uptake in experiments with *T. cruzi*.

Baker: As you already said, perhaps the coat is both trypanosome protein and host cell protein. Desowitz (1969) has suggested that host antibody may couple to the surface protein of the coat and so modify it that it causes an antigenic change. This idea might overcome some of the problems. The fuzzy coat that one sees on *T. cruzi* is perhaps just the host protein and not the trypanosome component, or *vice versa*. The evidence that host protein is absorbed onto *T. vivax* shows that there is certainly a host component there (Ketteridge 1970). It doesn't have to be 'either/or'.

Vickerman: If one washes bloodstream forms of *T. brucei* and *T. vivax* several times and then incubates them with an antiserum to host serum proteins, one can get agglutination to a very high titre with *T. vivax* but only to very low titres with *T. brucei*, and after fewer washings (D. S. Ketteridge, unpublished findings, 1971). So with *T. vivax* there obviously is a case for host serum protein being absorbed onto the surface of the trypanosome, but with *T. brucei* there is not.

Goodwin: I find some difficulty in believing that trypanosomes can't continue to make a coat if they can continue to divide. If they can make enough protein to pull themselves apart at great speed and increase their numbers, why can't a few of them continue to spin their threads?

Trager: I am also inclined to think that a trypanosome, or any cell, can do anything it pleases! Coats in *Leishmania* might be interesting too. Dr D. Dwyer, who is working with me, finds that the promastigotes of *Leishmania* have a very nice coat that stains with ruthenium red or violet for electron microscopy, and these are presumably mostly polysaccharide (unpublished results). When an amastigote changes into a promastigote *in vitro*, this coat appears within about the first half-hour, and it may help the promastigote to slough off that outer membrane which it had, at least under *in vitro* conditions. Dr Vickerman, have you looked for this type of a coat, which of course would show up in conditions different from the conditions of the bloodstream coats?

Vickerman: I found a similar sort of coat in *T. brucei* culture forms by fixing them first in osmium tetroxide vapour and then in glutaraldehyde. This procedure resulted in very heavy osmium staining of material outside the plasma membrane. I have not tried ruthenium red staining on the culture forms.

Newton: You said that the dyskinetoplastic strain you examined by electron microscopy still contained DNA which could be replicated. I know that electron-dense material can still be seen in the kinetoplast area of such strains but has anyone managed to extract it and show conclusively that it is DNA?

Vickerman: No, but whatever it is, the material replicates and it appears to be attached to the membrane, so it has characters in common with the DNA of normal kinetoplasts.

Bray: Is there any possibility for genetic lability in these organisms by DNA recombination between kinetoplast and nucleus?

Newton: I am sure that there is a possibility we should consider, and it is a very interesting one. Mühlpfordt (1964) proposed that an exchange of genetic material may occur between the kinetoplast and nucleus of members of the *T. brucei* group at certain stages of their life cycle. He published electron micrographs which appeared to show a breakdown of membranes between these two organelles and suggested that such an exchange may be essential to maintain a strain in a pleomorphic state. As far as I know nobody has ever confirmed these observations unequivocally but it is an interesting hypothesis which should be investigated further.

Vickerman: It was difficult to interpret the micrographs. They were of obliquely cut sections.

Baker: Maria Deane (Deane & Milder 1972) from Brazil published one or two micrographs showing a similar appearance to Mühlpfordt's, neither more nor less convincing.

Vickerman: As I have said, the outer mitochondrial envelope may be continuous with the endoplasmic reticulum which is in turn continuous with the outer nuclear membrane. If a very tiny bit of endoplasmic reticulum intervenes between the nuclear and mitochondrial envelopes, we could get the impression of continuity of nucleus and kinetoplast in an oblique section.

References

DEANE, M. P. & MILDER, R. (1972) Ultrastructure of the cyst-like bodies of *Trypanosoma conorhini*. *J. Protozool.* **19**, 28-42

DESOWITZ, R. S. (1969) African trypanosomes, in *Immunity to Parasitic Animals* (Jackson, G. L., Herman, R. & Singer, I., eds.), vol. 2, pp. 551-596, North Holland, Amsterdam; Appleton-Century-Crofts, New York

JONES, T. & HIRSCH, J. (1972) Interaction of *Toxoplasma gondii* with mammalian cells. II: The absence of lysosomal fusion with phagocytic vacuoles containing living parasites. *J. Exp. Med.* **136**, 1173-1194

KETTERIDGE, D. S. (1970) The presence of host serum components on the surface of rodent adapted *Trypanosoma vivax*. *J. Protozool*. **17** (Suppl.), 24

LAURENT, M. & STEINERT, M. (1970) Electron microscopy of kinetoplast DNA from *Trypanosoma mega*. *Proc. Natl Acad. Sci. U.S.A.* **66**, 419-424

MÜHLPFORDT, H. (1964) Über den Kinetoplasten der Flagellaten. *Z. Tropenmed. Parasitol*. **15**, 289-323

SANABRIA, A. & ARISTIMUÑO, J. (1969) Nuevas investigaciones acerca de la ultraestructura e histoquímica del *Tripanosoma cruzi* en el cerebro del ratón. *Acta Cient. Venez*. **20**, 32-39

SANABRIA, A. & ARISTIMUÑO, J. (1970) Nuevos estudios acerca de la ultraestructura del *Trypanosoma cruzi* en el miocardio del ratón. *Acta Cient. Venez*. **21**, 107-118

SANABRIA, A. & ARISTIMUÑO, J. (1972) Nuevos estudios ultraestructurales en la miocarditis chagásica aguda del ratón. *Acta Cient. Venez*. **23**, 22-33

Immunity and antigenic variation: clinical observations suggestive of immune phenomena in African trypanosomiasis

P. DE RAADT

Division of Malaria and Other Parasitic Diseases, World Health Organization, Geneva

Abstract In African human trypanosomiasis the early symptoms occur as a direct consequence of recurrent invasions of parasites into the general circulation. These symptoms are not specific, e.g. fever, general malaise, generalized lymphadenopathy. They are comparable to those observed in experimental infections in rodents. More specific symptoms such as meningoencephalitis and myocarditis develop slowly and are considered of immunopathological origin. This may also be the case with the generalized oedema and anaemia occurring later during the disease.

The surface or variant antigens elicit agglutinating, neutralizing and precipating IgM antibodies, which are specific for each parasitaemic population and are newly produced repeatedly during the infection. As trypanosome populations in the blood are antigenically heterogeneous and as differences in virulence occur amongst various antigenic types, it is suggested that biological competition between variants results in one, the most virulent type, predominating each time.

Common antigens elicit IgG antibodies as detected by fluorescent and complement fixation tests and indirect agglutination. They are released at the end of each parasitaemic wave and when trypanosomal treatment is started. On each occasion there is a temporary excess of antigens. Rheumatoid factor and heterophile and autologous antibodies have been reported. The pathology of sleeping sickness is probably related to immune-hypersensitivity reactions mediated by cells or by antigen–antibody complexes, possibly by combination of several processes at one time.

The immunological phenomena that occur when man is infected with pathogenic *Leishmania* or *Trypanosoma* have, since the discovery of protective antibodies against *Trypanosoma equiperdum* in experimental animals by Rouget (1896), provided an important challenge for the immunologist. In this paper I shall review the complicated antigenic challenges occurring during African trypanosomiasis in man, and the possible response by the host's immune defence system in the light of the clinical symptoms.

The symptoms observed in human patients need emphasis, because the characteristic lesions produced by parasites in man cannot be reproduced consistently in experimental animals. For instance, in sleeping sickness the most important histopathological lesion is meningoencephalitis. This can occur in experimental infections in monkeys, but its development cannot be guaranteed either by selecting a particular trypanosome stabilate, or by using the same host species each time.

As the lesions of the central nervous system are likely to be of immuno-pathological origin, the immune responses in man must be essentially different from those in experimental animals.

In rodents, virulent *Trypanosoma (Trypanozoon) brucei* strains can cause death within five days with terminal parasitaemia of up to 10^9 trypanosomes/ml blood. The rapid death of these animals must be due to metabolic disturbances comparable with the exhaustion of a nutrient medium. One may call this the immediate effect of trypanosome infections. It occurs in *T. rhodesiense* infections in man in the early stages, causing pronounced clinical symptoms without any histopathological lesions of importance. This is in contrast to the complicated interactions that result from the many different antigens that, during the course of infection, enter the circulation at intervals and cause the more important 'long-term' effect of the disease.

SLEEPING SICKNESS

The two forms of sleeping sickness are caused by closely related organisms, *T. rhodesiense* and *T. gambiense*, both nosodemes of the subspecies, *Trypanosoma (Trypanozoon) brucei gambiense*. The essential difference in their virulence towards mammalian hosts is reflected in their different reservoir hosts as well as in the symptoms they produce in man. However, the ultimate pathological effects, including the immunological effects during infection, are similar with either organism and the two will be treated here as, in essence, due to the same pathogenic process.

Trypanosomes are inoculated into the skin by infected *Glossina* and the characteristic chancre is formed as the parasites multiply in the subcutaneous tissues. From this primary focus trypanosomes invade the lymph, blood and tissues. The trypanosomes increase logarithmically in the blood for one to three days after they are first detected in the bloodstream. They then seem to disappear from the circulation altogether, but their remarkable properties of recovery in mammalian hosts allow the next population to develop in the blood; this population bypasses the earlier specific immune defence built up by the host by having antigens of a different constitution from those of the previous population (Ritz 1914). The interval between each parasitaemic wave in man may vary from one to eight days.

This recurrent parasitaemia means that the host is exposed to a continuous sequence of infections with practically the same microorganisms and to different but closely related antigen–antibody reactions each time. What occurs in influenza on a world scale over a period of years is condensed in trypanosomiasis to a single host and a period of several weeks or months.

The clinical symptoms which accompany each bout of parasitaemia are so unspecific that they are frequently mistaken for malaria or influenza. Patients complain of general malaise, headache and pains in the joints. No specific physical signs occur as an immediate effect of parasitaemia, except that the fever always exactly parallels the parasitaemic waves.

As the infection proceeds, symptoms related to the immediate effect become less prominent, in parallel with the parasitaemias, which tend to occur at longer intervals, with the numbers of organisms decreasing. The more typical symptoms develop gradually. These are a slowly progressing meningoencephalitis, myocarditis, generalized oedema—which can be severe—, anaemia and perhaps nephritis. As may be expected, malnutrition develops, which in turn aggravates the oedema and anaemia. In most patients the final cause of death is some concurrent infection, remarkably often pneumonia. The high incidence of pulmonary infections can be explained by underlying lung oedema, probably due to vascular leakage and heart failure at the same time.

Although, as already mentioned, the underlying pathological principles in the two forms of sleeping sickness must be the same, the clinical picture differs distinctly. East African sleeping sickness caused by *T. rhodesiense* is characterized by high parasitaemia with acute and severe symptoms during the first stage of infection. Most patients therefore seek medical treatment during this early stage, but with a limited chance of success, because the correct diagnosis can only be made when parasitaemia is present. The central nervous system symptoms become manifest between 3 and 12 weeks after infection, followed by oedema and cardiac symptoms. If untreated, the *T. rhodesiense* disease is usually fatal to man between three and nine months after infection.

Sleeping sickness due to *T. gambiense* occurs mainly in West and Central Africa and is a much more chronic disease. In particular, early symptoms are less severe and normally fail to alarm the patients seriously; an untreated patient with *T. gambiense* infection may survive for years with relatively few complaints.

In addition there are epidemiological differences between the two forms of sleeping sickness, such as vectors and reservoir hosts, which will not be discussed here.

THE ANTIGENIC CHALLENGE

The antigenic challenge to the host during an infection with blood trypanosomes is not only qualitatively complicated but also—due to the fluctuating parasitaemia—quantitatively inconstant, as the following calculations will illustrate. Trypanosomes have a cell volume of approximately 50 μm^3 and are probably the largest organisms which can infect human blood. Within 48 h, parasitaemia in a *T. rhodesiense* infection may rise from undetectable amounts to 10^7 trypanosomes/ml. If they are uniformly distributed in a total of about 10 litres of extracellular body fluids, including blood, the total number of trypanosomes present in the body will then be 10^{11}, each representing a surface of 100 μm^2 antigenic material. Most of these organisms are destroyed again within two or three days. For instance, Onyango *et al.* (1965) saw a reduction from 10^5 organisms/ml blood to less than 10/ml in man over a period of 48 h, as measured by the titration method of Lumsden (Lumsden *et al.* 1963). After each episode of parasitaemia, the cell contents—a different group of antigens—are discharged from the disintegrating trypanosomes into the circulation.

Before I discuss the host response to the different antigens introduced during trypanosomiasis, I shall describe the characteristics of the three main groups of trypanosomal antigens: variant or surface antigens, common or cytoplasmic and nuclear antigens, and free or exoantigens.

Surface or variant antigens

Variant antigens are population-specific and elicit protecting, agglutinating and lysing, as well as precipitating, antibodies. Vickerman (1969) demonstrated that bloodstream trypanosomes have a continuous coat on the cell pellicle and he assumed, and later provided the evidence, that the variant antigens were located in the surface layer (Vickerman & Luckins 1969). They consist of heterogeneous macromolecules—glycoproteins—the carbohydrate part of which acts as an antigenic determinant, with a protein component of inconstant structure being responsible for the chemical heterogeneity (Njogu & Humphryes 1972). According to Seed (1972) the variable antigens consist of two separate components, one connected with protective antibodies and the other being agglutinogens. This would imply that at each shift from one variant population to another, at least two groups of antigenic determinants are modified.

In accordance with the present view of cell biologists that the Golgi apparatus is the key organelle conducting the assembly of cellular secretion products

(Whaley *et al.* 1972), Vickerman (1971) succeeded in providing evidence suggesting that the surface layer in trypanosomes is a secretion product of the cell and that an elaborate secretory apparatus is present, consisting of a well developed Golgi apparatus with membrane-bound vesicles and tubules for transporting the excretion product to the flagellar pocket. The structures involved in secretion are thus reasonably well elucidated, but the question of how antigenic determinants can be modified during the course of infection remains unexplained.

Cantrell (1958) and Watkins (1964) have suggested that the mechanism is one based entirely on random mutation and selection. According to Watkins, mutation would take place independently of external stimuli such as host antibodies. Watkins' theory was based on observations in mice suggesting that new antigenic variants appeared as early as three days after inoculation, and he assumed that this was not long enough for antibody formation to have taken place. The objection against this theory is that from Gray's (1962) experiments it appeared that, for a given strain of trypanosomes, antigenic variation occurs according to a predictable pattern. Gray inoculated several animals with a certain parent strain and variants appeared in a similar sequence in each of the infections. In addition, Gray found that any variant developed from the same trypanosome strain, when inoculated in a new host, would reappear consistently as the same antigenic type, the 'basic strain antigenic type'. Reversion to this basic antigenic type takes place after transmission by flies as well as after passage by syringe (Gray 1965).

Ritz (1914, 1916) concluded that antigenic variation is due to the influences of the host's antibodies, and this was supported by several later observations. Gray (1965) and Vickerman (1969), assuming an adaptive property of the cell, suggested that the successive replacements of the surface coat are due to an organized process embedded in the cell's genetic constitution. By this hypothesis the regularity of the process can be explained satisfactorily. However, if we assume that individual trypanosomes are capable of shifting from one specific antigenic surface coat to another, there is no answer yet why apparently only a few individuals in each population succeed in using their genetically fixed device of escaping the defence mechanism of the host. It may be that the bloodstream trypanosomes are 'taken by surprise' whereas trypanosomes present in the tissues are relatively protected from the action of neutralizing antibodies. The inductive stimulant for the antigenic shift could then be either antibodies at low concentration, or other factors related to the immune response of the host, such as immune competent cells.

There is one other complication in the process of antigenic variation. Ritz (1914), Lourie & O'Connor (1937) and Broom & Brown (1940) had already concluded that trypanosome populations are antigenically heterogeneous mixtures. More recently McNeillage *et al.* (1969) confirmed that after single organisms had been inoculated the first relapse population contained more than one antigenic type at the same time. Recently Seed & Effron (1973), attempting to isolate trypanosomes from various sites of the brain of experimentally infected field mice (*Microtus montanus*) found that the antigenicity of these tissue trypanosomes differed from the bloodstream type, as well as from each other, in their agglutinating properties. Even if a distinction between tissue and bloodstream forms is not valid, this shows that several variants can occur at the same time. Hence, if a genetically pre-designed mechanism of the cell is involved, it must be easily disturbed, to make it work in a disorderly way.

A second unexplained point is that since different variants are present simultaneously in the host's blood and tissues, how do we explain the clear-cut interval which occurs between episodes of parasitaemia? One would expect several variant populations to overlap, continuously appearing and disappearing independently, synchronous appearance and disappearance of more than one variant during each wave of parasitaemia seeming highly improbable.

I feel that the possibility of biological competition occurring amongst different variants within each trypanosome population is one worth considering. In a slightly different context, Ritz (1914) suggested that one variant might dominate the others. Ecological interactions within the trypanosome population may be responsible for one variant predominating over others which are potentially or literally suppressed until the host has removed the predominant variety.

It is not clear what mechanism would enable one variant to do this, as it is not clear, for instance, why carriers of *Staphylococcus aureus* usually harbour one type, although ample opportunity exists for superinfection by other types of *S. aureus*. Similarly, in *Neisseria meningitidis* infections the isolation of more than one type at a time from one patient or carrier is extremely rare. According to the hypothesis proposed here, a few individuals of one population become an antigenically different type, for instance as a result of random mutation. Trypanosomes of any such variant could multiply or reappear continuously while remaining consistently suppressed in numbers by the more virulent, predominant variant. When a predominant variant of one population is eradicated by the host's antibodies, it is possible that the next most virulent variety in turn becomes predominant in the next wave of parasitaemia. In this way populations will appear in the order of virulence of subsequent antigenic variants, which is consistent with the regularity of the phenomenon. In support of this, the series of experiments by McNeillage and colleagues have also shown that differences in virulence occurred, associated with differences in antigenic type (McNeillage & Herbert 1968). In patients with sleeping sickness the level of parasitaemia commonly becomes lower and the intervals between peak levels more and more protracted during the course of infection, suggesting that the later variant populations are less virulent.

If we assume that each particular strain has a potential of a certain spectrum of antigenic variants, a fairly constant sequence can be expected. Transmission to a new host would mean that the most virulent variant would reappear as the predominant type of the first population, as random mutation may be rapidly reversed, i.e. it may occur both forwards and backwards. The theory of biological competition also provides an explanation for the phenomenon, reported by Gray (1962), that a certain anticipated variant can be bypassed in animals previously immunized against that specific variant.

Finally, according to Desowitz (1970) antigenic variation could also result from a cell-independent immunochemical reaction taking place at the cell surface as a part of the antigen–antibody reaction. Each time this happened new antigenic determinants would become exposed or be formed, thus excluding any specific participation by the trypanosomal cell. It is obvious that if one accepts that the surface material is produced by the cell itself, the later a variant appears during infection the more complex the series of chemical reactions that would be required to obtain the new variant. The occurrence of mixed populations cannot easily be fitted into this theory.

At present, whatever hypothesis one prefers, none is yet supported by conclusive evidence.

Common antigens

Common antigens are those within the cell, consisting of cytoplasmic and nuclear components. They seem to remain qualitatively unchanged during the course of infection. Common antigens elicit antibodies which are detectable by complement fixation (Schoenaers et al. 1953), indirect agglutination (Binz 1972), the fluorescent antibody technique (Sadun et al. 1963) and precipitation. According to Brown & Williamson (1964), at least two of the common antigens are nucleoproteins. The common antigens are typical but not specific for T. (T.) brucei. Cross-reactions with other species (Gray 1960) and even T. cruzi (Seah & Marsden 1970) occur.

The common antigens are released at the crisis of each parasitaemic wave, and their dynamics can be likened to those of an antigenic substance which is repeatedly brought into the circulation at intervals of several days.

Some idea about how frequently common antigens circulate freely in the blood was obtained when we tried (P. de Raadt, unpublished data) to detect them as a means of diagnosing sleeping sickness. Latex particles coated with rabbit IgG antibodies against *T. rhodesiense* common antigen were used for detecting free antigens in the sera of 60 patients infected with *T. gambiense*. In 26 cases free antigens could be demonstrated. Probably the antigens released in the blood are eliminated fairly quickly, either by action of antibodies or by rapid catabolism. The term 'stable antigen' as an alternative for 'common antigen' therefore has the disadvantage of suggesting a degree of chemical stability which may not exist.

Exoantigens

Weitz (1963) reported that soluble antigens in the serum of rats infected with *T. brucei* reacted with agglutinating, protecting and precipitating properties. In other words, their antigenic properties are similar to those of the variant antigens. Allsopp *et al.* (1971) recently provided evidence that surface antigens and exoantigens are chemically identical and that soluble antigens may not be present *in vivo* but may occur *in vitro* as a result of the disintegration of parasites in such conditions.

Apart from soluble material, the exoantigen may consist of loosened cell particles covered with surface material, the so-called plasmanemes, first described by Wright *et al.* (1970) as filopodia.

In addition, of course, free common antigens sometimes circulate in the blood, and metabolic products from trypanosomes, some of which are antigenic, have also been demonstrated in the blood (Desmet *et al.* 1970). Strictly speaking, these two should be included as part of the exoantigen. However, the term 'exoantigen' is usually associated only with the variant antigen material that is not attached to the cell.

Heterophile antigens

Houba & Allison (1966) discovered heterophile agglutinins in 85% of patients with *T. gambiense*. They suggested that a Forssmann-like antigen existed and, from the increased antibody titres observed after anti-trypanosomal treatment began, they assumed that this type of antigen was located within the trypanosomal cell.

THE HOST RESPONSE

Observations in man as well as animals have led to the assumption that immune phenomena play an important role in pathology. For instance, Fiennes (1950) suggested that the anaemia, nephrosis, liver degeneration and lung oedema seen in cattle with *T. congolense* infections were connected with hypersensitivity reactions of the host against trypanosomal antigens. Duke & Wallace (1930) reported red cell adhesion and platelet aggregation, and Goodwin (Goodwin & Hook 1968; Goodwin 1970) and Boreham (1968a, b, 1970) studied kinin activation in experimental infections in rabbits. Nagle *et al.* (1973) found glomerulonephritis and IgG immune complexes in the glomerular capillaries in rhesus monkeys infected with *T. rhodesiense*.

Several clinical symptoms in sleeping sickness also seem to hint at the part played by the immune response in pathology. For instance, urticaria is not uncommon during the early stages of the disease and, non-specific as they may be, symptoms like marked general lymphadenopathy and splenomegaly should be considered as signs of activation of the immune apparatus. The histopathological lesions of heart and brain, characterized by perivascular monocellular infiltrates (Koten & de Raadt 1969), are further signs, the histopathology of the brain being similar to that in experimental allergic encephalitis.

Except for the initial swelling during the first two days after the fly bite, the development of the chancre is not simply a local reaction to the presence of parasites and salivary components. The typical lesion develops after a 'silent' interval of several days, usually five. The secondary lesion is characterized by subcutaneous induration, concentric desquamation, oedema, erythema and eventually hyperpigmentation. Microscopically there are perivascular infiltrates of small round cells and occasional polymorphonuclear leucocytes (Fairbairn & Godfrey 1957). The multiplying trypanosomes in the skin thus become a continuing source of antigens, confined to one place. When antibodies start circulating in the blood immune complexes may be formed where the antigens are deposited in the tissue and immune complex-type hypersensitivity with increased vascular permeability may result (Gell & Coombs 1968). The way that the antigen is presented and the type of lesion that results are comparable with what occurred in the classical experiment of Arthus, except that antigens are produced on the spot instead of being inoculated.

As for the pathology of brain and heart, either cell-mediated immunity or increased vascular permeability resulting from complex-mediated hypersensitivity may cause the perivascular infiltration of cells. The marked preponderance of small mononuclear cells in these infiltrates could be an argument in favour of a cell-mediated immune process.

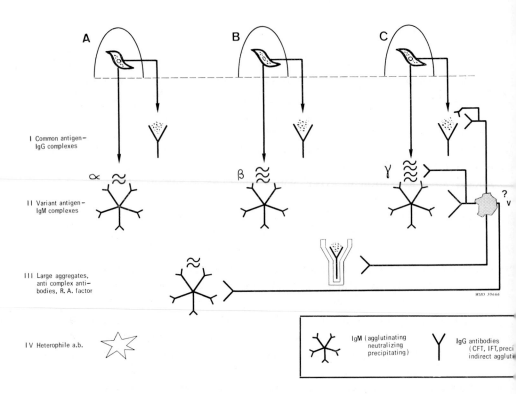

FIG. 1. Antigenic challenge and suggested points of impact of immune response during sleeping sickness.
A, B, C: Three successive relapse populations of bloodstream trypanosomes and their respective variant antigens ($\approx$ $\approx$ $\approx$) and common antigens ( ).
a, β, γ: Indicate the related IgM antibodies.

The two important questions are: which antigens would be involved in such a process, and by what mechanisms would they act? The various possible antigen-antibody reactions and suggested points of impact of cell-mediated immunity are drawn in Fig. 1. As autopsy material from patients with sleeping sickness is limited, few immunopathological studies have yet been carried out. Extensive serological studies, however, have been made, mainly with the purpose of improving diagnostic techniques.

IgM globulins

The most characteristic feature of the humoral response in sleeping sickness is the increased concentration of IgM in the serum, first reported by Mattern

(1963). Part of the IgM fraction consists of agglutinating, neutralizing, precipitating and lysing antibodies (Dupouey 1968) against the surface antigens. Since macroglobulins are usually connected with the early immune response, the exceptionally high levels of IgM could be explained by the sequential production of early antibodies against various surface antigens. However this is not necessarily the explanation, because in addition to anti-trypanosomal antibodies the IgM fraction contains heterophile and anti-immune complex antibodies, like the rheumatoid factor (Houba & Allison 1966; Houba *et al.* 1969; Klein & Mattern 1965). Mattern *et al.* (1967) found indications that part of the IgM in trypanosomiasis consists of 7S IgM. Klein *et al.* (1967) produced supportive evidence by comparing the results of IgM estimations by ultra-centrifugation with those obtained by precipitation with anti-IgM serum. The results suggested that the 7S IgM fraction contained the IgM antigenic determinants and that, since 7S globulins diffuse more easily in gel than 19S, the increase in IgM must be overestimated when measured by single diffusion and immune precipitation according to the method of Mancini *et al.* (1965).

Whether 19S IgM molecules are split into monomers under the influence of trypanosomes or their excretion products, or whether 7S IgM molecules are formed directly by plasma cells in trypanosomiasis, remain subjects for further investigations. One of the early observations in trypanosomiasis may be relevant here—the large strawberry-like cells, Mott cells, seen in tissues and cerebrospinal fluid. These cells are supposed to be derived from plasma cells, and may be associated with abnormal synthesis of antiglobulins.

IgG antibodies

The IgG antibodies which are directed against the common antigens may be of particular importance in the pathogenesis of trypanosomiasis in man since circulating antigen–IgG complexes seem to occur repeatedly during the infection. When we were evaluating the fluorescent antibody technique and the complement fixation test we observed that soon after the parasitaemic waves the antibody titre fell very low, sometimes down to undetectable levels, and later returned to the original titre, as shown in Fig. 2. Our explanation (de Raadt *et al.* 1966) of this phenomenon is that each time trypanosomes disappear from the circulation common antigens are released from the disintegrating organisms; the resulting temporary excess of antigens is then gradually compensated by stimulation of specific IgG production until antibody excess is re-established. As Dixon *et al.* (1961) have pointed out, soluble immune complexes occur at the turning points at which antigen and antibody concentrations are equal. With

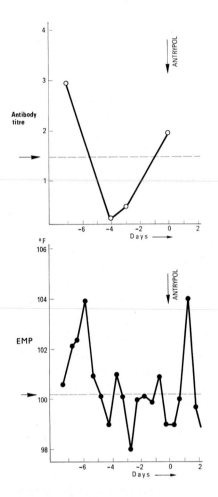

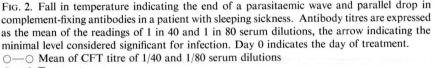

FIG. 2. Fall in temperature indicating the end of a parasitaemic wave and parallel drop in complement-fixing antibodies in a patient with sleeping sickness. Antibody titres are expressed as the mean of the readings of 1 in 40 and 1 in 80 serum dilutions, the arrow indicating the minimal level considered significant for infection. Day 0 indicates the day of treatment.
○—○ Mean of CFT titre of 1/40 and 1/80 serum dilutions
●—● Temperature

the common antigens and their antibodies these points are crossed in both directions several times during infection.

Similarly, when patients first received anti-trypanosomal treatment sharp falls in antibody titres were observed (de Raadt 1968). One such example is given in Fig. 3. In the same series of observations, we found that the number of eosinophilic polymorphonuclear leucocytes increased by two to four times

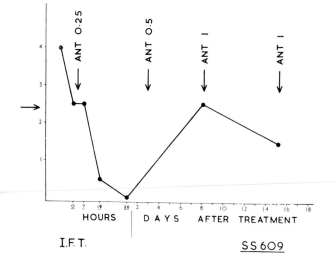

FIG. 3. The effect in a patient with sleeping sickness of the first dose of Antrypol on the fluorescent antibody titre, expressed (abscissa) as the mean of the readings of 1 in 40 and 1 in 80 serum dilutions. The arrow indicates the minimum level considered significant for infection. ANT 0.25 etc.: Antrypol 0.25 g i.v.

the original number in 43 out of 50 patients (de Raadt & Bakari 1966). According to Litt (1961) eosinophilia can be mediated by antigen–antibody complexes. In addition, some clinical symptoms (temperature peaks, enhanced enlargement of lymph glands and urticaria) were accelerated after treatment, comparable to the Herxheimer reaction in syphilis. The coincidence of the above complications with the release of common antigens supports the view that these antigens are important factors in the pathogenesis of the disease. In my opinion, the reactive encephalopathy which may develop some five to ten days after treatment begins belongs to the same type of reaction, rather than being due to the toxicity of arsenical drugs.

Cell-mediated immunity

Except for the indications from the histopathology of heart and brain, no substantial evidence has been obtained yet that cell-mediated immunity occurs. Tizard & Soltys (1971) demonstrated that skin hypersensitivity occurred in rabbits infected with *T. brucei*, and considered that this was due to cell-mediated immunity. In man, a series of experimental skin tests in *T. rhodesiense* infections in which we inoculated lysed trypanosomes, an antigen suspension rich in common antigens, and preparations of homologous organisms previously isolated from the same patient, were unsuccessful (de Raadt *et al.* 1967). Techniques such as the migration inhibition test and determination of pyroninophilic cells in lymph glands may provide useful information.

Autologous antibodies

Various autologous antibodies have been found in rabbits infected with *T. brucei* (Mackenzie *et al.* 1972). In a preliminary communication, Mackenzie *et al.* (1973) reported that anti-liver and anti-Wassermann antibodies are present in cattle and man. However, the search for anti-brain antibodies has remained unsuccessful (P. de Raadt & J. Feltkamp, unpublished data).

Immune suppression

Goodwin *et al.* (1972) showed that during *T. brucei* infections in rabbits the immune response against sheep erythrocytes was diminished. In sleeping sickness the general condition of patients is complicated a great deal by anaemia and malnutrition, which in themselves may cause a reduced immune response (WHO 1972). In contrast, resistance to concurrent infections seems strong rather than diminished, and if we assume that there is immune suppression, it is also surprising that the combination of malaria and trypanosomiasis is not seen more frequently. In fact, in 150 patients with sleeping sickness, we did not see a single case of malaria.

RECOMMENDATIONS

The key to the problem of immunity in trypanosomiasis is most certainly related to the mechanism of antigenic variation. There is little hope of success for a vaccination technique without the mechanism of antigenic variation being elucidated. Methods for the cultivation of bloodstream forms *in vitro* would mean a considerable step forward. Also studies on the interrelationship of mixed variant populations could provide useful information.

Concerning the role of antigen–antibody complexes in the pathogenic process, further research is needed on the detection of immune complexes in blood as well as tissues and on identification of their components. To this end biopsies of chancres might be useful, and easier than studies on autopsy material. The structure of lymph glands could provide important information, especially on the question of cell-mediated immunity, as indicated for instance by the occurrence of pyroninophilic cells in the paracortical region. Migration inhibition tests and elucidation of the nature and origin of 7S IgM globulins may also prove useful.

Once the antigens responsible for the pathological process have been determined, one could even look for means of providing protection against the harmful effects of the disease rather than against the infection itself, for instance immunization as a prophylactic against the reactive encephalopathy during treatment.

Further classification of factors may lead to a fragmentary approach and over-simplification of the problem. Neither the activation of the kinin system nor the demonstration of cell-mediated immunity or circulating immune complexes would exclude other mechanisms from playing a role at the same time. Presumably a complex interaction of different types of immune response leads to the pathological process as a whole.

ACKNOWLEDGEMENTS

I thank the Director of the East African Trypanosomiasis Research Organization for permission to publish data I collected while working at EATRO, the EATRO staff for their interest and assistance, Mrs I. Wevers-Prijs for her literature studies, and Dr H. Goodman for reading the manuscript.

References

ALLSOPP, B. A., NJOGU, A. R. & HUMPHRYES, K. C. (1971) Nature and location of *Trypanosoma brucei* subgroup exoantigen and its relationship to 4S antigen. *Exp. Parasitol.* **29**, 271-284

BINZ, G. (1972) An evaluation of the capillary and latex agglutination and heterophile antibody tests for the detection of *Trypanosoma rhodesiense* infections. *Bull. W.H.O.* **47**, 773-778

BOREHAM, P. F. L. (1968a) The possible role of kinins in the pathogenesis of chronic trypanosomiasis. *Trans. R. Soc. Trop. Med. Hyg.* **62**, 120-121

BOREHAM, P. F. L. (1968b) Immune reactions and kinin formation in chronic trypanosomiasis. *Br. J. Pharmacol.* **32**, 493-504

BOREHAM, P. F. L. (1970) Kinin release and the immune reaction in human trypanosomiasis caused by *Trypanosoma rhodesiense*. *Trans. R. Soc. Trop. Med. Hyg.* **64**, 395-400

BROOM, J. C. & BROWN, H. C. (1940) Studies in trypanosomiasis. IV. Notes on the serological characters of *Trypanosoma brucei* after cyclical development in *Glossina morsitans*. *Trans. R. Soc. Trop. Med. Hyg.* **34**, 53-64

BROWN, K. N. & WILLIAMSON, J. (1964) The chemical composition of trypanosomes. IV. Location of antigens in subcellular fractions of *Trypanosoma rhodesiense*. *Exp. Parasitol.* **15**, 69-86

CANTRELL, W. (1958) Mutation rate and antigenic variation in *Trypanosoma equiperdum*. *J. Infect. Dis.* **103**, 263-271

DESMET, G., WANE, A. & MATTERN, P. (1970) Antigènes somatiques et sériques mis en évidence au cours de la trypanosomiase à *Trypanosoma gambiense*. *C. R. Séances Soc. Biol. Fil.* **164**, 1879-1886

DESOWITZ, R. S. (1970) in *Immunity to Parasitic Animals* (Jackson, G. J., Herman, R. & Singer, I., eds.), vol. 2, pp. 551-596, Appleton-Century-Crofts, New York

DIXON, F. J., FELDMAN, J. D. & VAZQUEZ, J. J. (1961) Experimental glomerulonephritis: the pathogenesis of a laboratory model resembling the spectrum of a human glomerulonephritis. *J. Exp. Med.* **113**, 899-919

DUKE, H. L. & WALLACE, J. M. (1930) 'Red cell adhesion' in trypanosomiasis of man and animals. *Parasitology* **22**, 414-456

DUPOUEY, P. (1968) Structure antigénique de *T. gambiense*, in *VIII Int. Congr. Trop. Med. Malar.* 1968, Teheran, abstr. & rev. pp. 330-331

FAIRBAIRN, H. & GODFREY, D. G. (1957) The local reaction in man at the site of infection with *Trypanosoma rhodesiense*. *Ann. Trop. Med. Parasitol.* **51**, 464-470

FIENNES, R. N. T. W. (1950) The cattle trypanosomes: some considerations of pathology and immunity. *Ann. Trop. Med. Parasitol.* **44**, 42-54

GELL, P. G. H. & COOMBS, R. R. A. (1968) in *Clinical Aspects of Immunology* (Gell, P. G. H. & Coombs, R. R. A., eds.), Section IV, pp. 575-596, Blackwell Scientific Publications, Oxford

GOODWIN, L. G. (1970) The pathology of African trypanosomiasis. *Trans. R. Soc. Trop. Med. Hyg.* **64**, 797-812

GOODWIN, L. G. & HOOK, S. V. M. (1968) Vascular lesions in rabbits infected with *Trypanosoma (Trypanozoon) brucei*. *Br. J. Pharmacol.* **32**, 505-513

GOODWIN, L. G., GREEN, D. G., GUY, M. W. & VOLLER, A. (1972) Immunosuppression during trypanosomiasis. *Br. J. Exp. Pathol.* **53**, 40-43

GRAY, A. R. (1960) Precipitating antibody in trypanosomiasis of cattle and other animals. *Nature (Lond.)* **186**, 1058-1059

GRAY, A. R. (1962) The influence of antibody on serological variation in *Trypanosoma brucei*. *Ann. Trop. Med. Parasitol.* **56**, 4-13

GRAY, A. R. (1965) Antigenic variation in a strain of *Trypanosoma brucei* transmitted by *Glossina morsitans* and *G. palpalis*. *J. Gen. Microbiol.* **41**, 195-214

HOUBA, V. & ALLISON, A. C. (1966) M-Antiglobulins (rheumatoid-factor-like globulins) and other gammaglobulins in relation to tropical parasitic infections. *Lancet* **1**, 848-852

HOUBA, V., BROWN, K. N. & ALLISON, A. C. (1969) Heterophile antibodies, M-antiglobulins and immunoglobulins in experimental trypanosomiasis. *Clin. Exp. Immunol.* **4**, 113-123

KLEIN, F. & MATTERN, P. (1965) Rheumatoid factors in primary and reactive macroglobulinaemia. *Ann. Rheum. Dis.* **24**, 458-464

KLEIN, F., MATTERN, P., RADEMA, H. & VAN ZWET, T. L. (1967) Slowly sedimenting serum components reacting with anti-IgM sera. *Immunology* **13**, 641-647

KOTEN, J. W. & RAADT, P. DE (1969) Myocarditis in *Trypanosoma rhodesiense* infections. *Trans. R. Soc. Trop. Med. Hyg.* **63**, 485-489

LITT, M. (1961) Studies in experimental eosinophilia. III: The induction of peritoneal eosinophilia by the passive transfer of serum antibody. *J. Immunol.* **87**, 522-529

LOURIE, E. M. & O'CONNOR, R. J. (1937) A study of *Trypanosoma rhodesiense* relapse strains *in vitro*. *Ann. Trop. Med. Parasitol.* **31**, 319-340

LUMSDEN, W. H. R., CUNNINGHAM, M. P., WEBBER, W. A. F., VAN HOEVE, K. & WALKER, P. (1963) A method for the measurement of the infectivity of trypanosome suspensions. *Exp. Parasitol.* **14**, 269-279

MACKENZIE, A. R., BOREHAM, P. F. L. & FACER, C. A. (1972) Non-trypanosome specific components of the elevated IgM levels in rabbit trypanosomiasis. *Trans. R. Soc. Trop. Med. Hyg.* **66**, 344-345

MACKENZIE, A. R., BOREHAM, P. F. L. & FACER, C. A. (1973) Autoantibodies in African trypanosomiasis. *Trans. R. Soc. Trop. Med. Hyg.* **67**, 268

MANCINI, G., CARBONARA, A. O. & HEREMANS, J. F. (1965) Immunological quantitation of antigens by single radial immunodiffusion. *Immunochemistry* **2**, 235-254

MATTERN, P. (1963) L'hyper-β_2-macroglobulinémie et l'hyper-β_2-macroglobulinorachie, témoins constants de la perturbation protéinique humorale au cours de la trypanosomiase humaine, in *9th Meeting of the International Scientific Committee for Trypanosomiasis Research 1962*, Conakry, pp. 377-385

MATTERN, P., KLEIN, F., RADEMA, H. & VAN FURTH, R. (1967) Les γ-macroglobulines réactionnelles et paraprotéiniques dans le serum et dans le liquide céphalo-rachidien humain. *Ann. Inst. Pasteur (Paris)* **113**, 656-866

MCNEILLAGE, G. J. C. & HERBERT, W. J. (1968) Infectivity and virulence of *Trypanosoma (Trypanozoon) brucei* for mice. II: Comparison of closely related trypanosome antigenic types. *J. Comp. Pathol.* **78**, 345-349

MCNEILLAGE, G. J. C., HERBERT, W. J. & LUMSDEN, W. H. R. (1969) Antigenic type of first relapse variants arising from a strain of *Trypanosoma (Trypanozoon) brucei*. *Exp. Parasitol.* **25**, 1-7

NAGLE, R. B., WARD, P. A., SADUN, E. H., BERKAW, R. E., JOHNSON, A. J., DUXBURY, R. E. & HILDEBRANDT, P. K. (1973) Glomerulonephritis in experimental African trypanosomiasis. *Fed. Proc.* **32**, 3433

NJOGU, A. R. & HUMPHRYES, K. C. (1972) The nature of the 4S antigens of the *brucei* subgroup trypanosomes. *Exp. Parasitol.* **31**, 178-187

ONYANGO, R. J., RAADT, P. DE, CUNNINGHAM, M. P. & HOEVE, K. VAN (1965) Periodicity and infectivity of trypanosomes in a man infected with *T. rhodesiense*. *East Afr. Trypanosomiasis Res. Organ. Rep.* 1964, 32-34

RAADT, P. DE (1968) The Herxheimer reaction during treatment of *T. rhodesiense* infections, in *VIII Int. Congr. Trop. Med. Malar.*, 1968, Teheran, abstr. & rev., pp. 336-337

RAADT, P. DE & BAKARI, N. (1966) Evidence of an increase of eosinophilic leucocytes after initial administration of antitrypanosomal drugs. *East Afr. Trypanosomiasis Res. Organ. Rep.* 1965, 54-55

RAADT, P. DE, CUNNINGHAM, M. P., KIMBER, C. D. & GRAINGE, E. B. (1966) Trials of a skin test for sleeping sickness. *East Afr. Trypanosomiasis Res. Organ. Rep.* 1965, 33

RAADT, P. DE, HART, G., GRAINGE, E. B., MBWABI, D. & KWEYAMYA (1967) Serological tests in *T. rhodesiense* infections. *East Afr. Trypanosomiasis Res. Organ. Rep.* 1966, 39-42

RITZ, H. (1914) Über Rezidive bei experimenteller Trypanosomiasis. *Dtsch. Med. Wochenschr.* **27**, 1355-1358

RITZ, H. (1916) Über Rezidive bei experimenteller Trypanosomiasis II. *Arch. Schiffs- & Tropenhyg.* **20**, 397-422

ROUGET, J. (1896) Contribution à l'étude du trypanosome des mammifères. *Ann. Inst. Pasteur (Paris)* **10**, 716-728

SADUN, E. H., DUXBURY, R. E., WILLIAMS, J. S. & ANDERSON, R. I. (1963) Fluorescent antibody test for the serodiagnosis of African and American trypanosomiasis in man. *J. Parasitol.* **49**, 385-388

SCHOENAERS, F., NEUJEAN, G. & EVENS, F. (1953) Valeur pratique de la réaction de fixation du complément dans la maladie du sommeil à *T. gambiense*. 1ère partie: Le diagnostic de la maladie. *Ann. Soc. Belge Méd. Trop.* **33**, 141-169

SEAH, S. & MARSDEN, P. D. (1970) Complement fixation test in *Trypanosoma rhodesiense* infection with cultured *Trypanosoma cruzi* as antigen. *Trans. R. Soc. Trop. Med. Hyg.* **64**, 279-283

SEED, J. R. (1972) *Trypanosoma gambiense* and *T. equiperdum*: characterization of variant specific antigens. *Exp. Parasitol.* **31**, 98-108

SEED, J. R. & EFFRON, H. G. (1973) Simultaneous presence of different antigenic populations of *Trypanosoma brucei gambiense* in *Microtus montanus*. *Parasitology* **66**, 269-278

TIZARD, I. R. & SOLTYS, M. A. (1971) Cell-mediated hypersensitivity in rabbits infected with *Trypanosoma brucei* and *Trypanosoma rhodesiense*. *Infect. Immun.* **4**, 674-677
VICKERMAN, K. (1969) On the surface coat and flagella adhesions in trypanosomes. *J. Cell Sci.* **5**, 163-193
VICKERMAN, K. (1971) in *Ecology and Physiology of Parasites* (Fallis, A. M., ed.), pp. 58-89, University of Toronto Press, Toronto
VICKERMAN, K. & LUCKINS, A. G. (1969) Localization of variable antigens in the surface coat on *Trypanosoma brucei* using ferritin conjugated antibody. *Nature (Lond.)* **224**, 1125-1126
WATKINS, J. F. (1964) Observations on antigenic variation in a strain of *Trypanosoma brucei* growing in mice. *J. Hyg.* **62**, 69-80
WEITZ, B. (1963) Immunological relationships between African trypanosomes and their hosts. *Ann. N.Y. Acad. Sci.* **113**, 400-408
WHALEY, W. G., DAUWALDER, M. & KEPHART, J. E. (1972) Golgi apparatus: influence on cell surfaces. *Science* **175**, 596-599
WHO (1972) A survey of nutritional-immunological interactions. *Bull. W. H. O.* **46**, 537-546
WRIGHT, K. A., LUMSDEN, W. H. R. & HALES, H. (1970) The formation of filopodium-like processes by *Trypanosoma (Trypanozoon) brucei*. *J. Cell Sci.* **6**, 285-297

Discussion

Baker: I don't entirely see the force of your argument that there would be too few trypanosomes for abrupt antigenic variation to occur as a result of some sort of cell-regulated mechanism, Dr de Raadt.

de Raadt: If it happened in the blood, it would have to be a complicated procedure because otherwise one would expect that most trypanosomes would have the capacity to undergo this process. There would be too many, and hence the next population could follow after a much shorter interval than it does in reality.

Baker: Surely the point is that most of them are killed and only a few, for some reason, can change. Then one has to wait for those few to multiply up to a detectable level, so the change appears abrupt because one can't measure it when very small numbers are present.

de Raadt: If it is a cell-regulated process, why are so few taking part?

Baker: Because the rest are killed.

de Raadt: Yes, but why? That would be selection, if the rest are killed. It means that only a few of each population are capable of taking part.

Baker: I wouldn't have thought they were capable in the sense of being different from the ones that are killed, but perhaps they escape the antibody because they are in the tissue spaces (Ormerod & Venkatesan 1971*a*)?

de Raadt: If they are in the tissues, the antibodies would reach the trypanosomes unless the organism were intracellular.

Vickerman: I don't think anyone has succeeded in initiating a new infection with stumpy forms, which seem to be quite incapable of changing their antigens and forming a new parasitaemic wave. Maybe just a certain fraction of the multiplying slender forms are capable of going on to the next variant.

de Raadt: I quite agree, but if the trypanosomes are brought to fresh surroundings, such as a new host, where there are no antibodies against the existing antigenic variants, one of the essential stimuli to the process is lacking.

Vickerman: My point is that the trypanosome may be capable of switching over to synthesis of a new variant antigen only at a certain stage in its cell cycle.

de Raadt: One needs evidence; of course this may well be what happens, but the presence of several variants in a population at the same time, with one variant always predominating, seems to indicate that there is some mechanism by which the population is organized rather than a genetically predisposed pattern for each cell.

Vickerman: The evidence against the mutation–selection theory is not overwhelming but it is fairly persuasive. One can get antigenic variation occurring in clones, and if one stretches the mutation rate a bit it could just about account for the appearance of variants at intervals of two to three days (Watkins 1964) in a clone. But Gray's (1965) observations on the reversion back to a basic antigen and the appearance of variants in a particular sequence argues heavily against mutation and selection.

de Raadt: I quite agree, but if one accepts the concept of biological competition, differences in virulence amongst the variants will allow one specific, most virulent variant to appear first in each new host inoculated with a certain strain.

Vickerman: But if a particular genetic mutant has been eliminated, how can the trypanosome population revert to producing the basic antigen? One would have to have back mutation on a very predictable basis.

de Raadt: I think that every strain of trypanosomes has a certain spectrum of variants which can occur. This is genetically fixed in their constitution and the chances for a particular variant occurring are about the same. After a certain period of infection all the variants will be present. However, as soon as a former variant reappears by mutation, the antibodies already existing will wipe it out. The variant that will prevail at any time during infection will always be the most virulent one to which the host has never yet produced antibodies.

Vickerman: Are you suggesting not so much mutation and selection, as selection of those that have adapted in a particular way?

de Raadt: I suggest there is random mutation plus different levels of virulence of each particular variant, and as soon as the most virulent variant has disappeared the next most virulent variant will overcome the rest.

Bray: But, if I understood you correctly, you say that each trypanosome has within it a predetermined sequential development of variants and then you talk about random mutation. It doesn't seem to me that one can have predetermination and randomness at the same time.

de Raadt: No; I assume that each trypanosome has a certain spectrum of diverse variants which can occur as a result of random mutation. But the spectrum is limited because of the genetic constitution of each trypanosome of that particular strain.

Bray: Random mutation is random—it occurs by accident.

de Raadt: Yes, but it occurs within certain limits and certain frequencies in each case. When there is random mutation in bacteria one does not get *Pseudomonas* from *E. coli*.

Peters: Professor Beale's work (1953) on the genetics of *Paramecium* shows that a protozoon can very well carry within it this entire spectrum. This is a significant difference between the genetics of bacteria and the genetics of protozoa. The genes for the spectrum of antigenic variants are present in a given clone of *Paramecium*; in suitable conditions one can expose these because they are built into the genetic mechanism. This is surely the situation in trypanosomes.

Baker: Could there be a concentration effect of antibody? If there is enough antibody it kills the trypanosomes but a certain minimal amount might act as a trigger and switch the other genes on (if that is the controlling mechanism). The trypanosomes in tissue spaces may be protected from some of the antibody and may just receive enough to switch something else in, rather than actually being killed by it.

Goodwin: In the tissue spaces the trypanosomes would get about a fifth of the dose they would experience in the blood.

Baker: That might be just enough to switch on the next gene.

Trager: In *Paramecium* serotypes can be brought out by various kinds of environmental changes. One such change is exposure of the paramecium to its original immobilization antiserum; when this happens most of the paramecia are immobilized but some of them begin producing another serotype and then these are able to swim around again. But the situation in this organism seems very complex. I don't think that we could immediately extrapolate from one to the other, but paramecia and trypanosomes certainly appear to be parallel in this matter.

Peters: We are perhaps taking a rather too simplistic view of the genetic make-up of an organism such as a trypanosome. There is much more in the genome than is actually expressed at a given moment and we tend to forget this.

Lumsden: I don't see anything difficult in supposing that the population of organisms is decimated at each turnover. By continuous titration and organism counts through the course of infection in rats, we showed (Cunningham *et al.*

1963) that infectivity corresponds closely to the numbers of organisms in the crescendo part of a curve. But as soon as the curve starts going down there may be wide differences—four logs or more—between the numbers of organisms and the infectivity titration. We interpreted this as indicating that although those organisms seem active and undamaged, they are in fact coated with antibody and are going to be phagocytosed in the host animal. We should not forget that in some parts of the body the organisms may be protected from the antibody to a given antigenic type. Ormerod & Venkatesan (1971a, b) have suggested that the shunt vessels in the choroid plexus are such an area in man. Immunologists seem very uncertain about whether this is likely to happen or not. There is also the Millipore filtration work in which infectivity was found in filtrates of organ suspensions at pore sizes that seemed unlikely to let through whole organisms, but not in similar filtrates of blood (Soltys et al. 1969). So there may be tissue forms that differ from the blood forms.

Targett & Wilson (1972) have recently shown that after *T. lewisi* infections in mice there seems to be a completely sterile immunity, with no organisms anywhere in the body, but with *T. musculi* one can find the organisms in the similar shunt vessels of the kidney. Kidney suspensions are infective to other animals as much as a year after the end of the natural period of the infection. We shouldn't disregard the possibility that the organisms may be walled away and protected from the host's immune response.

de Raadt: That would mean there were few in the tissues, or that their initial cell division may be delayed after antigenic variation has taken place. It is very difficult to understand why parasitaemia levels become lower during the later stages of infection. One would expect the trypanosomes to take advantage of immunosuppression and that the levels of parasitaemia would become higher as the infection proceeds. Possibly the immune suppression which occurs is related to the production of different antibodies rather than to neutralizing antibodies against trypanosomes. A more likely explanation would be that the trypanosomes which appear during the later stages of infection are less virulent than the preceding populations.

Lumsden: What I was saying was that at the end of infection one can still show organisms in the kidney. They survive for long periods after the natural end of the infection, presumably protected from whatever immune mechanism the host can bring to bear.

Goodwin: In the rabbit the parasitaemia gets higher as it goes along. The parasites seem to make use of the lowered resistance of the host.

One of the problems of the disease is the way in which the host makes useless immunoglobulin. About 95% of the globulins in infected monkeys are not trypanosome-specific (Freeman et al. 1970).

Lumsden: Yes, people have tried to absorb the IgM out with all sorts of things. It includes rheumatoid factor and antibodies to heterophile antigens, as well as anti-trypanosomal antibodies.

Goodwin: Terry *et al.* (1973) suggested that T cells normally control B cells and that in certain circumstances the B cells may break out and make antigens on their own without being triggered. The trypanosome infection may in some way dissociate the control of one over the other, so that there are B cells all over the place, making rubbish.

Peters: Is this the same situation as occurs in visceral leishmaniasis, with vast outpourings of IgG?

Goodwin: I think it is the same.

Bray: The whole question of B cell modulation of T cell function and T cell modulation of B cell function has only come up in the last two years. Something of this nature may occur, but no one knows yet whether, for instance, T cell breakdown leads to something like 95% of rubbish antibody being produced by uncontrolled B cells.

Antigen–antibody complexes of course do give delayed hypersensitivity in people who are specifically antigen-sensitive. Soluble antigen–antibody complexes also give immediate and Arthus-type reactions in non-sensitized people. So delayed hypersensitivity may well be seen even in the presence of a great deal of antibody.

de Raadt: Malnutrition plays an important role in trypanosomiasis, which in itself may be the cause of immunosuppression. Another possible reason for immunosuppression could be increased secretion of cortisone. We know that patients with a long-standing trypanosome infection tend to look like patients with Cushing's syndrome. However, clinically one would expect secondary infections with opportunistic organisms like *Candida albicans* and *E. coli* to occur, as in patients treated with immunosuppressive drugs, but we have not seen this in patients with sleeping sickness. One would also expect recrudescences of malaria, which I have never seen in a trypanosomiasis patient, so I don't know how important the role of immunosuppression is in humans. It would be worth investigating.

Bray: Do you see any symptoms of interstitial pneumonia, for instance? *Pneumocystis carinii* is the organism which most often seems to appear in immunosuppressed individuals in heart transplant and similar cases.

de Raadt: Pneumonia often occurs, but circumstances did not allow us to identify its cause.

Baker: Surely your biological competition hypothesis could be tested quite easily by putting each successive variant into a mouse and measuring its generation time? On that hypothesis, the first one should have the shortest generation time, and so on.

de Raadt: It should be quite easy but it has not yet been done. I don't think that the generation time is all-important. It is the interrelationship between organisms belonging to the same strain but of different antigenic types that matters. Experiments with mixtures of isolates from the same strains could therefore provide useful information. In contrast, different subspecies seem to tolerate each other, as for example infections with more than one trypanosome species in cattle.

Baker: Is it true that there is no antigenic variation of *T. cruzi* within the host?

Goble: I don't think we know.

Pulido: The antigen that Dr Maekelt and his group are using in serology comes from the whole parasite. It is a mosaic. Some preliminary experiments we are doing on its purification have shown that there are at least seven or eight protein fractions, of which two proteins of high molecular weight, above 200 000, are important antigenically. We tested these fractions in the complement fixation test and the indirect haemagglutination test. So there is a family of antigens inside *T. cruzi*, and there are some other protein fractions that have nothing to do with the antigen–antibody reaction.

Baker: But do you get an actual variation in the surface antigen? If you don't, how can trypomastigotes of *T. cruzi* appear in the bloodstream repeatedly, time after time, as they seem to do for years?

Bray: From the intracellular form.

Baker: They should be knocked off by antibody when they come out. Didn't Michael Miles obtain some evidence (unpublished) that there was variation?

Lumsden: I don't think there is much evidence for antigenic variation in *T. cruzi*; the continuous parasitaemia may be a matter of release of the organisms from the protected intracellular situation from time to time.

Pulido: As Dr Newton said earlier, there are several stages of the same parasite. The heterogeneous antigen we have is a mixture of several phases of the same trypanosomes.

Peters: Didn't one of Brener's students do some work on antigenic variation?

Martinez-Silva: Brener & Chiari (1963) and Brener (1969) worked with the stumpy and the slender forms. We observed that when *T. cruzi* is treated with hyperimmune serum its ability to penetrate the cells *in vitro* is not neutralized. We inoculated *T. cruzi* into cells maintained with growth medium to which hyperimmune serum was added and observed that the growth rate was the same as that in the control group treated with normal serum.

Goble: We did some work on antigenic analyses that some of you will consider to be very unsophisticated but it has not been subsequently contradicted by any more sophisticated work. We started this after von Brand *et al.* (1949) had reported that they couldn't find any difference between the physiology and biochemistry of several different strains of trypanosomes. This was before Brener & Chiari (1963) had pointed out the morphological differences between strains. We already knew from many studies that virulence in animals was a poor way of classifying these strains, so we thought we should try to do serological tests which would show up differences and perhaps put them into different categories. Of course it had been known for some time that when an antiserum against *T. cruzi* in the rabbit was tested in Ouchterlony tests against various strains, it gave nine, ten or eleven lines, all of which coalesced badly and depended on the concentration of antigen used. This did not lead to very much differentiation. Then Nussenzweig (1963) started using, instead of rabbit serum, horse serum immunized against Brazilian strains with what we now call the A type antigen. He found that only three lines normally appeared, and that the dozen or so strains that he tested could be separated into three categories, A, B, and C, C being more closely related to A than to B. When Nussenzweig came to work in the United States he tested more strains and by 1966 about 36 had been classified (Nussenzweig & Goble 1966). Subsequent work (see Table 1) brought the total to 53 strains, examined by roughly the same method, which depends on getting the organisms into culture and growing antigen in liquid medium. Table 1 shows the geographical distribution and the host distribution of these strains. The only generalization we can make is that there are more of the B type than of the others. So far it doesn't make any pattern. Within these groups there is a great deal of cross-immunity, and this is not only serological cross-immunity but also protective immunity, if the whole organism is being used as an antigen (Goble 1961).

Lumsden: Hadn't all the strains used by González Cappa *et al.* (1968) been kept for rather long periods in the laboratory?

Goble: They were of various ages, from maybe 15 or 17 years down to just long enough to get them into culture. Some strains still fell into the same categories when they were rechecked by the same person or by someone else, either at the same time or maybe two years later, after being kept continuously in culture.

Maekelt: Have you any information about the chemical composition of these different antigens? Soluble antigens used in the immune-precipitation tests of Ouchterlony are mostly somatic or endoantigens and not surface antigens. Generally in African trypanosomes the strain-specificity is related to the surface antigen and not to the common endo- or somatic antigen.

Goble: Surface materials were not separated from somatic materials. The antigen was undoubtedly heterogeneous.

TABLE 1 (Goble)

Geographical and host distribution of strains of *Trypanosoma cruzi*, typed according to the antigenic classes proposed by Nussenzweig (1963)*

Hosts	Antigenic types		
	A	*B*	*C*
Primates			
Homo sapiens		USA (2)	
		Salvador	
	Brazil (6)	Venezuela (2)	
	Peru	Brazil	
	Argentina	Argentina (2)	Argentina (2)
Callithrix jacchus		Brazil	
Saimiri sciureus		Brazil	
Carnivora			
Mephitis mephitis		USA	
Procyon lotor	USA (6)	USA	
Tayra barbata			Brazil
Chiroptera			
Eumops abrasus		Brazil (2)	
Rodentia			
Nectomys squamipes		Brazil	
Marsupialia			
Didelphis marsupialis		USA (6)	
Didelphis marsupialis		Venezuela (7)	
Didelphis paraguayensis		Brazil (3)	
Hemiptera			
Triatoma spp.	Chile	Mexico	
Unknown			
	Venezuela	Argentina	Argentina
Total number of strains characterized	16	33	4

* Compiled from information from the following authors: Nussenzweig & Goble (1966), González Cappa *et al.* (1968) and Medina & Chaves (1970). Where more than one strain was tested the total number is shown in parentheses.

Maekelt: Another important question is what kind of antibodies are detected using the different trypanosome antigens, i.e. exo-, surface or endoantigens? What class of immunoglobulins are they?

Goble: We haven't done anything with that. This scheme was based on Ouchterlony precipitation tests and confirmatory tests by absorption and electrophoresis.

References

BEALE, G. H. (1953) Adaptation in *Paramecium*, in *Adaptation in Microorganisms* (Davis, R. & Gale, E., eds.), *Symp. Soc. Gen. Microbiol.* **3**, 294-305, Cambridge University Press, London

BRENER, Z. (1969) The behaviour of slender and stout forms of *Trypanosoma cruzi* in the blood-stream of normal and immune mice. *Ann. Trop. Med. Parasitol.* **63** (2), 215-220

BRENER, Z. & CHIARI, E. (1963) Variações morfológicas observadas em diferentes amostras de *Trypanosoma cruzi. Rev. Inst. Med. Trop. São Paulo* **5** (5), 220-224

CUNNINGHAM, M. D., VAN HOEVE, K. & LUMSDEN, W. H. R. (1963) Variable infectivity of organisms of the *T. brucei* subgroup during acute relapsing infections in rats related to parasitaemia, morphology and antibody response, in *East African Trypanosomiasis Research Organization Report, 1962-1963*, English Press, Nairobi, Kenya

FREEMAN, T., SMITHERS, S. R., TARGETT, G. A. T. & WALKER, P. J. (1970). Specificity of immunoglobulin G in rhesus monkeys infected with *Schistosoma mansoni, Plasmodium knowlesi* and *Trypanosoma brucei. J. Infect. Dis.* **121**, 401-406

GOBLE, F. C. (1961) Observations on cross-immunity in experimental Chagas disease in dogs, in *An. Cong. Int. Doença Chagas (Rio de Janeiro, 1959)*, **2**, 603-611

GONZÁLEZ CAPPA, S. M., SCHMUNIS, G. A. & TRAVERSA, O. C. (1968) Complement-fixation tests, skin tests, and experimental immunization with antigens of *Trypanosoma cruzi* prepared under pressure. *Am. J. Trop. Med. Hyg.* **17**, 709-715

GRAY, A. R. (1965) Antigenic variation in a strain of *Trypanosoma brucei* transmitted by *Glossina morsitans* and *G. palpalis. J. Gen. Microbiol.* **41**, 195-214

MEDINA, M. & CHAVES, J. (1970) Gel diffusion and immunoelectrophoretic analysis of some Venezuelan *Trypanosoma cruzi* strains. *Acta. Cient. Venez.* **21**, 65-67

NUSSENZWEIG, V. (1963) Immunological types of *Trypanosoma cruzi*, in *VII Int. Congr. Trop. Med. Malaria, Rio de Janeiro*, Abstracts of papers, p. 131

NUSSENZWEIG, V. & GOBLE, F. C. (1966) Further studies on the antigenic constitution of strains of *Trypanosoma (Schizotrypanum) cruzi. Exp. Parasitol.* **18**, 224-230

ORMEROD, W. E. & VENKATESAN, S. (1971a) The occult visceral phase of mammalian trypano-somes with special reference to the life cycle of *Trypanosoma (Trypanozoon) brucei. Trans. R. Soc. Trop. Med. Hyg.* **65**, 722-735

ORMEROD, W. E. & VENKATESAN, S. (1971b) An amastigote phase of the sleeping sickness trypanosome. *Trans. R. Soc. Trop. Med. Hyg.*, **65**, 736-741

SOLTYS, M. A., WOO, P. & GILLICK, A. C. (1969) A preliminary note on the separation and infectivity of tissue forms of *Trypanosoma brucei. Trans. R. Soc. Trop. Med. Hyg.* **63**, 495-496

TARGETT, G. A. T. & WILSON, V. C. L. C. (1972) The persistence of *Trypanosoma (Herpeto-soma) musculi* in the kidneys of immune CBA mice. *Trans. R. Soc. Trop. Med. Hyg.* **66**, 669-670

TERRY, R. J., FREEMAN, J., HUDSON, K. M. & LONGSTAFFE, J. A. (1973) Immunoglobulin M production and immunosuppression in trypanosomiasis: a linking hypothesis. *Trans. R. Soc. Trop. Med. Hyg.* **67**, 263

VON BRAND, T., TOBIE, E. J., KISSLING, R. E. & ADAMS, G. (1949) Physiological and patho-logical observations on four strains of *Trypanosoma cruzi. J. Infect. Dis.* **85**, 5-16

WATKINS, J. F. (1964) Observations on antigenic variation in a strain of *Trypanosoma brucei* growing in mice. *J. Hyg.* **62**, 69-80

Nutrition and biosynthetic capabilities of flagellates: problems of *in vitro* cultivation and differentiation

WILLIAM TRAGER

The Rockefeller University, New York

Abstract   The trypanosomes and leishmanias undergo remarkable changes in morphology and especially in physiology as they pass from their vertebrate host to their invertebrate vector and back again. Cultivation *in vitro* provides a powerful approach to determining the nature of the factors concerned in these morphogenetic transformations. At the same time it provides a way of establishing the nutritional requirements of each stage, in this way giving a basis for a rational chemotherapy. Until recently only the stages developing in the invertebrate, and not always all of these, had been cultivated *in vitro*. Only a few species of haemoflagellates have been grown in a chemically defined medium. Of these the most studied are *Crithidia fasciculata*, a parasite of mosquitoes, and the promastigote stage of *Leishmania tarentolae* from lizards. These organisms require an energy source (proline and glutamic acid being superior to carbohydrate), an array of amino acids, inorganic nutrients, haemin, the usual B vitamins, and an unconjugated pteridine such as biopterin. Indications are that the invertebrate stages of the pathogenic trypanosomes and leishmanias require at least these materials and probably others in addition. In the morphogenesis of *Leishmania donovani* some of the factors controlling the change from amastigote to promastigote are now known, but the reverse change occurs only in living host cells. With *Trypanosoma cruzi* all of the forms of the cycles in both the mammal and the bug have been recently obtained in complex media *in vitro*, so that the stage seems set for determination of the factors involved in these cycles. With the salivarian trypanosomes not even all the forms of the invertebrate cycle occur in culture, so that cultures are typically non-infective. Only limited multiplication of the blood forms has so far been obtained *in vitro*. Finally, recent observations on phenomena interpretable as providing for genetic interchange reopen the old question of sex in the haemoflagellates.

The trypanosomes and leishmanias provide remarkable examples of cellular differentiation (Bishop 1967; Honigberg 1967; Newton 1968; Trager 1970; Cosgrove 1971; Zeledón 1971). As they pass from their vertebrate host to their invertebrate vector and back again to the vertebrate they undergo striking changes in morphology and especially in physiology. These changes evidently are in part evoked by, and constitute a response to, the changed environment. Furthermore, within each host these protozoa exhibit cyclic changes, some of which result in the production of forms preadapted for transfer to the other host. We would like to know in some detail the physical and chemical nature of the factors controlling these cellular differentiations. A powerful approach to such understanding is provided by culture methods (Trager 1968). If we could duplicate in *in vitro* culture the entire life cycle we would have a direct way of testing the morphogenetic factors, particularly if the culture media were chemically defined or nearly so. At the same time we would be able to establish the nutritional requirements of each stage and begin to devise a rational chemotherapy.

The truth of the matter is, as we all know, that we are still rather far from this goal. Until recently only the stages found in the invertebrate host had been obtained in culture. Except for a few species from cold-blooded hosts, even these invertebrate stages had not been grown in a chemically defined medium. For the pathogenic trypanosomes and leishmanias it has been necessary to infer their biosynthetic capabilities from experiments of an indirect nature and from work with haemoflagellate parasites of insects or with the invertebrate stages of the few species from cold-blooded vertebrates for which a defined medium was available.

Accordingly I shall first consider the few species for which we have definite information about their nutritional requirements. I shall proceed to see how much of this information applies to the pathogenic species, both in their stages in the vector and especially their stages in the vertebrate host. I shall then discuss the morphogenetic changes in the life cycles of three typical pathogenic forms and see what is known as to control of these changes by nutritional and other environmental factors. Finally, I shall refer briefly to some recent work suggesting the possibility of exchange of genetic material among trypanosomes.

NUTRITIONAL REQUIREMENTS OF CRITHIDIA FASCICULATA AND LEISHMANIA TARENTOLAE

The two species of haemoflagellates first grown in defined media are *Crithidia fasciculata* (see Guttman & Wallace 1964), a choanomastigote parasitic in the gut of mosquitoes, and *Leishmania tarentolae* (see Trager 1968), the promastigote forms of which were originally derived in culture from North African lizards. These are also the two species whose nutritional requirements have been most thoroughly studied. They grow in media containing inorganic salts,

TABLE 1

Amino acid requirements of *Crithidia fasciculata* (data from Kidder & Dutta 1958)

Amino acid	Concentration (μg/ml)	
	In defined medium in absence of any non-essential amino acids	For maximal growth in presence of non-essential amino acids[a]
L-Histidine-HCl	210	80
L-Phenylalanine	500	80
DL-Isoleucine	630	320
DL-Valine	660	200
L-Leucine	970	160
L-Lysine	760	160
L-Arginine-HCl	430	350
L-Tyrosine	200	60
DL-Methionine	340	180
L-Tryptophan	120	24
DL-Threonine	440	80

[a] There were present (in μg/ml): DL-alanine, 550; L-aspartic acid, 610; glycine, 50; L-glutamic acid, 1165; L-proline, 770; DL-serine, 440

a carbon source, amino acids, haemin and vitamins. Some of these requirements are interrelated and dependent on the other nutrients available. This is notably so for the amino acids.

Table 1 summarizes the amino acid requirements of *C. fasciculata*. These are like those of rats with an additional requirement for tyrosine. Although *C. fasciculata* requires threonine for optimal growth, it can synthesize this amino acid by either of two pathways: (1) from methionine; (2) in the absence of methionine in the medium, from phosphenolpyruvate via α-keto-γ-hydroxybutyrate and the β-carbon of serine (Kidder & Dewey 1972). In the latter situation methionine is formed from cysteine.

For *Leishmania tarentolae* promastigotes proline has been found to play a key role (Table 2) (Krassner & Flory 1971). If glucose was omitted, both proline and glutamic acid were essential in addition to the ten amino acids required under all conditions. Most interesting was the finding that with glucose present but proline omitted *L. tarentolae* required 15 amino acids—the ten required in all circumstances and in addition glutamic acid, methionine, isoleucine, alanine and aspartic acid. Thus proline not only can replace glucose as an energy source (Krassner 1969) but in addition it enables the organism to synthesize adequate amounts of methionine, isoleucine, alanine and aspartic

TABLE 2

Effects of amino acid and glucose deletion on growth of *Leishmania tarentolae* in defined Medium C (data from Krassner & Flory 1971)

Amino acid	Concentration (μg/ml)	Growth[a]		
		In absence of amino acid[b]	In absence of both amino acid and proline[b]	In absence of both amino acid and glucose
L-Histidine	150	—	—	—
DL-Phenylalanine	400	—	—	—
L-Valine	500	—	—	—
L-Leucine	1500	—	—	—
L-Lysine	1250	—	—	—
L-Arginine	300	—	—	—
L-Tyrosine	400	—	—	—
L-Tryptophan	200	—	—	—
L-Threonine	500	—	—	—
DL-Serine	400	—	—	—
L-Proline	500	+		—
L-Glutamic acid	1900	+	—	—
L-Methionine	300	+	—	+
L-Isoleucine	600	+	—	+
L-Alanine	700	+	—	+
L-Aspartic acid	1200	+	—	+
Glycine	100	+	+	+

[a] + = Continuous growth through at least 6 successive subcultures.
[b] Glucose present at 5 mg/ml.

acid, as well as of glutamic acid, but this last only if both glucose and proline are present. The special significance of proline in the metabolism of the insect stages of haemoflagellates will be discussed again later.

The ability of *L. tarentolae* to grow in the absence of methionine or any other source of organic sulphur, providing that proline is present, is of special interest. This seems to hold only for one culture strain; this strain has been clearly shown able to grow continuously with inorganic sulphate as its sole sulphur source, though not surprisingly growth is less abundant than with methionine or cystine (Da Cruz & Krassner 1971).

Both *C. fasciculata* and *L. tarentolae* require haemin. For *L. tarentolae* the minimum effective concentration is 200 ng/ml (Simpson 1968a). The haemin could be replaced by catalase or peroxidase but not by cytochrome *c* or protoporphyrin IX (Gaughan & Krassner 1971). The haemin requirement of *L.*

tarentolae was markedly influenced by, and affected the response to, acriflavin (Strauss 1972). A strain selected for resistance to acriflavin required haemin at a concentration of 31 mM in the presence of acriflavine at 470 ng/ml, but at only 0.6 mM (200 ng/ml) in the absence of the drug. This relationship may well deserve much further study; it may have a bearing on the nature of drug resistance in strains resistant to drugs such as Ethidium bromide and others acting on the kinetoplast.

Besides haemin, the growth factors required by haemoflagellates are not unusual except in one other respect. *C. fasciculata* and *L. tarentolae* require not only the usual B vitamins—thiamin, riboflavin, pantothenic acid, nicotinamide, pyridoxamine, biotin and folic acid—but also an unconjugated pteridine. This requirement can however be met by supplying folic acid at an exceptionally high level. For *L. tarentolae* folic acid had to be present at a concentration of at least 1.7 ng/ml to support growth in the absence of an unconjugated pteridine. In the presence of biopterin at 1.7 ng/ml the folic acid could be reduced to a concentration of only 0.34 ng/ml (Trager 1969). Unconjugated pteridines are cofactors in the hydroxylation of phenylalanine, tyrosine, tryptophan and sterols and are widely distributed in nature (Blakeley 1969). *L. tarentolae* and *C. fasciculata* and some other haemoflagellates of insects are the only organisms so far known to require an exogenous source. Thus *C. fasciculata* has provided a sensitive bioassay for biopterin and closely related pteridines (Guttman 1969). Since pteridines are especially abundant in insects one wonders whether this might have some connection with a pteridine requirement in these parasites of insects. One wonders, also, whether the stages in the vertebrate host have a similar biosynthetic defect and, if they do, whether this could provide another approach to finding effective chemotherapeutic agents.

When *L. tarentolae* is grown with minimal concentrations of certain required growth factors the organisms tend to lack a flagellum, even though the populations attained are as great as with higher concentrations of the factors. Thus with 0.34 ng folic acid/ml and 1.7 ng biopterin/ml only 22% of the organisms had a flagellum at least as long as the body. With the same concentration of folic acid but with 170 ng biopterin/ml 52% of the organisms had a flagellum as long as the body or longer (Trager 1969).

Of the purines and pyrimidines only adenine is required by the insect flagellates grown in defined medium (Kidder 1967). Similarly, adenosine can replace the mixture of purines and pyrimidines originally used in the defined medium for *L. tarentolae* (L. Simpson, personal communication).

Often neglected, because difficult to work with, are the requirements for metals and other inorganic nutrients. *L. tarentolae* could be shown to require at least calcium, magnesium and a mixture of other inorganic salts (Trager

1968), but little other work seems to have been done on this aspect of haemo-flagellate nutrition. Yet it is perfectly clear that as one replaces natural media such as blood with defined mixtures it will be essential to supply not only metals but also appropriate chelating agents that help to make these available to the cell (Hutner 1972).

NUTRITIONAL REQUIREMENTS OF INVERTEBRATE STAGES OF OTHER LEISHMANIAS AND OF TRYPANOSOMES

Trypanosoma ranarum and *T. mega*, both from amphibia, have been grown in defined media, the former in the same medium used for *Crithidia* (Guttman 1963) and the latter in a more complex medium that has not been published (G. Boné & M. Steinert, I Int. Congr. Parasitology, Rome, 1964). One strain of *T. cruzi* and numerous strains of *L. tropica* have been grown in a nearly defined medium (Citri & Grossowicz 1955) of such a nature as to indicate growth requirements at least similar to those of *L. tarentolae*. *T. rotatorium*, also from amphibia, has been reported to grow through five subcultures over a period of 20 days in tissue culture Medium 199 supplemented with haematin, ribulose-5-phosphate, ribose-5-phosphate, NADP, ATP and ADP (Fromentin 1971).

Fromentin (1971) obtained some growth of *T. theileri* and also *T. gambiense* in Medium 199 supplemented with 5% by volume of the liquid portion of Tobie's medium, or with an extract made by allowing erythrocytes to stand in Hanks' solution at 35 °C overnight and then centrifuging. Using this medium she found that growth of *T. gambiense* was favoured by the presence of proline and inhibited by omission of glutamine, arginine or lysine. Glucose was essential for *T. gambiense* but not for *T. theileri*. For neither of these species could the erythrocyte extract be replaced by known substances. It may be significant, however, that an extract of human red blood cells genetically deficient in glucose-6-phosphate dehydrogenase (G-6-PDH) did not support growth of *T. gambiense*, whereas a similar extract from normal erythrocytes did. It may be that supplying this enzyme is one of the functions of the red cell extract; certainly it is not the only one, for partially purified G-6-PDH preparations could not replace the extract. A medium giving exceptionally heavy growth of African trypanosomes contained in Hanks' solution 0.5% lactalbumin hydro-lysate, 10% by volume calf serum and 15% by volume of a 3% haemoglobin solution (Jadin & LeRay 1969a).

In general one may predict that the invertebrate stages of pathogenic trypan-osomes and leishmanias have at least the following nutritional requirements:

at least ten but often more amino acids, depending in part on other constituents of the medium; a mixture of inorganic nutrients; haemin; a purine; thiamin, riboflavin, pantothenic acid, nicotinamide, pyridoxamine, biotin, folic acid and biopterin. They may also turn out to have specific lipid requirements. Thus one strain of *T. cruzi* could be grown in a Bactotryptone medium only if this was supplemented with stearate (Boné & Parent 1963). Other strains however did not grow even with stearate. It is of interest in this connection to mention the favourable effect of stearate on the intraerythrocytic development of the malaria parasite *Plasmodium knowlesi* in a medium free from plasma (Siddiqui *et al.* 1967).

It is very encouraging that Cross (1973) has recently reported development of a newly defined medium for culture forms of *T. brucei* strains, including one of *T. rhodesiense*. Cross first obtained multiplication in a medium consisting of tissue culture Medium 199 plus (in mg/ml): haemin 10, adenine 20, adenosine 20, guanine 20, guanosine 20, L-methionine 20, folic acid 10, EDTA 80, glucose 2000, acid hydrolysate of casein (Oxoid) 5000, and a linoleic acid–bovine serum albumin complex. The pH had to be carefully maintained between 7.2 and 7.4 by the use of HEPES buffer (N-2-hydroxyethylpiperazine-N'-2 2-ethane sulphonic acid). Growth was improved by the further addition of D(+)-glucosamine-HCl (216), L-proline (576), sodium acetate (544), succinate (272), citrate (588) and bicarbonate (800 mg/l) with phosphate at 10 mM. It will be of the greatest interest to see whether such a medium will also support *T. cruzi* or *Leishmania donovani*. If it does, and particularly if it permits development of infective stages of *T. brucei*, we shall be in a position to analyse fully the environmental factors controlling the developmental cycle in the invertebrate vector. There will still remain a large area of ignorance—the vertebrate stages, none of which has yet with any certainty been grown apart from a living host or host cell. Such development of the vertebrate stages as has been obtained *in vitro* can conveniently be discussed in relation to studies on factors affecting morphogenesis.

MORPHOGENESIS IN PATHOGENIC TRYPANOSOMATIDAE

The morphogenetic changes occurring in the life cycle of haemoflagellates are analogous to cellular differentiation in metazoa. The genome remains unchanged; only certain portions of it are activated or repressed in response to changes in either intracellular or extracellular factors. In considering these morphogenetic changes as they occur in nature and in relation to attempts to duplicate and control them *in vitro*, it will be convenient to treat separately each

of the three main types of trypanosomatids of pathogenic significance:
(*a*) *Leishmania donovani;* (*b*) *Trypanosoma cruzi;* (*c*) the salivarian trypanosomes.

(*a*) *Leishmania donovani*

This parasite has two main forms, an intracellular amastigote in macrophages
of the spleen and other organs of the mammalian host and a promastigote form
found in the phlebotomine vector. The amastigote form can be propagated
indefinitely in tissue cultures of a dog sarcoma line (Lamy *et al.* 1964; Frothingham & Lehtimoki 1969). When infected cell cultures were grown at 36 °C only
intracellular amastigotes were present and the parasites multiplied as such
within the host cells.

The promastigotes are easily maintained in continuous culture at temperatures of 23–30 °C in any of various media containing vertebrate blood. Constituents of both cells and serum are essential. A convenient monophasic
medium giving large populations has been recently described (Dwyer 1972).

The transformation from amastigote to promastigote is readily obtained *in
vitro*. It suffices to disrupt infected cells, as by grinding the spleen of an infected
hamster, and to suspend the amastigotes in an appropriate medium at about
28 °C. The cells increase in size, become more elongate, and the flagellum
grows out. These changes, visible by light microscopy, are complete in about
a day. By electron microscopy significant changes are evident after only 5 h:
the kinetoplast–mitochondrion is enlarged and the two nucleoli characteristic
of the amastigote fuse into one (Rudzinska *et al.* 1963). By this time also an
increase in oxygen uptake per cell begins, in keeping with the increased
mitochondrial material (Simpson 1968*b*).

For transformation to occur the medium must contain an energy source and
at least certain combinations of amino acids (Table 3). In considering these
results we have to remember that the experiments were done with organisms
prepared from a spleen suspension, so that despite extensive washing there
would probably be some carry-over of materials from the spleen. Such
materials could include additional factors essential to the transformation.

The reverse transformation, from promastigote to amastigote, can be observed if cells in tissue culture are exposed to promastigotes. Upon entry into
a suitable host cell the promastigote may change to an amastigote; it then
multiplies as such intracellularly. The change occurs even at a temperature
of 25 °C (Lamy 1970). However, at 33 °C or below extracellular promastigotes
are also present, whereas at 36 °C there are only intracellular amastigotes
(Frothingham & Lehtimoki 1969).

TABLE 3

Effects of amino acids on amastigote–promastigote transformation of *L. donovani* (data from Simpson 1968*b*)

Exp.	Medium[a]	% transformation of control
A	SBG + 17 amino acids (control)	100
	SBG	4
	SBG + glutamic acid	12
	SBG + aspartic acid	15
	SBG + lysine	10
	SBG + arginine	10
	SBG + histidine	19
B	SBG + 17 amino acids (control)	100
	SBG + aspartic acid + glutamic acid	75
	SBG + lysine + histidine + arginine	70

[a] SBG = 0.15 M-NaCl, 0.02 M-phosphate buffer pH 7.9, 0.02 M-glucose. Amino acids were used at the concentrations at which they occur in Medium C for *L. tarentolae*. (See Trager 1968.)

Hence, though temperature alone does not determine the form, it ordinarily restricts the growth of promastigotes. Either promastigotes or extracellular amastigotes soon die if placed abruptly at 38 or 37 °C, unless the medium contains living cells or special ingredients (Trager 1953). Cultures may be adapted to growth at higher temperatures in cell-free media (Lemma & Schiller 1964; Wonde & Honigberg 1971). Even so, for vigorous growth with retention of infectivity it is essential to supplement the medium with 5 or 10 % by volume of a chick embryo extract. Very significant is the fact that at all temperatures, including 37 °C, such cultures consisted mostly of active promastigotes (Wonde & Honigberg 1971). Furthermore, when such lines adapted to growth as promastigotes at 37 °C were passed through hamsters and then recovered in culture they were capable from the start of growth at 37 °C. Clearly a process of selection had occurred for a strain genetically endowed with ability to grow *in vitro* at 37 °C as promastigotes.

This is a different situation from that occurring when promastigotes infect host cells and, with a genetic endowment permitting promastigote growth only at lower temperatures, are nevertheless then able to multiply at the higher temperature as intracellular amastigotes. The living cell must provide factors that enable the parasites to withstand the otherwise lethal effect of the higher temperature.

Since promastigotes of *Leishmania* will grow in an aflagellate form when placed in suboptimal conditions (as shown for *L. tarentolae* grown with limiting concentrations of certain vitamins), it is important to have more than morphological criteria with which to define the intracellular amastigote form. Ability to grow at 37 °C without prior adaptation would be one such criterion, but perhaps the best criteria will be antigenic characterization of the two forms. That they differ was first noted by D'Alesandro (1954) and confirmed by Simpson (1968*b*). D. M. Dwyer (unpublished) is now carrying out a detailed analysis of antigens separated by disc electrophoresis. It is clear that the promastigote and amastigote forms of *L. donovani* have certain common antigens, as one would expect, but also numerous stage-specific antigens.

We have already alluded to the plasticity of form of haemoflagellates in culture. *L. donovani* shows obvious differences in form in different media and at different times during the cycle of growth in a culture tube. These have never been correlated with infectivity, though it was clear from Stauber's work (1955) that in an average culture of promastigotes only 10 % as many organisms were infective to hamsters as in a suspension of amastigotes. In keeping with this are observations by electron microscopy on the fate of promastigotes of *L. donovani* placed with hamster macrophages and incubated at 37 °C (Akiyama & McQuillen 1972). It was noted that many of the promastigotes were ingested by the macrophages into food vacuoles and digested. Only a small proportion established themselves in a viable state within the macrophage. Possibly only these were competent to initiate infection. Recent work by J. Keithly (unpublished) shows that the infectivity of cultures of *L. donovani*, in proportion to number of organisms, is low during the exponential phase of growth but reaches a peak at the start of the plateau phase. This is correlated with the presence of long slender forms.

(b) *Trypanosoma cruzi*

The complex developmental cycles of this important parasite have been well summarized in diagrams by Petana (1972). Both cycles, in the bug and in the mammal, include the same series of forms. When a reduviid bug takes blood from a host in which bloodstream trypomastigotes of *T. cruzi* are circulating these forms become rounded, lose their external flagellum and undergo in the gut of the insect a multiplicative phase as amastigotes. Intermediate spherical forms with a short flagellum have been called sphaeromastigotes by Brack (1968). The amastigote phase is followed by another multiplicative phase as epimastigotes, characterized by a kinetoplast just anterior to the nucleus. Finally the epimastigotes transform either directly or via sphaeromastigotes

(Brack 1968) into metacyclic trypomastigotes resembling bloodstream forms, though smaller. These forms probably do not multiply. They are excreted in faecal droplets and are infective through minute abrasions in the skin of a host animal. In this new host the trypomastigotes enter cells of various types, including those of the heart and other muscles. They become amastigotes and multiply intracellularly in this form. As cells become filled with the parasites, the amastigotes transform to epimastigotes and then to trypomastigotes, which break out of the cell. As bloodstream trypomastigotes these can either infect other cells or serve for infection of a vector. Like the metacyclic forms in the bug they do not multiply. This cycle of intracellular development can be easily reproduced in cell culture, as first shown by Meyer (1942) and later elaborated by others (Neva *et al.* 1961). In ordinary culture media at 28 °C morphologically similar forms are obtained. These dividing amastigotes probably represent amastigotes corresponding to those in the vector, since they do not survive at 37 °C. The majority of organisms grow as epimastigotes, which again cannot survive at 37 °C and are not infective to the mammalian host. Usually only a small proportion of infective metatrypomastigotes are seen in the typical cultures in blood-containing media.

Several new types of culture media, however, have not only given large yields of trypomastigotes but have also provided some measure of control over the various forms. Wood & Pipkin (1969) found that Grace's insect tissue culture medium (see Hink 1972) supplemented with 10% fetal bovine serum and 0.5% moth pupal haemolymph, supported a developmental cycle (at 28 °C) very similar to that in the vector bug. If this medium was inoculated with bloodstream trypomastigotes (6000 in 5 ml) these became amastigotes in 48–72 h and multiplied actively to give rise to large masses of adherent amastigotes. These then began to change to epimastigotes until by about five days this form predominated. The epimastigotes likewise multiplied actively to reach a peak population of about 40×10^6/ml at 14 days. On the tenth day there were about 10% trypomastigotes; their proportion rose rapidly to a maximum of 75% on the 16th day. If the medium contained 20% fetal bovine serum rather than 10%, growth was the same but very few trypomastigotes ever developed. Changes in pH in these cultures were not followed; they would be of interest in view of the observation of Fernandes *et al.* (1969) that in a heart infusion–lactalbumin hydrolysate medium an initial pH of 6.7 fell to 5.6 during the cycle of growth of epimastigotes, and in such cultures 80% of the organisms changed into trypomastigotes. In the same medium adjusted to an initial pH of 7.2 the growth of the epimastigotes was the same but the pH did not go below 6.3 and no differentiation occurred.

Whereas the studies just discussed were concerned with duplicating the devel-

TABLE 4

Growth of *Trypanosoma cruzi* in two different media at two different temperatures: series of 10 subcultures begun with an inoculum of epimastigotes grown in Medium F-29 at 29.5 °C and passed every fourth day (data from Pan 1971)

Temp. of incubation	Average figures for 6th to 10th subcultures at 96 h					
	In Medium F-29 (10% bovine fetal serum)			In Medium F-32 (5% bovine fetal serum, 5% chicken plasma)		
	Increase	% epimastigotes	% amastigotes	Increase	% epimastigotes	% amastigotes
29.5 °C	6 ×	97	1[a]	5 ×	0	99[a]
35.5 °C	6 ×	0	94[a]	6 ×	0	95[a]

[a] Remainder chiefly promastigotes.

opmental cycle in the vector, with special reference to the morphogenesis of infective trypomastigotes, Pan (1971) has attempted duplication of the vertebrate cycle in cell-free media. He has used ability to grow at 35.5 °C as a distinguishing characteristic since, as already noted, the same morphological types occur in both the vertebrate and invertebrate cycles. Two media were prepared, both with the same base: tissue culture Medium 199 (10 × concentrate) 10 ml; 0.8% glucose 25 ml; 5% aqueous trypticase solution 10 ml; 2.8% $NaHCO_3$ solution 1.5 ml; distilled water 53.5 ml. The first modification (F-29) contained 85 ml of the base, 10 ml heat-inactivated bovine fetal serum, and 5 ml haemin solution (0.5 mg/ml in 0.04% NaOH, sterilized by filtration). The second (F-32) contained 85 ml of the base, 5 ml inactivated bovine fetal serum, 5 ml of the haemin solution, and 5 ml freshly prepared chicken plasma. Each medium was tested at two temperatures, 29.5 and 35.5 °C, giving four series of cultures inoculated from an initial culture in F-29 at 29.5 °C and maintained through ten subcultures. The results (Table 4) showed a clear morphogenetic effect of temperature when the organisms were grown in F-29. Whereas nearly all were epimastigotes at 29.5 °C, at 35.5 °C amastigotes predominated already in the second subculture and by the sixth over 90% were in this form. The rate of multiplication was the same at both temperatures. The result in F-32 was quite different. The initial subculture at 29.5 °C showed mostly epimastigotes but with a transient phase with abundant trypomastigotes. In all subsequent subcultures at both temperatures virtually all the organisms were amastigotes. The chicken plasma here seems to exert a morphogenetic effect independent of temperature.

Space does not permit any discussion of much significant work done on cultivation and morphogenesis of other stercorarian trypanosomes and of trypanosomes parasitic in vertebrates other than mammals. Cultures of such trypanosomes usually duplicate the entire cycle of the invertebrate vector. With a few exceptions, however, as in *T. mega* (Steinert 1958), *T. avium* (Baker 1966), *T. lewisi* (D'Alesandro 1962; Dougherty *et al.* 1972), *T. theileri* (Splitter & Soulsby 1967) and *T. conorhini* (Deane & Kirchner 1963; Desowitz 1963), bloodstream forms have not been obtained in culture.

(c) The salivarian trypanosomes

These organisms, of the subgenera *Duttonella*, *Nannomonas*, *Trypanozoon* and *Pycnomonas* (Hoare 1972), show a situation still more interesting than that of *T. cruzi*. Not only has it so far been impossible to get continuous cultures of the bloodstream forms (although they can be passaged continuously in animals by syringe), but in addition it has been difficult to duplicate *in vitro* the complete cycle occurring in the vector insect, so that cultures have in general been non-infective (Thomson & Sinton 1912).

Trypanosoma (Duttonella) vivax is considered by Hoare to represent the most primitive of the salivarian trypanosomes. It gives the highest percentage of infection in appropriate species of *Glossina* and its entire invertebrate developmental cycle occurs in the proboscis of the fly. Here it multiplies as epimastigotes that later transform to infective trypomastigotes. Bloodstream forms of *T. vivax* ingested into the gut of the fly die off after a few days. It is therefore not surprising that cultures of *T. vivax* usually cannot be started on blood agar media, since these represent an approximation to conditions in a fly gut soon after ingestion of a blood meal. Cultures of *T. vivax*, however, were initiated in an insect tissue culture medium in the presence of living tissues of *Glossina palpalis* (Trager 1959). It was essential to start the cultures with bloodstream forms from a sheep with a long-standing chronic infection and to incubate them at 30–32 °C. Thus the change from blood trypomastigote to epimastigote and the multiplication of the latter depended not only on a medium with factors from living insect tissue but also on temperature and, perhaps most interesting, on the vertebrate host from which the inoculum was derived. In the *Glossina* tissue culture *T. vivax* showed all its developmental stages including metatrypomastigotes. Two cultures that survived exposure for 19 h to 38 °C were infective to sheep. Cultures established in fly tissue culture were successfully subcultured on Tobie's medium. Jadin & Wery (1963) also make passing mention of a strain of *T. vivax* maintained in culture.

In the next more advanced group of the Salivaria, represented by *T. (Nan-nomonas) congolense*, the developmental cycle in tsetse flies begins in the midgut. Here we find for the first time a multiplicative phase as trypomastigotes in the insect host. It is worth emphasizing, in view of some confusion in the recent literature, that midgut forms of *T. congolense* (as well as of *T. brucei*) are not epimastigotes. They are trypomastigotes, since the kinetoplast is clearly posterior to the nucleus. But they differ from bloodstream trypomastigotes in being larger and more elongate, and in having the kinetoplast about midway between the centrally located nucleus and the posterior end of the body, rather than at the posterior tip. They also differ in their much more extensive mitochondrial development accompanied by an active respiratory metabolism (Newton 1968; Vickerman 1971). Since these midgut or culture trypomastigotes have been more widely used for experimental purposes than any other form of trypanosome it would be convenient to have a special term for them. I suggest *midmastigote*, connoting both their normal presence in the midgut of the tsetse and the position of the kinetoplast midway between nucleus and posterior end. As with *T. vivax*, the ability of *T. congolense* to grow in culture is influenced by the vertebrate host from which the cultures are inoculated (Yesufu 1970). Of six strains infective for rats, mice, rabbits, sheep, goats and dogs, five grew when isolated in culture from rats or rabbits, only three from mice or dogs, two from sheep, and one from goats. These results bore no relation to the severity of infection in the host or to the species of blood used in the blood agar–yeast extract medium. Cultures of *T. congolense* contain only midmastigotes. They lack the epimastigote forms that multiply in the food canal of the fly and that then transform to infective metatrypomastigotes. Accordingly, they are not infective to mammalian hosts. Indeed Tobie (1958) noted loss of infectivity after only one day *in vitro* at 25 °C.

We come now to consideration of the *T. (Trypanozoon) brucei* group, fascinating for its complex developmental physiology and its intricate ecological relationships. In the mammalian host multiplication occurs as slender trypomastigotes, with the stumpy forms probably representing a phase preadapted for initiation of the cycle in *Glossina* (Hoare 1972). There may also be an occult visceral amastigote phase (Ormerod & Venkatesan 1971). Although it is now clear that immunological factors are not responsible for appearance of the stumpy forms (see Balber 1972), we do not know what is responsible. Generally the stumpy forms are more infective to *Glossina* (see Hoare 1972, p. 481) and they also more readily establish themselves as cultures in the usual blood–agar media.

As for *T. congolense*, such cultures typically contain elongate midmastigotes corresponding to the first multiplicative phase in the midgut of the tsetse fly. It is noteworthy that *T. brucei* does not readily infect any species of tsetse fly, though here again this may depend on the vertebrate host (Corson 1936). Usually, in the best conditions about 20 to 30% will develop gut infections and perhaps half of these will then show infection in the salivary glands, male flies being more suitable for this than female (Harley 1971). Since there is some parallelism between establishment in culture and in the midgut of the vector, studies on the former might help to disclose conditions affecting the latter. A. E. Balber (unpublished) has found that the transformation of slender forms of *T. brucei* into culture forms and their subsequent growth was particularly sensitive to inhibition by glucose. Glucose was inhibitory at 16 mM and even at only 2.5 mM. These findings emphasize the somewhat anomalous situation that most media used for cultivation of trypanosomes are based on vertebrate blood, yet the stages actually grown are those in the insect host. For these glucose may be not only inessential but actually inhibitory, especially at high concentrations. In view of the special role of proline in the nutrition of promastigotes of *L. tarentolae*, and since proline is an important metabolite in insects (Sacktor & Childress 1967), it might make sense to get away from glucose in media designed for the insect stages and to substitute proline and perhaps glutamic acid as energy sources. In support of such a move is the recent finding that culture forms of *T. rhodesiense* show a higher rate of oxidation of proline than of any other substrate tried (Srivastava & Bowman 1971; Bowman *et al.* 1972). Moreover, Harton (1972) has reported that small morphological differences between culture and midgut forms of *T. brucei* disappear if the cultures are grown in a proline-enriched medium. The non-essentiality of carbohydrate has already been shown not only for promastigotes of *L. tarentolae* (see above, p. 227) but also for *Crithidia fasciculata* (Tamburro & Hutner 1971).

A change in temperature has always been considered as one of the factors initiating morphogenesis; in haemoflagellate parasites of warm-blooded hosts lowering the temperature from that of the vertebrate host to about 28°C would initiate change to the insect stage. Even this firm pillar of our knowledge has now been undermined. Honigberg & Gabre (1972) have just reported that a strain of *T. rhodesiense* not only grew well at 37°C in Tobie's medium + 10% (by volume) chick embryo extract + 2% β-glycerophosphate, but cultures could be initiated from bloodstream forms at 37°C in this supplemented medium. Most disappointing was the fact that these cultures again consisted only of midmastigotes. They were not infective. Indeed, bloodstream forms inoculated to the medium and incubated at 37°C transformed to midmastigotes and lost their infectivity even faster than at 28°C.

Forms resembling metatrypomastigotes do, however, appear when *T. brucei* is grown at 24°C or 28°C in Weinman's medium, and infective cultures are obtained sporadically (Weinman 1960; Geigy & Kauffmann 1964). Weinman's medium consists of three parts of nutrient agar with one part reconstituted human blood. The latter is prepared from saline-washed red cells resuspended in their original citrated plasma after this has been treated for 30 min at 56 °C and cooled. The agar slants are inoculated with blood drawn into polyvinyl sulphuric acid as anticoagulant. Amrein et al. (1965) noted that in these conditions occasional cultures incubated at 24 °C were infective to mice after 18 days but not before. Results were not reproducible and the individual blood donor played a major role. Amrein & Hanneman (1969) then tried substituting blood from animals of different species for human blood. They again found a low percentage of cultures infective after 17–18 days. The best results were obtained with cattle blood, but the individual blood donor was far more important than the species. Further work is needed for clarification of this situation.

If the full tsetse cycle of T. brucei could be duplicated in vitro, with multiplication of epimastigotes as well as midmastigotes and with formation of metatrypomastigotes, there would still remain the problem of continuous culture of the bloodstream forms. Initial growth of these forms at 37 °C was obtained by Le Page (1967) in tissue cultures of mouse L cells. The L cells were allowed to form a monolayer in a medium of NCTC-109 with 10% presucking calf serum before inoculation of blood trypanosomes at a level of $2–6 \times 10^5$/ml medium. The trypanosomes multiplied about fivefold in 24 h but subcultures were unsuccessful. Without the L cells there was no growth (see also Hawking 1971). Equivalent initial multiplication of T. brucei at 37 °C for a 24 h period has been obtained with merely 1% whole mouse blood in NCTC-109 plus 10% fetal bovine serum (Chaloner 1972).

Since bloodstream forms live and multiply in the plasma, it could well be that labile constituents of this complex fluid, perhaps lipoproteins, are essential for them. That they can ingest both particulate fat (Wotten & Halsey 1957) and protein has been demonstrated. T. rhodesiense and T. brucei bloodstream forms ingest protein by pinocytosis from the flagellar reservoir (Brown et al. 1965; Geigy et al. 1970). Culture forms of other species, such as T. raiae (Preston 1969), T. mega (Steinert & Novikoff 1960) and C. fasciculata (Brooker 1971), have in addition a cytostome or cytopharynx from which endocytic vesicles containing ingested protein are formed. In keeping with this mechanism of ingestion of protein is the localization of digestive enzymes (as indicated by acid phosphatase) in the same cellular regions (Seed et al. 1967; Brooker 1971). The uptake of exogenous sterols by haemoflagellates has also been demonstrated experimentally; the blood forms of T. rhodesiense cannot synthesize sterols and they depend on the cholesterol of their habitat (Dixon et al. 1972). It is of interest that the culture forms of *T. rhodesiense*, in which the mitochondrial membranes are much more extensive, are capable of sterol biosynthesis, the principal sterol being then ergosterol. Perhaps application of these newly discovered relationships may facilitate development of a culture medium for the bloodstream trypomastigotes of the salivarian group.

SEX IN TRYPANOSOMATIDS?

I am tempted to put several question marks after this heading. The Trypanosomatidae are the only large group of protozoa in which sex has never been demonstrated. Recently, however, phenomena have been described that could be connected in some way with interchange of genetic material. Deane & Milder (1972) have analysed the fine structure of the 'cyst-like bodies' previously noted by them in cultures of *T. conorhini* and resembling structures seen by Iralu (1964) and years earlier by Muniz (1927) in cultures of *T. cruzi*, and also noted in cultures of *T. brucei* by Jadin & LeRay (1969b). Seven-day cultures of *T. conorhini* in LIT medium (liver infusion, tryptose, salts, dextrose, haemoglobin solution and calf serum) frequently show hollow spheres that seem to consist of a number of fused flagellates surrounding a fluid-filled space. Sometimes flagellates may be seen within the space. Electron microscopy shows narrow cytoplasmic bridges between epimastigotes. The hollow space results from fused and much-enlarged flagellar pockets of the associated organisms. Some flagellates are multinucleate and have several kinetoplasts. Deane and Milder believe these cyst-like bodies are formed by fusion of a number of organisms. The same interpretation is applied by Brener (1972) to similar structures seen by him in the gut of *Triatoma infestans* infected three or four days previously with *T. cruzi*. By light microscopy amastigotes were seen apparently fused in pairs or in much larger clusters. All had an unusually large flagellar reservoir and the large masses seemed to have a clear hollow centre resembling the cyst-like bodies of *T. conorhini*. For both *T. cruzi* and, especially, *T. conorhini* individual organisms appear to bud off from the mass, either from the outer surface or into the hollow interior. Electron microscope observations on *T. conorhini* showing several nuclei and kinetoplasts within the same cytoplasmic mass could be interpreted to indicate that a nucleus from one cell might later bud off with a kinetoplast from another, permitting at least this type of genetic interchange. There is, however, no proof that these masses arise from fusion. They could equally well result from incomplete division. The phenomenon undoubtedly deserves intensive further study.

References

AKIYAMA, H. J. & McQUILLEN, N. K. (1972) Interaction and transformation of *Leishmania donovani* within *in vitro* cultured cells. An electron microscopical study. *Am. J. Trop. Med. Hyg.* **21**, 873-879

AMREIN, Y. U. & HANNEMAN, R. B. (1969) Suitable blood sources permitting reacquisition of infectivity by culture-form *Trypanosoma (Trypanozoon) brucei. Acta Trop.* **26**, 70-75

AMREIN, Y. U., GEIGY, R. & KAUFFMANN, M. (1965) On the reacquisition of virulence in trypanosomes of the Brucei-group. *Acta Trop.* **22**, 193-203

BAKER, J. R. (1966) Studies on *Trypanosoma avium.* IV: The development of infective meta-cyclic trypanosomes in cultures grown *in vitro. Parasitology* **56**, 15-19

BALBER, A. E. (1972) *Trypanosoma brucei:* Fluxes of the morphological variants in intact and X-irradiated mice. *Exp. Parasitol.* **31**, 307-319

BISHOP, A. (1967) Problems in the cultivation of some parasitic protozoa, in *Advances in Parasitology* (Dawes, B., ed.), pp. 93-138, Academic Press, London & New York

BLAKELEY, R. L. (1969) *The Biochemistry of Folic Acid and Related Pteridines*, North-Holland, Amsterdam

BONÉ, G. J. & PARENT, G. (1963) Stearic acid, an essential growth factor for *Trypanosoma cruzi. J. Gen. Microbiol.* **31**, 261-266

BOWMAN, I. B. R., SRIVASTAVA, H. K. & FLYNN, I. W. (1972) Adaptations in oxidative metab-olism during the transformation of *Trypanosoma rhodesiense* from bloodstream into culture form, in *Comparative Biochemistry of Parasites* (Van den Bossche, H., ed), pp. 329-342, Academic Press, New York

BRACK, C. (1968) Elektronenmikroskopische Untersuchungen zum Lebenszyklus von *Try-panosoma cruzi. Acta Trop.* **25**, 289-356

BRENER, Z. (1972) A new aspect of *Trypanosoma cruzi* life-cycle in the invertebrate host. *J. Protozool.* **19**, 23-27

BROOKER, R. E. (1971) The fine structure of *Crithidia fasciculata* with special reference to the organelles involved in the ingestion and digestion of protein. *Z. Zellforsch. Mikrosk. Anat.* **116**, 532-563

BROWN, K. N., ARMSTRONG, J. A. & VALENTINE, R. C. (1965) The ingestion of protein mole-cules by blood forms of *Trypanosoma rhodesiense. Exp. Cell Res.* **39**, 129-135

CHALONER, L. A. (1972) Multiplication of bloodstream forms of *Trypanosoma brucei in vitro* at 37° in the presence of mouse blood. *Trans R. Soc. Trop. Med. Hyg.* **66**, 527

CITRI, M. & GROSSOWICZ, N. (1955) A partially defined culture medium for *Trypanosoma cruzi* and some other haemoflagellates. *J. Gen. Microbiol.* **13**, 273-278

CORSON, J. F. (1936) A second note on a high rate of infection of the salivary glands of *Glossina morsitans* after feeding on a reedbuck infected with *Trypanosoma rhodesiense. Trans. R. Soc. Trop. Med. Hyg.* **30**, 207-212

COSGROVE, W. B. (1971) The cell cycle and cell differentiation in Trypanosomatids, in *Develop-mental Aspects of the Cell Cycle* (Cameron, I. L., Padilla, G. M. & Zimmerman, A. M., eds.), pp. 1-21, Academic Press, New York

CROSS, G. A. M. (1973) Development of defined media for growth of *Trypanosoma brucei* spp. *Trans. R. Soc. Trop. Med. Hyg.* **67**, 255-256

DA CRUZ, F. S. & KRASSNER, S. M. (1971) Assimilatory sulfate reduction by the hemo-flagellate *Leishmania tarentolae. J. Protozool.* **18**, 718-722

D'ALESANDRO, P. A. (1954) A serological comparison of the leishmaniform and the lepto-monad stages of *Leishmania donovani.* Thesis, Rutgers University Graduate School

D'ALESANDRO, P. A. (1962) *In vitro* studies of ablastin, the reproduction-inhibiting antibody to *Trypanosoma lewisi. J. Protozool.* **9**, 351-358

DEANE, M. P. & KIRCHNER, E. (1963) Life cycle of *Trypanosoma conorhini.* Influence of temperature and other factors on growth and morphogenesis. *J. Protozool.* **10**, 391-400

DEANE, M. P. & MILDER, R. (1972) Ultrastructure of the 'cyst-like bodies' of *Trypanosoma conorhini*. *J. Protozool.* **19**, 28-42

DESOWITZ, R. S. (1963) The development and survival of the bloodstream forms of *Trypanosoma conorhini* in culture. *J. Protozool.* **10**, 390-391

DIXON, H., GINGER, C. D. & WILLIAMSON, J. (1972) Trypanosome sterols and their metabolic origin. *Comp. Biochem. Physiol.* **41B**, 1-18

DOUGHERTY, J., RABSON, A. S. & TYRRELL, S. A. (1972) *Trypanosoma lewisi: in vitro* growth in mammalian cell culture media. *Exp. Parasitol.* **31**, 225-231

DWYER, D. M. (1972) A monophasic medium for cultivating *Leishmania donovani* in large numbers. *J. Parasitol.* **58**, 847-848

FERNANDES, J. F., CASTELLANI, O. & KIMURA, E. (1969) Physiological events in the course of the growth and differentiation of *Trypanosoma cruzi*. *Genetics* (suppl.) **61**, 213-226

FROMENTIN, H. (1971) Contribution à l'étude comparée des besoins nutritifs chez diverses espèces du genre *Trypanosoma*. *Ann. Parasitol. Hum. Comp.* **46**, 337-445

FROTHINGHAM, T. E. & LEHTIMOKI, E. (1969) Prolonged growth of *Leishmania* species in cell culture. *J. Parasitol.* **55**, 196-199

GAUGHAN, P. L. Z. & KRASSNER, S. M. (1971) Hemin deprivation in culture stages of the hemoflagellate *Leishmania tarentolae*. *Comp. Biochem. Physiol.* **39B**, 5-18

GEIGY, R. & KAUFFMANN, M. (1964) On the effect of substances found in *Glossina* tissues on culture trypanosomes of the *brucei*-subgroup. *Acta Trop.* **21**, 169-173

GEIGY, R., STEIGER, R. & HECKER, H. (1970) Beiträge zur Pinocytose von *Trypanosoma (Trypanozoon) brucei*, Plimmer & Bradfort, 1899. *Acta Trop.* **27**, 271-277

GUTTMAN, H. N. (1963) Experimental glimpses at the lower Trypanosomatidae. *Exp. Parasitol.* **13**, 129-142

GUTTMAN, H. N. (1969) Assays for unconjugated pteridines, in *Analytical Microbiology* (Kavanaugh, F., ed.), vol. 2, pp. 527-550, Academic Press, New York

GUTTMAN, H. N. & WALLACE, F. G. (1964) in *Biochemistry and Physiology of Protozoa* (Hutner, S. H., ed.), pp. 459-494, Academic Press, New York

HARLEY, J. M. B. (1971) Comparison of the susceptibility to infection with *Trypanosoma rhodesiense* of *Glossina pallidipes*, *G. morsitans*, *G. fuscipes* and *G. brevipalpis*. *Ann. Trop. Med. Parasitol.* **65**, 185-189

HARTON, W. S. (1972) Development of *Trypanosoma brucei* in the gut of *Glossina morsitans*. *Trans. R. Soc. Trop. Med. Hyg.* **66**, 548

HAWKING, F. (1971) The propagation and survival of *Trypanosoma brucei* in vitro at 37 °C. *Trans. R. Soc. Trop. Med. Hyg.* **65**, 672-675

HINK, W. F. (1972) A catalog of invertebrate cell lines, in *Invertebrate Tissue Culture* (Vago, C., ed.), vol. 2, pp. 363-387, Academic Press, New York

HOARE, C. A. (1972) *The Trypanosomes of Mammals*, Blackwell Scientific Publications, Oxford

HONIGBERG, B. M. (1967) in *Chemical Zoology* (Florkin, M. & Scheer, B. T., eds.), vol. 1: *Protozoa* (Kidder, G. W., ed.), pp. 695-814, Academic Press, New York

HONIGBERG, B. M. & GABRE, B. (1972) Cultivation of *Trypanosoma rhodesiense* at 37°. *J. Protozool.* **19**, (suppl.), Abstr. no. 32

HUTNER, S. H. (1972) Inorganic nutrition. *Annu. Rev. Microbiol.* **26**, 313-346

IRALU, V. (1964) Production of *Trypanosoma cruzi* cysts *in vitro*. *Nature (Lond.)* **204**, 486-487

JADIN, J. & LeRAY, D. (1969a) Acquisitions récentes dans les techniques de culture des trypanosomes africains. *Ann. Soc. Belge Méd. Trop.* **49**, 331-340

JADIN, J. & LeRAY, D. (1969b) Présence des formes kystiques dans les cultures de *Trypanosoma brucei*. *Protistologica* **5**, 381-382

JADIN, J. & WERY, M. (1963) La culture des trypanosomidae. *Ann. Soc. Belge Méd. Trop.* **43**, 831-842

KIDDER, G. W. (1967) in *Chemical Zoology* (Florkin, M. & Scheer, B. T., eds.), vol. 1: *Protozoa* (Kidder, G. W., ed.), pp. 93-159, Academic Press, New York

KIDDER, G. W. & DEWEY, V. C. (1972) Methionine or folate and phosphenolpyruvate in the biosynthesis of threonine in *Crithidia fasciculata*. *J. Protozool.* **19**, 93-98

KIDDER, G. W. & DUTTA, B. M. (1958) The growth and nutrition of *Crithidia fasciculata*. *J. Gen. Microbiol.* **18**, 621-638

KRASSNER, S. M. (1969) Proline metabolism in *Leishmania tarentolae*. *Exp. Parasitol.* **24**, 348-363

KRASSNER, S. M. & FLORY, B. (1971) Essential amino acids in the culture of *Leishmania tarentolae*. *J. Parasitol.* **57**, 917-920

LAMY, L. H. (1970) Transformation intracellulaire des formes amastigotes de *Leishmania donovani* et *Trypanosoma cruzi* en formes mastigotes. *Protistologica* **6**, 457-466

LAMY, L., SAMSO, A. & LAMY, H. (1964) Installation, multiplication et entretien d'une souche de *Leishmania donovani* en culture cellulaire. *Bull. Soc. Pathol. Exot.* **57**, 16-21

LEMMA, A. & SCHILLER, E. L. (1964) Extracellular cultivation of the leishmanial bodies of species belonging to the protozoan genus *Leishmania*. *Exp. Parasitol.* **15**, 503-513

LE PAGE, R. W. F. (1967) Short term cultivation of *Trypanosoma brucei in vitro* at 37 °C. *Nature (Lond.)* **216**, 1141-1142

MEYER, H. (1942) Culturas de tecido nervoso infectados por *Schizotrypanum cruzi*. *An. Acad. Bras. Cienc.* **14**, 253-255

MUNIZ, J. (1927) Quelques formes intéressantes trouvées dans des cultures de *Trypanosoma cruzi*. *C. R. Séances Soc. Biol. Fil.* **97**, 831-833

NEVA, F. A., MALONE, M. F. & MYERS, B. R. (1961) Factors influencing the intracellular growth of *Trypanosoma cruzi in vitro*. *Am. J. Trop. Med. Hyg.* **10**, 140-154

NEWTON, B. A. (1968) Biochemical peculiarities of trypanosomatid flagellates. *Annu. Rev. Microbiol.* **22**, 109-130

ORMEROD, W. E. & VENKATESAN, S. (1971) The occult visceral phase of mammalian trypanosomes with special reference to the life cycle of *Trypanosoma (Trypanozoon) brucei*. *Trans. R. Soc. Trop. Med. Hyg.* **65**, 722-735

PAN, C-T. (1971) Cultivation and morphogenesis of *Trypanosoma cruzi* in improved liquid media. *J. Protozool.* **18**, 556-560

PETANA, W. B. (1972) A revision of *Trypanosoma (Schizotrypanum) cruzi* strains from British Honduras, and the importance of strain characteristics in experimental chemotherapy of Chagas' disease. *Trans. R. Soc. Trop. Med. Hyg.* **66**, 463-470

PRESTON, T. M. (1969) The form and function of the cytostome-cytopharynx of the culture forms of the elasmobranch hemoflagellate *Trypanosoma raiae* Laveran and Mesnil. *J. Protozool.* **16**, 320-333

RUDZINSKA, M. A., TRAGER, W. & D'ALESANDRO, P. A. (1963) The fine structure of *Leishmania donovani* and the role of the kinetoplast in the leishmania-leptomonad transformation. *J. Protozool.* **11**, 166-191

SACKTOR, B. & CHILDRESS, C. C. (1967) Metabolism of proline in insect flight muscle and its significance in stimulating the oxidation of pyruvate. *Arch. Biochem. Biophys.* **120**, 583-588

SEED, J. R., BYRAM, J. & GAM, A. A. (1967) Characterization and localization of acid phosphatase activity of *Trypanosoma gambiense*. *J. Protozool.* **14**, 117-125

SIDDIQUI, W. A., SCHNELL, J. V. & GEIMAN, Q. M. (1967) Stearic acid as plasma replacement for intracellular *in vitro* culture of *Plasmodium knowlesi*. *Science* **156**, 1623-1625

SIMPSON, L. (1968a) Effect of acriflavin on the kinetoplast of *Leishmania tarentolae*. Mode of action and physiological correlates of the loss of kinetoplast DNA. *J. Cell Biol.* **37**, 660-682

SIMPSON, L. (1968b) The leishmania-leptomonad transformation of *Leishmania donovani*: nutritional requirements, respiration changes and antigenic changes. *J. Protozool.* **15**, 201-207

SPLITTER, E. J. & SOULSBY, E. J. L. (1967) Isolation and continuous cultivation of *Trypanosoma theileri* in media containing tissue culture fluids. *Exp. Parasitol.* **21**, 137-148

SRIVASTAVA, H. K. & BOWMAN, I. B. R. (1971) Adaptation in oxidative metabolism of *Trypanosoma rhodesiense* during transformation in culture. *Comp. Biochem. Physiol.* **40B**, 973-981

STAUBER, L. A. (1955) Leishmaniasis in the hamster, in *Some Physiological Aspects and Consequences of Parasitism* (Cole, W. H., ed.), pp. 76-90, Rutgers University Press, New Brunswick, N.J.

STEINERT, M. (1958) Etudes sur la déterminisme de la morphogenèse d'un trypanosome. *Exp. Cell Res.* **15**, 560-569

STEINERT, M. & NOVIKOFF, A. B. (1960) The existence of a cytostome and the occurrence of pinocytosis in the trypanosome *Trypanosoma mega*. *J. Biophys. Biochem. Cytol.* **8**, 563-569

STRAUSS, P. R. (1972) Acriflavin resistance in the hemoflagellate, *Leishmania tarentolae*. *J. Cell Biol.* **53**, 312-334

TAMBURRO, K. M. & HUTNER, S. H. (1971) Carbohydrate-free media for *Crithidia*. *J. Protozool.* **18**, 667-672

THOMSON, J. G. & SINTON, J. A. (1912) The morphology of *Trypanosoma gambiense* and *Trypanosoma rhodesiense* in cultures: and a comparison with the developmental forms described in *Glossina palpalis*. *Ann. Trop. Med. Parasitol.* **6**, 331-359

TOBIE, E. J. (1958) The cultivation of *Trypanosoma congolense in vitro*. *J. Parasitol.* **44**, 241-242

TRAGER, W. (1953) The development of *Leishmania donovani in vitro* at 37°. Effects of the kind of serum. *J. Exp. Med.* **97**, 177-188

TRAGER, W. (1959) Tsetse fly tissue culture and the development of trypanosomes to the infective stage. *Ann. Trop. Med. Parasitol.* **53**, 473-491

TRAGER, W. (1968) in *Infectious Blood Diseases of Man and Animals* (Weinman, D. & Ristic, M., eds.), pp. 149-174, Academic Press, New York

TRAGER, W. (1969) Pteridine requirement of the hemoflagellate *Leishmania tarentolae*. *J. Protozool.* **16**, 372-375

TRAGER, W. (1970) Recent progress in some aspects of the physiology of parasitic protozoa. *J. Parasitol.* **56**, 627-633

VICKERMAN, K. (1971) Morphological and physiological considerations of extracellular blood protozoa, in *Ecology and Physiology of Parasites* (Fallis, A. M., ed.), pp. 58-89, University of Toronto Press, Toronto

WEINMAN, D. (1960) Cultivation of the African sleeping sickness trypanosomes from the blood and cerebrospinal fluid of patients and suspects. *Trans. R. Soc. Trop. Med. Hyg.* **54**, 180-190

WONDE, T. & HONIGBERG, B. M. (1971) Morphology and infectivity of *Leishmania donovani* cultivated in nonliving media at elevated temperatures. *Am. J. Trop. Med. Hyg.* **20**, 828-838

WOOD, D. T. & PIPKIN, A. C. (1969) Multiplication and differentiation of *Trypanosoma cruzi* in an insect cell culture system. *Exp. Parasitol.* **24**, 176-183

WOTTON, R. M. & HALSEY, H. R. (1957) The ingestion of particulate fat from the blood by *Trypanosoma lewisi* and *Trypanosoma equiperdum*. *Parasitology* **47**, 427-431

YESUFU, H. M. (1970) Influence of different vertebrate hosts on the ability of *Trypanosoma congolense* to grow in culture. *J. Comp. Pathol.* **80**, 1-7

ZELEDÓN, R. (1971) Cultivation and transformation of hemoflagellates. A review. *Rev. Biol. Trop.* **19**, 197-210

Discussion

Newton: The loss of infectivity of salivarian trypanosomes in culture is particularly interesting and I hope it will soon be possible to investigate this under defined conditions. The semi-defined medium used by G. A. M. Cross in my laboratory has given rise to infective forms of *T. brucei* after months of subculture. This medium no longer contains crude blood constituents so I think the idea that only certain blood types give rise to infective cells really doesn't stand up. It seems more likely that the critical (and as yet unknown) conditions required for the production of infective stages may develop in some cultures by chance, perhaps as a result of the metabolic activity of trypanosomes during their growth.

Trager: How long will the organisms grow in the defined medium? Does it allow continuous cultivation?

Newton: The medium at present being used by Cross allows continuous cultivation of *T. brucei* (strain S42) and this strain has now been maintained in the medium for about 15 weeks (30 subcultures). The medium is still being modified. It was semi-defined about 18 months ago; at that stage Cross was unable to replace a commercial casein digest preparation by an amino acid mixture, but later this was achieved by increasing the concentration of vitamins in the medium (Cross 1973).

Trager: Is the infectivity still unpredictable?

Newton: Yes, but on the other hand not every culture is put into mice to see whether infective organisms are there. A lot of work remains to be done.

Trager: As I said, I think this medium will really enable us to analyse the factors responsible for appearance of infectivity.

Baker: You suggested the term 'midmastigote' for the so-called midgut forms of *T. brucei*, Professor Trager. Dr Newton, Dr Cross and I (Newton *et al.* 1973) have called these forms 'procyclic' trypomastigotes, to contrast them with the metacyclic trypomastigotes that occur at the end of the cycle in the insect vector.

When people talk about infective cultures of *T. brucei*, they always carefully avoid any reference to the development of metacyclic trypomastigotes in them. In neither Amrein's nor Cross's infective cultures has anyone ever seen anything that looks like a metacyclic trypomastigote, but that may be because they are present only in very small numbers.

Trager: I think Weinman (1968) said he saw them.

Baker: There is no evidence that the process Brener (1972) described in the gut of bugs infected with *T. cruzi* was anything other than either fusion or degenerative agglomeration.

In Cambridge a strain of *T. cruzi* growing in ordinary liquid medium at 28 or 30 °C developed initially almost entirely as amastigotes, in great big clumps. In the electron microscope we could not see evidence of anything other than division, resulting in adherence of the organisms to each other (Baker & Price 1973).

Maria Deane (1969) has suggested that morphological differentiation into, say, bloodstream trypomastigotes or metacyclic trypomastigotes seems to be contrasted to division. In other words, a trypanosome growing in culture or anywhere else can either go on dividing or stop dividing and differentiate. At any stage of the trypanosome life cycle, Maria Deane rightly contrasts the division forms with the differentiated forms. In the *T. brucei* group this would be the long slender form versus the stumpy form in the vertebrate; in the invertebrate host it would be the procyclic trypomastigote versus the metacyclic trypomastigote. This concept that there is *either* division *or* differentiation seems useful. I think the same sort of thing occurs in mammalian cells to some extent.

Newton: This concept is also consistent with the observations of infectivity developing in culture, because I believe infective stages have only been observed in old stationary phase cultures in which cell division has ceased.

Trager: This is another way in which the situation is similar to cellular differentiation in metazoa. The embryologists think that in general a cell which is differentiating cannot at the same time be busy dividing, but this doesn't hold up of course. I think the same thing would probably be true with trypanosomes: in general differentiating forms would not be multiplying. But there would be exceptions.

Vickerman: You said that the Trypanosomatidae were the only protozoa without a sexual process, but aren't most flagellates and amoebae asexual?

Trager: One can find examples which have a sexual process. The trichomonads, at least those that are parasites of vertebrates, are not known to have any sexual phenomena; on the other hand the related polymastigote and hypermastigote flagellates of the wood-feeding roach *Cryptocercus*, as shown by Cleveland (1956), have a whole variety of sexual phenomena. Nothing has been found with *Entamoebae* or with soil amoebae, but nuclear fusion of one kind or another has been demonstrated in various other kinds of related amoebae.

Vickerman: But these are sporadic examples and their existence lends support to the idea that protozoa may all have had a sexual process at one time but many have given it up because it was not much use to them. Provided the fission rate is sufficiently high in a haploid organism, mutation should give sufficient variation for natural selection to act upon.

Trager: We should always remember the example of bacteria. Many years ago when some Russian workers claimed that they had found something indicating nuclear fusion in bacteria, everybody was rather scornful, but now nuclear interchange in *E. coli* has become one of the most powerful tools in genetics.

Vickerman: But isn't sex in bacteria largely a device put up by viruses for getting around?

Trager: Sex in *E. coli* is probably a good opportunity for nuclear interchange.

Vickerman: Prokaryotes just exchange part of the genome, whereas eukaryotes go in for recombination of whole genomes.

Trager: I don't think there is any evidence in the trypanosomes. Perhaps they are perfectly happy without sex. On the other hand we really should look for it during the insect cycle that Brener (1972) was working on.

Vickerman: One needs stable marker characters in trying to find genetic recombination.

Bowman: Sexual conjugation in the bloodstream forms of trypanosomes would probably help the immunologists who are trying to account for antigenic variation.

Baker: Everyone's desperate attempts to find a sex life for trypanosomes must arise out of sympathy for their deprivation. Fairbairn & Culwick (1946) years ago suggested that there was sexual combination in the bloodstream forms but no convincing evidence has ever been published. However sorry we feel for the poor beasts, maybe one has to accept that they are deprived.

Bowman: Fulton's work (1960) on attempted transformation of trypanosomes also failed.

Newton: Inoki & Matsushiro (1960) and Inoki *et al.* (1961) reported transformation of drug resistance in *T. gambiense* and *T. evansi* but I don't know of anyone who has confirmed these findings.

Trager: That was under a special set of conditions, and peculiar criteria were used.

Bowman: Did they try to account for this by conjugation or simple transformation?

Newton: By transformation. Cell lysates were used and the transforming activity of these was destroyed by treatment with DNase.

Peters: There was some negative evidence from Amrein (1965).

Martinez-Silva: It is an accepted dogma that the epimastigote stage of *T. cruzi* is non-infective for mammalian cells, but our evidence is contrary to this. We found (Martinez-Silva *et al.* 1970) that single epimastigotes from virulent strains of *T. cruzi* were able to infect cells in tissue culture and produce trypomastigotes of intracellular origin. Using fibroblasts in a perfusion chamber we observed penetration of cells by epimastigotes and the intracellular events that followed. In some cases the epimastigote becomes an amastigote, which divides by binary fission and fills up the cell; the parasites transform themselves into trypomastigotes and begin to move very actively, so disrupting the cell and liberating themselves into the medium, from whence they can invade new cells. In other cases the epimastigote is surrounded in the cell by a vacuole, moves very actively and divides into two new epimastigotes; these two forms may become amastigotes and start the cycle just described, or they may transform into trypomastigotes which escape from the cell without disrupting it; in some cases the two epimastigotes divide again and transform themselves into trypomastigotes.

Njogu: Do the trypanosomes that become infective in infective cultures continue being infective if you put them back in culture, after they have infected mice, Dr Newton, or do they lose infectivity immediately you get them back from the mice to the culture?

Newton: This hasn't been investigated.

de Raadt: In what proportion did infective organisms occur?

Newton: I don't know. Infectivity of cultures was tested by inoculating mice with a large number of trypanosomes and it is quite possible that only a small proportion of those injected were infective. Cross has not investigated this aspect.

Lumsden: I was very interested in what you said about infectivity not being related to the donor blood. After looking at the evidence recently, I was unsatisfied that there had been sufficiently extensive testing to be sure of this.

I admit it would spoil Dr Vickerman's argument if tsetse forms show infectivity before the coat actually appears; and Dr Baker has referred to as heretical the suggestion that regurgitated proventricular forms can be infective, which was suggested by Ward & Bell (1971) as a way of explaining the higher infectivity found in flies after they had been feeding as compared to the infection rate found by gland dissection. But I wonder whether we should entirely close our minds to this possibility. We are dealing with large numbers of organisms but there could well be differentiation of very small numbers which might never be detected.

Baker: There is quite a lot of early evidence from members of the Royal Society's Sleeping Sickness Commission (e.g. Gray & Tulloch 1905) in Uganda, who tried repeatedly to infect various mammals with gut forms because they thought that was the end of the life cycle.

Vickerman: This raises the important point of how strictly programmed are these sequential changes in the trypanosome life cycle? Can we go backwards or can we miss out a stage?

I would be very surprised if the proventricular forms were infective. Their mitochondria are very different from the bloodstream forms.

Trager: This sort of thing is more applicable to the difference between slender and stumpy forms. There are indications that the slender form can initiate the invertebrate cycle, although the stumpy form does it better. Maybe the slender form has to be given a chance to survive long enough to effect this change in its biochemical machinery, whereas the stumpy form is ready to go.

Vickerman: This is quite true. The slender form can infect the tsetse fly and can initiate a culture. It does so by becoming a stumpy form first (D. A. Evans, unpublished observations, 1972).

Newton: We have heard that transformation of amastigotes to promastigotes occurs *in vitro* whereas the reverse transformation only occurs intracellularly, but didn't you once report, Professor Trager, that this latter transformation could be induced *in vitro* when cells were grown in limiting concentrations of certain vitamins?

Trager: I was relying on temperature as a differentiating condition. Mostly I started with amastigotes from the hamster spleen which were washed free from cells and put in a cell-free medium (Trager 1953). They then developed as amastigotes but not typical amastigotes; they did not have a flagellum but they were larger than the normal amastigote. I called them intermediate forms. They were capable of growing for about four days and increasing in number at 37 °C. The more recent evidence indicates that physiologically they were probably closer to promastigotes growing without a flagellum . With *Leishmania tarentolae*, for example, if we reduce the vitamin level low enough we can get a culture growing as amastigotes. The population is as great as with a high level of, say, riboflavin but they are all aflagellate (Trager & Rudzinska 1964). Wonde & Honigberg (1971) have got *Leishmania donovani* to adapt to growing at high temperature. Once they are adapted, they grow as promastigotes and not really as amastigotes. So we really can't consider temperature as such a sharply distinctive factor as we did some years ago.

Newton: This effect of limiting vitamins is most interesting and clearly should be investigated further.

Bray: Quite a lot of what Lemma & Schiller (1964) described as amastigotes were in fact fairly degenerate sphaeromastigotes. When Wonde & Honigberg (1971) used tissue culture Medium 199 instead of Hanks' as an overlay on the blood agar, they got perfectly healthy promastigotes growing at 34 and 37 °C. This was part of the proof that nutrition and not temperature was the deciding factor. With *Leishmania* the transformation back to promastigotes also changes from strain to strain. *L. enriettii* in culture at about 22 °C still continues to divide as an apparent amastigote for some two days before it starts to grow even the stumpiest of visible flagella. Most of the others, particularly *L. aethiopica* with which we are dealing, convert extremely quickly to promastigotes in the gut of the sandfly. According to Shortt (1927), *L. donovani* was likely to divide for up to two days as an apparent amastigote in the sandfly, so there is a very large variation.

Zeledón: Pan (1968) obtained transformation of *T. cruzi* epimastigotes into amastigotes *in vitro* by experimenting with temperature and nutritional conditions. Is there any physiological or electron microscopic evidence that these forms are really amastigotes, or are we dealing here with sphaeromastigotes or promastigotes with very short free flagella?

Newton: Has Dr Krassner investigated this in his leishmanial system?

Trager: No. I think Professor Zeledón is perfectly right. Pan (1971) was relying on the ability to grow at high temperature as an indication that these amastigotes were equivalent to those in the mammalian host, but that was the only criterion. I believe that is insufficient, and morphology is obviously insufficient too. We may need a detailed knowledge of the antigenic differences between the different forms. In *L. donovani* there is evidence of some antigenic differences between promastigotes and amastigotes and we may be able to characterize the true intracellular amastigote in this way. Or we might find some biochemical activity which would specifically characterize the intracellular amastigote.

Peters: Would proline be useful in the medium if we are trying to grow even promastigotes of the slow-growing *L. braziliensis*-type strains?

Trager: I would certainly add proline and glutamate.

Goodwin: The mammalian host forms of the *T. brucei* subgroup, growing as they do in connective tissue, are surrounded by proteins containing hydroxyproline. Perhaps that is why the trypanosomes like to live there. Could hydroxyproline replace proline in the cultures?

Bowman: I have no information on hydroxyproline but at least the bloodstream forms of the salivarians do not oxidize proline. Since hydroxyproline oxidation is generally considered to follow the usual route of proline oxidation I would not have thought your idea was right, if one considers bloodstream forms and not the interstitial forms.

Goodwin: I don't think there would be any difference between the interstitial tissue and the bloodstream forms.

Maekelt: What are the minimum nutritional requirements for the culture medium, Professor Trager? One *T. cruzi* culture may show an excellent growth curve but may not be able to maintain multiplication in continuous culture. Are you trying to find the optimum conditions for continuous culture?

Secondly, what about the oxygen tension and oxygen consumption needed for the different trypanosomes? We observed that a high oxygen tension may inhibit the growth of *T. cruzi*. We also found that growth curves are generally steeper in darkness than in daytime (G. A. Maekelt, unpublished, 1972).

Does immune serum influence growth of different trypanosomes? For example, in experimental xenodiagnosis we have observed that when blood from antibody carriers is ingested by insects, the growth of trypanosomes in the insect gut seems to be partially inhibited in comparison to the growth that occurs when normal blood without specific antibodies is ingested (G. A. Maekelt, unpublished, 1971).

Trager: I would define an adequate medium as one which supports continuous cultivation. For practical purposes, growing the organisms through six successive subcultures is a good criterion. This is very important. For example, if we omit biotin, *L. tarentolae* will still grow very well in the first and second transfers, and only in the third transfer would we begin to see an effect. Evidently the biotin requirement is so low that the organisms store up enough for a number of generations.

Your observation on immune serum is interesting. I don't know of much work done with immune serum added to defined media. In a study with *L. tarentolae* my student, Phyllis Strauss (1971), added immune serum prepared in rabbits. The organisms then grew in great clumps in the manner that Adler (1964) described for a number of species. In fact, we had hoped to be able to get fusion of organisms in this way, because Adler talked about these clumps being syncytia. But on electron microscopy we saw there were boundaries between every cell and they were just stuck together.

The haemoflagellates grown in defined media and the insect stages in general seem to do better with a rather good exposure to air. For the blood forms the situation might be quite different. With a defined medium a number of growth factors, such as riboflavin and folic acid, are light-sensitive, so that one would expect any appreciable amount of illumination to interfere. Typically the cultures are kept in darkness but are brought out for examination.

Goble: You referred (p. 240) to Amrein's suspicion that blood from different individuals or different animals differed in their effects on growth or other phenomena. When we were trying to scale up the production of large amounts of *T. cruzi* for a vaccine, we went from rabbit blood to sheep blood. When the blood was not pooled, we found great differences in the productivity of the media which could apparently be attributed only to the blood being from different sheep.

Again in relation to scaling up the *T. cruzi* production, after finding that we got better growth in flasks which had been moved around the laboratory, either accidentally or purposely, during eight or ten days growth, we finally started using an oscillating shaker. This greatly increased the production of organisms, although we never determined whether this was due to oxygenation or whether it was perhaps breaking up the rosettes so that the individual organisms had a chance to start multiplying a little more rapidly than if they were attached to each other.

Lumsden: I was not completely convinced by Amrein's data about the specific relation of effect to particular donors (Amrein & Hanneman 1969). I don't think each donor was tested enough to show whether the effect was related specifically to himself or to when he had last had a meal or something of this sort.

Peters: I am not at all surprised to find that individual donors make a big difference. Some years ago when we were using short-term cultures of mouse macrophages, we collected batches of calf serum from a local abattoir. Serum collected one day might be a very good admixture for the medium, whereas on the next day it was quite useless and toxic to the macrophages. I think this is fairly common.

Newton: I agree. Those of us who have used 'time-expired' human blood from blood banks in culture media have frequently found that some batches are highly toxic to trypanosomes whereas others are not. I have never been able to correlate this with anything obvious, such as blood type. This variability might well result from such unknown factors as what the donor had for breakfast! Certainly I have observed big differences in the lipid content of different batches of blood.

References

ADLER, S. (1964) Leishmania. *Adv. Parasitol.* **2**, 35-97

AMREIN, Y. U. (1965) Genetic transfer in trypanosomes, II: Genetic transformation in *Trypanosoma equiperdum. Exp. Parasitol.* **17**, 264-267

AMREIN, Y. U. & HANNEMAN, R. B. (1969) Suitable blood sources permitting reacquisition of virulence by culture from *Trypanosoma (Trypanozoon) brucei. Acta Trop.* **26**, 70-75

BAKER, J. R. & PRICE, J. (1973) Growth in vitro of *Trypanosoma cruzi* as amastigotes at temperatures below 37 °C. *Int. J. Parasitol.* **3**, 549-551

BRENER, Z. (1972) A new aspect of *Trypanosoma cruzi:* life-cycle in the vertebrate host. *J. Protozool.* **19**, 23-27

CLEVELAND, L. R. (1956) Brief accounts of the sexual cycles of the flagellates of *Cryptocercus. J. Protozool.* **3**, 161-180

CROSS, G. A. M. (1973) Development of defined media for growth of *Trypanosoma brucei* spp. *Trans. R. Soc. Trop. Med. Hyg.* **67**, 255-256

DEANE, M. P. (1969) On the life cycle of trypanosomes of the *lewisi* group and their relationships to other mammalian trypanosomes. *Rev. Inst. Med. Trop. São Paulo* **11**, 34-43

FAIRBAIRN, H. & CULWICK, A. T. (1946) A new approach to trypanosomiasis. *Ann. Trop. Med. Parasitol.* **40**, 421-452

FULTON, J. D. (1960) in *Host Influence on Parasite Physiology* (Stauber, L., ed.), pp. 11-23, Rutgers University Press, New Brunswick, N.J.

GRAY, A. C. H. & TULLOCH, F. M. G. (1905) The multiplication of *Trypanosoma gambiense* in the alimentary canal of *Glossina palpalis. Rep. Sleeping Sickness Comm. R. Soc. (Lond.)* **6**, 282-287

INOKI, S. & MATSUSHIRO, A. (1960) Transformation of drug resistance in *Trypanosoma. Biken J.* **3**, 101-106

INOKI, S., TANINCHI, Y., SAKAMOTO, H., OMO, T. & KUBO, R. (1961) Interspecific transformation of drug resistance between *Trypanosoma gambiense* and *T. evansi. Biken J.* **4**, 111-119

LEMMA, A. & SCHILLER, E. L. (1964) Extracellular cultivation of the leishmanial bodies of species belonging to the protozoan genus *Leishmania. Exp. Parasitol.* **15**, 503-513

MARTINEZ-SILVA, R., LOPEZ, V. A., ARAUJO, G. P. & CHIRIBOGA, J. (1970) Infectividad del estadío critidia de cepas virulentas de *T. cruzi*, in *II Congr. Lat. Americano Parasitol.*, Abstract 74, p. 16

NEWTON, B. A., CROSS, G. A. M. & BAKER, J. R. (1973) Differentiation in Trypanosomatidae, in *Microbial Differentiation* (Ashworth, J. M. & Smith J. E., eds.), *Symp. Soc. Gen. Microbiol.* **23**, 339-373), London, Cambridge University Press

PAN, C-T. (1968) Cultivation of the leishmaniform stage of *Trypanosoma cruzi* in cell free media at different temperatures. *Am. J. Trop. Med. Hyg.* **17**, 823-832

PAN, C-T. (1971) Cultivation and morphogenesis of *Trypanosoma cruzi* in improved liquid media. *J. Protozool.* **18**, 556-560

SHORTT, H. E. (1927) The life-history of *Leishmania donovani* in its insect and mammalian hosts. *Trans. F.E.A.T.M. VII Congr.* **3**, 12-18

STRAUSS, P. R. (1971) The effect of homologous rabbit antiserum on the growth of *Leishmania tarentolae*—a fine structure study. *J. Protozool.* **18**, 147-156

TRAGER, W. (1953) The development of *Leishmania donovani in vitro* at 37 °C. *J. Exp. Med.* **97**, 177-188

TRAGER, W. & RUDZINSKA, M. A. (1964) The riboflavin requirement and the effects of acriflavin on the fine structure of the kinetoplast of *Leishmania tarentolae. J. Protozool.* **11**, 133-145

WARD, R. A. & BELL, L. H. (1971) Transmission of *Trypanosoma brucei* by colonized *Glossina austeni* and *G. morsitans. Trans. R. Soc. Trop. Med. Hyg.* **65**, 236-237

WEINMAN, D. (1968) The human trypanosomiases, in *Infectious Blood Diseases of Man and Animals* (Weinman, D. & Ristic, M., eds.), vol. 2, pp. 97-173, Academic Press, New York

WONDE, T. & HONIGBERG, B. M. (1971) Morphology and infectivity of *Leishmania donovani* cultivated in nonliving media at elevated temperatures. *Am. J. Trop. Med. Hyg.* **20**, 828-838

Intermediary metabolism of pathogenic flagellates

I. B. R. BOWMAN

Department of Biochemistry, Edinburgh University Medical School

Abstract   *Trypanosoma* possess a variety of pathways for the reoxidation of NADH produced during the oxidation of glucose and related substrates. These mechanisms and the metabolism of carbohydrate, amino acids and lipids are reviewed with reference to the subgenera *Trypanozoon* and *Schizotrypanum*.

   The bloodstream forms of *T. rhodesiense, gambiense* and *brucei* oxidize NADH by means of a complex L-glycerol-3-phosphate oxidase which is cyanide-insensitive and cytochrome-independent. *T. cruzi* differs in that NADH oxidation is mediated by a cytochrome electron transport system which is cyanide-sensitive. However, the salivarian and stercorarian trypanosomes are not so dissimilar in their terminal oxidation systems as this would suggest, since the salivarians show great biochemical adaptability. This can be seen in their culture (insect midgut) forms which oxidize a wider range of substrates by means of a terminal pathway of electron transport which is cytochrome-dependent. The culture forms of *Trypanozoon* and *Schizotrypanum* species, in addition, appear to be much more similar in respect of succinate oxidation or synthesis under anaerobic conditions and both groups of trypanosomes incompletely oxidize substrates such as glucose, pyruvate, α-oxoglutarate and certain amino acids. Although the bloodstream and culture forms of *T. cruzi* do not differ in their oxidative metabolism as radically as those of the *Trypanozoon* species, it remains to be determined whether the tissue stages show extremes of metabolic variation.

It is an old adage of parasitology that the more specialized the form of parasitism, the more simplified or reduced is the parasite's metabolic apparatus (Sagan 1967). This holds true in the genus *Trypanosoma* in which the oxidation of carbohydrate, fatty acids and amino acids is incomplete or absent. The African salivarian trypanosomes causing human or animal trypanosomiasis are metabolically highly adapted in both their mammalian and their insect vector hosts, while the stercorarian *Trypanosoma cruzi*, the causative organism of American trypanosomiasis, appears to be more primitive and less metabolically modified by its host–parasite relationship. It is possibly for these reasons of metabolic simplification that *T. rhodesiense*, *T. gambiense* and *T. brucei* can be controlled chemotherapeutically, whereas there is still no useful drug against *T. cruzi*, whose metabolism is not very dissimilar from that of its host.

There is, then, considerable diversity among the different subgenera not only in their life cycles but also in their biochemical properties, for example in their pathways of terminal oxidation. I shall attempt here to compare and contrast the metabolism of the African salivarian trypanosomes of the subgenus *Trypanozoon* with that of the stercorarian American trypanosome *T. (Schizotrypanum) cruzi*. These represent two extremes of the spectrum of biochemical specialization, but it will be shown that the culture (insect midgut) forms of *Trypanozoon* are transformed metabolically so that they closely resemble *Schizotrypanum*, suggesting a fairly close phylogenetic relationship (see Baker 1963).

TERMINAL RESPIRATORY SYSTEMS

At least two different hydrogen transport systems are present in the family Trypanosomatidae. This is illustrated in Table 1, in which it can be seen that the bloodstream forms of *Trypanozoon* species have no detectable cytochromes, their oxygen uptake is cyanide-insensitive and they possess a unique terminal oxidase, L-glycerol-3-phosphate oxidase (GP oxidase). In contrast the oxygen uptake of the bloodstream form of *T. cruzi* is cyanide-sensitive, has been assumed to possess a cytochrome system and to lack a GP oxidase of the cytochrome-independent type. The culture form of *T. cruzi* has been more closely investigated, no doubt because it is easy to cultivate. This form shows cyanide sensitivity, the presence of a cytochrome system and no GP oxidase of the type described by Grant & Sargent (1960). Ryley (1956) showed spectroscopically that *T. cruzi* had an intense α-band at 553–565 nm, a weaker β-band at 525–535 nm and a very weak band at 608 nm due to cytochrome *a*. Baernstein (1953) reported similar absorption bands and both he and Ryley suggested that cytochromes *a* and *b* were present, but since bands characteristic of cytochrome *c* were absent, even at liquid nitrogen temperature, they were forced to conclude that it was absent. However, as will be seen later, trypanosomatids have an unusual cytochrome *c* with an α-band at 555 nm in the reduced form, such that the spectrum of this cytochrome would not be resolved from that of cytochrome *b* by the methods used.

Kallinikova (1968*a*, *b*), using cytochemical methods, has demonstrated the presence of cytochrome oxidase, NADH, and NADPH tetrazolium reductases

TABLE 1

Terminal respiratory systems of trypanosomes

Subgenus	Species	Form	Cytochromes	GP oxidase	Cyanide inhibition	References[a]
Trypanozoon	rhodesiense	B	−	+	−	1, 2, 3
		C	+	−	+	1, 2, 3
Trypanozoon	gambiense	B	−	+	−	2, 3
		C	+	−	+	4, 2, 3
Trypanozoon	brucei	B	−	+	−	5, 3
Trypanozoon	equiperdum	B	−	+	−	4, 6
Nannomonas	congolense	B	0	−	±	2, 3
		C	+	−	+	
Megatrypanum	conorhini		+		+	7, 6
Schizotrypanum	cruzi	B	0	0	+	3
		C	+	−	+	8, 9, 4, 2, 3

B: bloodstream form; C: culture form; GP oxidase: L-glycerol-3-phosphate oxidase; 0: not determined.

[a] References:

1: Bowman et al. (1972); 2: Grant et al. (1961); 3: von Brand & Tobie (1948); 4: Fulton & Spooner (1959); 5: Flynn & Bowman (1973); 6: Bayne et al. (1969a); 7: von Brand & Johnson (1947); 8: Ryley (1956); 9: Baernstein (1953).

in the trypanosomal and leishmanial forms *in vivo* and the leptomonad, crithidial and metacyclic forms *in vitro*. During log phase growth in culture there was high cytochrome oxidase activity which decreased during the stationary phase.

This difference between the African and American trypanosomes in the mechanism of terminal electron transfer to oxygen is not so clear-cut as the above account would suggest, as it can be seen from Table 1 that *T. rhodesiense* and *T. gambiense* culture forms have switched from a cytochrome-independent GP oxidase to a cytochrome-mediated electron transport system and oxygen uptake has become sensitive to inhibition by cyanide. It should be noted that the concentration of cyanide is in the millimolar range, suggestive of an atypical cytochrome oxidase. Rotenone, Amytal and antimycin A inhibit the oxidation of α-oxoglutarate in culture forms (Srivastava & Bowman 1971). It now seems likely that before *T. brucei* can establish itself in blood lysate broth culture it may pass through a cyanide-insensitive phase before developing into the sensitive form which will grow in medium containing a lower concentration of blood lysate (Evans & Brown 1971). Data for *T. equiperdum, T. congolense* and *T. conorhini*, included in Table 1 for comparative purposes, show that the *T. congolense* bloodstream form has partial cyanide sensitivity and this may contain both terminal oxidative pathways although there was no marked GP oxidase activity (Grant *et al.* 1961).

The African salivarian trypanosomes seem more adaptable than *T. cruzi* in the mammalian bloodstream; they are able to develop non-mitochondrial oxidation while retaining their ability to transform to mitochondria-centred oxidative metabolism for the more complete oxidation of carbohydrate in the insect midgut form (Vickerman 1970; Bowman *et al.* 1972).

GLYCEROPHOSPHATE OXIDASE

Grant & Sargent (1960, 1961) discovered in the bloodstream form of *T. rhodesiense* a particulate L-glycerol-3-phosphate oxidase which reacts with oxygen without the intervention of either pyridine nucleotide coenzymes or cytochromes. The high activity and substrate specificity of this oxidase is sufficient to account for the respiration of trypanosomes *in vitro*. This enzyme complex is insensitive to inhibitors of the mammalian respiratory system such as cyanide, azide, Amytal and antimycin A, and it is not coupled to the phosphorylation of ADP. Iron, thiol groups and possibly FAD are components of the oxidase (Bide & Grant 1964) which may consist of two coupled enzymes, an oxygen–oxidoreductase and a substrate-specific peroxidase catalysing specifically:

$$\text{L-}\alpha\text{-glycerophosphate} \;+\; O_2 \rightarrow \text{dihydroxyacetonephosphate} \;+\; H_2O_2$$
$$\text{L-}\alpha\text{-glycerophosphate} \;+\; H_2O_2 \rightarrow \text{dihydroxyacetonephosphate} + 2H_2O$$

$$2\text{L-}\alpha\text{-glycerophosphate} + O_2 \rightarrow 2 \text{ dihydroxyacetonephosphate} \;+\; 2H_2O$$

This coupled reaction would account for the stoichiometry of the overall reaction (Grant & Bowman 1963; Grant 1966). The oxidase is functionally linked to glycolysis for the oxidation of NADH. Catalytic amounts of dihydroxyacetonephosphate are reduced by NADH to form glycerophosphate which is in turn reoxidized back to dihydroxyacetonephosphate by the oxidase. Bayne *et al.* (1969*a*) have demonstrated that this oxidase is associated with microbodies isolated from *T. equiperdum*. The same workers (1969*b*) proposed a possible mechanism for the reciprocal regulation of the synthesis of GP oxidase in the bloodstream forms and its replacement by a mitochondrial cytochrome system in the insect midgut or culture forms. Kinetoplast DNA is likely to be involved in the regulation of this process since acriflavin-induced dyskinetoplastic cells are unable to synthesize a mitochondrion (see papers by Newton and Vickerman, this symposium).

The long slender bloodstream trypanosomes have a single simple tubular mitochondrion with few cristae (Mühlpfordt & Bayer 1961). The short stumpy bloodstream trypanosomes seem to be intermediate developmental forms between the long slender and the insect midgut forms in that although they are still GP oxidase-dependent, ultrastructural studies have shown that they have developed cristae in their mitochondria. Unlike the long slender forms, these stain histochemically for NADH–tetrazolium reductase and the formazan deposit is located in the tubular mitochondrion (Vickerman 1965). However there are no detectable cytochromes in the short stumpy forms (Flynn & Bowman 1973). This suggests that mitochondrial biogenesis is initiated in the mammalian bloodstream but is not completed until transfer to the insect vector or to culture. The tissue stages of *T. cruzi* studied by Sanabria (1963) showed incomplete cristae in the mitochondria and proliferation of the mitochondrial apparatus in the stages in the insect hindgut (Sanabria 1966). There may be some similarity in cristae development with the blood and insect forms of salivarians.

CYTOCHROMES OF TRYPANOSOMATIDS

In contrast to the bloodstream forms of the salivarian trypanosomes in which NADH is reoxidized by the glycerophosphate oxidase, the culture forms

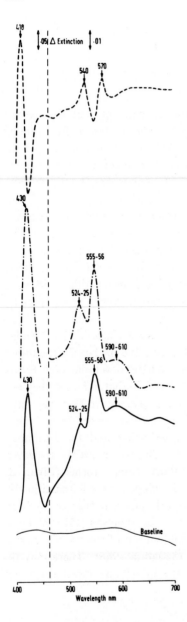

Fig. 1. Difference spectra of a mitochondrial preparation of *T. rhodesiense* culture form. Lower solid curve: dithionite reduced minus oxidized spectrum. Middle broken curve: the reduced sample treated with cyanide minus oxidized spectrum. Upper dashed line: sample reduced with dithionite and saturated with carbon monoxide minus a dithionite reduced sample. (From Bowman *et al.* 1972.)

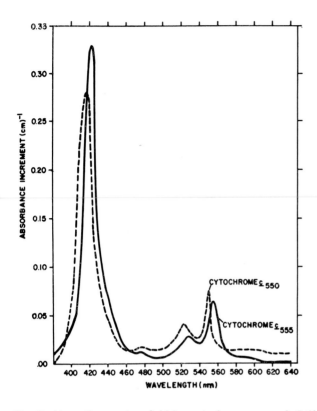

FIG. 2. Absorption spectra of chicken cytochrome c_{550} and *Crithidia fasciculata* cytochrome c_{555} in the reduced forms. (From Hill *et al.* 1971*a*.)

of these and the bloodstream and culture forms of *T. cruzi* reoxidize NADH by a cytochrome electron transport system. The difference spectra of culture *T. rhodesiense* are shown in Fig. 1 (Bowman *et al.* 1972). The carbon monoxide difference spectrum suggests the presence of cytochrome *o*, which may be the terminal oxidase, and there is no evidence in the spectrum of cytochrome a_3. The reduced minus oxidized spectrum indicates the presence of cytochromes *b* and *c* and that cytochrome aa_3 is absent. It should be noted that, unlike the mammalian cytochrome *c*, the trypanosomatid cytochrome *c* has an α-band at 555 nm as opposed to 550 nm. The spectrum of this reduced cytochrome c_{555} from *Crithidia fasciculata* is illustrated in Fig. 2 (Hill *et al.* 1971*a*). Similar cytochromes c_{555} have been identified in *T. rhodesiense* and *T. cruzi* by Hill *et al.* (1971*b*) in *Crithidia oncopelti* (Pettigrew 1972) and *C. fasciculata* (Hill & White 1968; Kusel *et al.* 1969). Cytochrome *c* from Kinetoplastida differs from that of mammalian origin in a number of respects—in being less basic, in the spectral

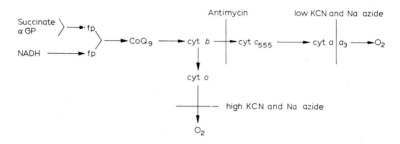

Fig. 3. The proposed branched electron transport system in *Crithidia fasciculata*. (From Hill 1972.)

shift to longer wavelengths, and in containing two moles of trimethyllysine (Hill *et al.* 1971*b*). The haem is probably bound through only one cysteine residue, leaving one vinyl side chain of the haem free and this unusual attachment of the prosthetic group could account for the distinctive spectral shift (Pettigrew 1972). Hill (1972) suggests that *Crithidia fasciculata* has a branched electron transport system containing both cytochrome *o* and cytochrome aa_3 (Fig. 3). A similar branched cytochrome chain involving cytochromes *o* and aa_3 has been postulated for *T. mega* (Ray & Cross 1972) and *Crithidia oncopelti* (Srivastava 1971). Interestingly, in this latter organism cytochrome *o* is present only in log phase growth and both oxidases are present in stationary phase cells. The failure to demonstrate cytochrome a_3 in *T. rhodesiense* may have been due to the use of log phase cells and it is possible that in stationary phase *T. rhodesiense* may have both cytochrome aa_3 and cytochrome *o*.

ALTERNATIVE PATHWAYS OF NADH OXIDATION

Although GP oxidase or cytochrome systems are aerobically the principal mechanism of reoxidation of NADH, a number of reduced end products act as electron acceptors. With *T. rhodesiense* the long slender form accumulates about 9% of the glucose carbon used as glycerol (presumably by dephosphorylation of glycerophosphate) and about 1% as succinate, while in the short stumpy form of *T. rhodesiense* significantly more succinate (7%) is formed (Flynn & Bowman 1973). However, anaerobically equimolar amounts of pyruvate and glycerol are produced for every mole of glucose used, dihydroxyacetonephosphate being the terminal electron acceptor (Grant & Fulton 1957). No lactic acid is produced aerobically or anaerobically as the *Trypanozoon* spp. lack lactate dehydrogenase. The culture form of *T. gambiense* produced about

TABLE 2

Distribution of radioactivity in succinate and acetate formed during the incubation of *T. cruzi* with $^{14}CO_2$, [1-^{14}C]glucose or [U-^{14}C]glucose

Compound		Radioactivity $\mu Ci/mole*$			
		Carbon atom	$^{14}CO_2$	[1-^{14}C]glucose	[U-^{14}C]glucose
N$_2$/5% CO$_2$	Succinate	1 + 2 + 3 + 4	55.5	94.1	388
	BaCO$_3$	2 + 3	0.00	87.2	231
	BaCO$_3$	1 + 4	53.8	0.56	169
	Acetate	1 + 2		38.2	
	BaCO$_3$	2		34.9	
	BaCO$_3$	1		3.6	
Air/5% CO$_2$	Succinate	1 + 2 + 3 + 4	3.25	97.6	283
	BaCO$_3$	2 + 3	0.00	64.6	164
	BaCO$_3$	1 + 4	3.58	27.0	135

* The results are expressed as the molar activity of the undegraded acid calculated from the molar activity of the part.

Suspensions (5 ml) of organisms in Ringer-phosphate containing NaHCO$_3$ or NaH^{14}CO$_3$ (16.66 μmole) and [1-^{14}C]glucose (77.32 μCi/g) or [U-^{14}C]glucose (79.95 μCi/g) (55.5 μmole) were incubated in air/5% CO$_2$ for 2 h at 30 °C. One ml metaphosphoric acid (10%) containing succinic acid (1 mmole) or acetic acid (1 mmole) as carriers was added after the incubation. The acids were isolated and degraded as described. (From Bowman *et al.* 1963.)

15% of glucose carbon as succinate (von Brand *et al.* 1955), though Ryley (1962) was unable to show more than 1% of succinate in *T. rhodesiense*. The *T. cruzi* bloodstream form accumulates 12% of glucose carbon as succinate aerobically and 20% anaerobically and in the culture form 30% of glucose carbon accumulates as succinate aerobically and 70% anaerobically. This suggests that aerobically the cytochrome system is inefficient and some of the reducing equivalents are diverted to a pathway of production of succinate which acts as an electron sink for *T. cruzi* (Ryley 1956; Bowman *et al.* 1963). Bowman *et al.* (1963) showed that succinate formation aerobically and anaerobically involved $^{14}CO_2$ fixation. Table 2 shows that the labelling patterns in carboxyl or methylene carbons are consistent with $^{14}CO_2$ fixation. The presence of possible enzymes of this process in *T. cruzi* has been demonstrated. Raw (1959) identified malic enzyme, Baernstein (1953) found malate dehydrogenase and fumarase while Seaman (1953) and Agosin & von Brand (1955) have characterized succinate dehydrogenase. It is important to distinguish between succinate dehydrogenase and fumarate reductase in this context (see Singer 1965) and this has yet to be achieved, as has a definite identification of the CO$_2$ fixation reaction.

TABLE 3

Carbohydrate degradation by bloodstream forms of *T. rhodesiense* and *T. cruzi*. The figures represent the percentage of carbon of glucose utilized, in the products examined

	T. rhodesiense[a] Long slender	*T. rhodesiense*[b] Short stumpy	*T. cruzi*[c]
Pyruvate	83	60	1
CO_2	1	10	55
Succinate	1	7	12
Glycerol	9	7	0
Acetate	–	9	17
Citrate	–	<1	0
Lactate	0	0	6

[a] From Grant & Fulton 1957; [b] from Flynn & Bowman 1973; [c] from Ryley 1956; – denotes not determined.

CARBOHYDRATE CATABOLISM

All the trypanosomes under consideration are, in von Brand's (1967) terminology 'partial aerobic fermenters', or incomplete oxidizers. The end products of glucose catabolism of *T. rhodesiense* and *T. cruzi* bloodstream forms are shown in Table 3. The long slender form of *T. rhodesiense* oxidizes glucose to pyruvate which is not further metabolized, and little CO_2 is produced. A small amount (9%) of glycerol accumulates as a degradation product of glycerophosphate. The short stumpy stage accumulates much less pyruvate from glucose but significant amounts of CO_2, acetate, and succinate are formed. Extracellular pyruvate is not oxidatively decarboxylated, presumably because of a membrane permeability barrier, since it is decarboxylated to CO_2 and acetate by broken cell preparations. The related acid, α-oxoglutarate, is readily oxidatively decarboxylated to succinate and CO_2 by intact short stumpy trypanosomes (Flynn & Bowman 1973). This acid has previously been shown to maintain the motility of short stumpy forms preferentially (Balis 1964; Vickerman 1965). These results support the finding that the long slender form lacks a functional mitochondrion and tricarboxylic acid cycle. Several enzymes of the tricarboxylic acid cycle have been detected in those forms (Ryley 1962) and their failure to metabolize glucose further than pyruvate has been ascribed to the absence of pyruvate decarboxylase (Shaw *et al.* 1964). However in the stumpy forms a mitochondrion has started to develop and with it the oxidative decarboxylases of pyruvate and α-oxoglutarate, but the cycle is still not functional, due to the low activity of citrate synthase and succinate dehydro-

TABLE 4

Carbohydrate degradation by culture forms of *T. rhodesiense* and *T. cruzi*. The figures represent the percentage of carbon of glucose utilized in the products examined

	T. rhodesiense[a]	*T. cruzi*[b]
Pyruvate	0	1
CO_2	55	32
Succinate	3	34
Glycerol	0	–
Acetate	5	20
Citrate	–	0
Lactate	0	0

[a] From Ryley 1962; [b] from Bowman *et al.* 1963; – denotes not determined.

genase (Flynn & Bowman 1973). In contrast, the bloodstream form of *T. cruzi* is capable of oxidizing about half of the glucose to CO_2 with accumulations of acetate, succinate and, unlike the salivarian trypanosomes, some lactate. These results suggest that the metabolism of glucose in *T. cruzi* is much more complete than in *T. rhodesiense*.

Table 4 shows the end products of glucose catabolism in the culture forms of *T. rhodesiense* and *T. cruzi*. The most striking feature is the similarity between the *T. rhodesiense* culture form and the *T. cruzi* bloodstream form, about half the carbon appearing as CO_2 and 8% as acetate and succinate. Clearly succinate is not such a useful electron trap in *T. rhodesiense* as in *T. cruzi* and the carbon balance is far from complete. The metabolism of this form of *T. rhodesiense* deserves further investigation. Unlike the bloodstream form congener of *T. rhodesiense*, no glycerol accumulates in the culture form, possibly because of a cytochrome system having replaced the glycerophosphate oxidase.

The culture form of *T. cruzi* differs from its bloodstream counterpart in producing less CO_2 and about three times as much succinate, which is accumulated to maintain the redox balance of the pyridine nucleotide coenzymes. It is generally agreed that the culture form of *T. cruzi* can oxidize all tricarboxylic acid cycle intermediates when they are supplied at pH 5.0 to facilitate entry into the organism (von Brand & Agosin 1955; Zeledón 1960a).

Grant & Fulton (1957) have clearly demonstrated that in long slender forms of *T. rhodesiense*, glucose is metabolized by a classical glycolytic pathway. The distribution of isotopic carbon in the carbon skeleton of pyruvate derived from specifically labelled [^14C]glucose is that predicted by the glycolytic scheme. The pentose phosphate pathway in which C-1 of glucose is evolved as CO_2 does

TABLE 5

Production of $^{14}CO_2$ by *T. cruzi* from [^{14}C]glucose

Glucose added	Gas phase	Inhibitor	Glucose utilized mg	Radioactivity nCi		Radiochemical yield CO_2
				In glucose utilized (A)	In $BaCO_3$ (B)	$\dfrac{B}{A} \times 100$
[1-^{14}C]	$N_2/5\% CO_2$	—	3.45	267	5.39	2.04
	Air/5% CO_2	—	7.31	565	158.5	28.0
[6-^{14}C]	$N_2/5\% CO_2$	—	11.27	412	2.71	0.65
	Air/5% CO_2	—	18.68	684	35.4	5.2
[U-^{14}C]	$N_2/5\% CO_2$	—	10.52	840	106	12.6
	$N_2/5\% CO_2$	Fluoroacetate	8.22	660	85	12.8
[U-^{14}C]	Air/5% CO_2	—	3.42	274	98.2	36
	Air/5% CO_2	Fluoroacetate	2.23	178	37	20.8
[U-^{14}C]	Air/5% CO_2	—	3.75	300	116	38.5
	Air/5% CO_2	Malonate	4.4	350	115	33

Suspension of flagellates (5 ml) was incubated with [^{14}C]glucose (55.5 μmole) in Ringer-phosphate containing 16.66 μmol $NaHCO_3$. All suspensions were equilibrated with the appropriate gas mixture. The concentrations of inhibitors were 20 mM. Since the organisms contained no detectable reducing sugar it was assumed that the specific radioactivity of the glucose utilized was the same as that of the glucose added. (From Bowman *et al.* 1963.)

not operate to a significant extent under the experimental conditions used, since only 0.6% of [1-^{14}C]glucose and 0.7% of [3,4-^{14}C]glucose was found as $^{14}CO_2$. In similar experiments in which we used [1-^{14}C]glucose and [6-^{14}C]glucose with short stumpy forms of *T. rhodesiense* there was no preferential release of $^{14}CO_2$ from C-1, showing that in resting cells at least the pentose phosphate pathway is not functioning (Peng Lee Yap & I. B. R. Bowman, unpublished results). In *T. cruzi* culture forms the major pathway of glucose catabolism is again glycolysis (Bowman *et al.* 1963). This can be inferred from the distribution of label in succinate produced under aerobic conditions, as shown in Table 2. The ratio of ^{14}C in methylene (C–2+3) to carboxyl carbon (C–1+4) should be 2:1 from the operation of the combined glycolytic and tricarboxylic acid systems when [1-^{14}C]glucose gives rise to [3-^{14}C]pyruvate. The observed ratio is close to that predicted, the dilution of radioactivity in the carboxyl groups being due to CO_2 fixation. Table 5 shows that aerobically the yields of $^{14}CO_2$ from [1-^{14}C]glucose and [6-^{14}C]glucose are 28% and 5.2%

respectively, indicating that the pentose phosphate pathway contributes significantly to the metabolism of glucose by *T. cruzi* (Bowman *et al.* 1963). Mancilla & Naquira (1964) confirmed this observation and on the basis of the radioactivity in glycerol produced from [6-^{14}C]glucose and [U-^{14}C]glucose they calculated, from the method of Katz & Wood (1960), that the pentose phosphate pathway contributed 40% towards glucose catabolism in the Tulahuen strain and 28% in the Peruvian strain of *T. cruzi*.

LIPID METABOLISM

Dixon *et al.* (1971) have shown that radioactive acetate and glycerol are incorporated into total lipids and acetate into saturated and unsaturated fatty acids in the culture form of *T. rhodesiense*. There was no incorporation of these lipid precursors in the bloodstream forms of *T. rhodesiense* but preformed C_{16} and C_{18} saturated and unsaturated fatty acids were absorbed, interconverted and esterified by both bloodstream and culture forms. The blood parasite is therefore dependent on the host for preformed fatty acids and *de novo* fatty acid synthesis is either inhibited or repressed by some negative feedback control which is relieved after transformation in culture. Palmitic acid (C_{16}) oxidation is insignificant in both blood and culture forms. This is not surprising in the blood form which lacks a mitochondrion, but in the culture form this shows that fatty acid oxidation provides little of the energy needs of the cell. The *T. cruzi* culture form was shown by Halevy (1962) to incorporate appreciable amounts of acetate into total lipids, predominantly phospholipids. Cholesterol is the main sterol (von Brand *et al.* 1959), with traces of ergosterol (Halevy 1962). In *T. rhodesiense*, the main sterol in the bloodstream form was cholesterol, and in the culture form it was ergosterol (Threlfall *et al.* 1965). It was suggested that cholesterol was absorbed intact from the host blood whereas ergosterol might be formed endogenously by the culture form.

AMINO ACID METABOLISM

Little is known of the amino acid metabolism of trypanosomes. Oxygen uptake of the bloodstream form of *T. equiperdum*, a monomorphic long and slender organism, is not stimulated by glutamate, aspartate or alanine (Thurston 1958). Neither the long slender nor the stumpy bloodstream forms of *T. rhodesiense* are able to oxidize glutamate, aspartate, alanine or proline (I. W. Flynn & I. B. R. Bowman, unpublished). However, when *T. rhodesiense*

TABLE 6

Products of [U-^{14}C]proline metabolism by the culture (midgut) form of *T. rhodesiense*

	% Proline specific activity	% of [^{14}C]proline utilized		
		Uninhibited	+ Malonate	+ Arsenite
'Carboxylic acids'	–	27.5	55.4	42.6
Aspartic acid	65.0	2.9	<1.0	<1.0
'Compound A'	–	<1.0	<1.0	1.1
Glutamic acid	92	19.0	41.2	54.5
Alanine	73	21.8	<1.0	1.5
Carbon dioxide	46	23.0	1.7	0.2
Protein	–	3.0	1.0	<1.0
'Wash off'	–	<1.0	<1.0	<1.0
% ^{14}C accounted for		97.2	99.3	99.9

Cell suspension (about 10 mg protein) in 3 ml saline was incubated at 26 °C for 120 minutes in air with [U-^{14}C]proline (10 μmol, 2 μCi). Results were corrected for incorporation occurring in a preincubation period of 10 min before sampling. The concentration of malonate was 16.6 mM and that of arsenite 0.5 mM. The specific activity of proline in the above experiment was 0.037 μCi/μg atom carbon.

adapts to culture conditions it is characterized by high rates of proline and glutamate-supported oxidation (Srivastava & Bowman 1971). Table 6 shows some figures for the metabolism of [U-^{14}C]proline (W. C. L. Ford & I. B. R. Bowman, unpublished) which are consistent with its metabolism by a conventional pathway involving cleavage to glutamate. Compound A has the chromatographic characteristics of Δ^1-pyrroline-5-carboxylate, an intermediate in the oxidation of proline to glutamate. The carboxylic acids are probably tricarboxylic acid cycle intermediates. The specific activity of glutamate approached that of proline but alanine, aspartate and CO_2 have somewhat lower activities, showing that they are derived in part from an unlabelled pool. It is likely that glutamate is transaminated to α-oxoglutarate and that aspartate and alanine are formed in the process, the activities of glutamate–pyruvate and glutamate–oxaloacetate transaminases being sufficient to account for the observed labelled products. Inhibition by malonate and arsenite lead to the expected decrease in CO_2 production and an increase of ^{14}C in carboxylic acids and glutamate. The results can be ascribed to inhibition of succinate dehydrogenase and keto acid decarboxylase enzymes, respectively. It is significant that this route of metabolism of proline by the culture (insect midgut) form parallels that of the tsetse fly vector which is dependent on proline oxidation for energy supply during flight, and which is considered to rely on amino acids produced by digestion of blood proteins after a blood meal (Bursell 1966).

The culture form of *T. cruzi* likewise shows considerable stimulation of oxygen uptake with glutamate, aspartate and alanine although proline was not tested (Zeledón 1960*b*). It would be of interest to compare the amino acid metabolism of *T. cruzi* with that of its triatomine host, which like the tsetse fly is a blood feeder.

CONCLUSION

In comparing and contrasting the biochemical changes occurring during the different transitional stages of trypanosomes I have tried to review the more recent developments in the field (for more complete reviews see von Brand 1966, 1967). It can be seen that the energy-trapping metabolism of blood-stream forms of *Trypanozoon* spp. differs radically from that of the culture or insect midgut forms, and the enzymic changes occurring during this trans-formation are associated with the development of a mitochondrion controlled by kinetoplast DNA. The bloodstream form depends on carbohydrate for its energy supply while the culture form seems to depend on amino acid catabolism. It can be assumed that within a few hours of the tsetse fly taking a blood meal there will be a lack of glucose in its intestine which could be responsible for the rapid transition from an energetically inefficient process of glycolysis to the more complete degradation of pyruvate and amino acids which characterizes the metabolism of the culture forms. Carbohydrate metabolism of *T. cruzi* resembles that of *T. rhodesiense* culture forms, but the bloodstream and culture forms of *T. cruzi* do not show the radical differences in terminal oxidases of the *Trypanozoon* spp. It is significant that neither the bloodstream nor culture forms of *T. rhodesiense* oxidize fatty acids, but not enough is known about fatty acid metabolism in *T. cruzi*. It is possible that some of the tissue stages may be fatty acid dependent. A more detailed study of the terminal oxidases, fatty acid and amino acid metabolism of *T. cruzi* at various stages would be rewarding since it is possible that, as with the African trypanosomes, much biochemical variation occurs especially in the tissue stages. It is this variation in the African species controlled by the kinetoplast–mitochondrion complex which is exploited chemotherapeutically. *Schizotrypanum* strains are less highly evolved to the parasitic mode, thus differing less from the host's me-tabolism and making effective chemotherapy more difficult. While *T. cruzi* appears more primitive than the *Trypanozoon* spp., the redundancy intrinsic in both parasitic relationships has been selected against so that the parasite has '... relegated all dispensable metabolic functions to the host' (Sagan 1967).

References

AGOSIN, M. & BRAND, T. VON (1955) *Exp. Parasitol.* **4**, 548-563
BAERNSTEIN, H. D. (1953) *Ann. N.Y. Acad. Sci.* **56**, 982-994
BAKER, J. R. (1963) *Exp. Parasitol.* **13**, 219-233
BALIS, J. (1964) *Proc. Int. Congr. Parasitol.* p. 41, Pergamon Press, Oxford
BAYNE, R. A., MUSE, K. E. & ROBERTS, J. F. (1969a) *Comp. Biochem. Physiol.* **30**, 1049-1054
BAYNE, R. A., MUSE, K. E. & ROBERTS, J. F. (1969b) *Comp. Biochem. Physiol.* **30**, 61-72
BIDE, R. W. & GRANT, P. T. (1964) *Abstr. 1st Meeting, Fed. Eur. Biochem. Soc.*, p. 72
BOWMAN, I. B. R., TOBIE, E. J. & BRAND, T. VON (1963) *Comp. Biochem. Physiol.* **9**, 105-114
BOWMAN, I. B. R., SRIVASTAVA, H. K. & FLYNN, I. W. (1972) in *Comparative Biochemistry of Parasites* (Van den Bossche, H., ed.), pp. 329-342, Academic Press, New York
BRAND, T. VON (1966) *The Biochemistry of Parasites*, Academic Press, New York
BRAND, T. VON (1967) in *Medicina Tropical* (Anselmi, A., ed.), pp. 261-275, Editorial Fournier, Mexico
BRAND, T. VON & AGOSIN, M. (1955) *J. Infect. Dis.* **97**, 274-279
BRAND, T. VON & JOHNSON, E. (1947) *J. Cell. Comp. Physiol.* **29**, 33-49
BRAND, T. VON & TOBIE, E. J. (1948) *J. Cell. Comp. Physiol.* **31**, 49-68
BRAND, T. VON, WEINBACH, E. C. & TOBIE, E. J. (1955) *J. Cell. Comp. Physiol.* **45**, 421-434
BRAND, T. VON, MCMAHON, P., TOBIE, E. J., THOMPSON, M. J. & MOSETTIG, E. (1959) *Exp. Parasitol.* **8**, 171-181
BURSELL, E. (1966) *Comp. Biochem. Physiol.* **19**, 809-812
DIXON, H., GINGER, C. D. & WILLIAMSON, J. (1971) *Comp. Biochem. Physiol.* **39B**, 247-266
EVANS, D. A. & BROWN, R. C. (1971) *Nature (Lond.)* **230**, 251-252
FLYNN, I. W. & BOWMAN, I. B. R. (1973) *Comp. Biochem. Physiol.* **45B**, 25-42
FULTON, J. D. & SPOONER, D. F. (1959) *Exp. Parasitol.* **8**, 137-162
GRANT, P. T. (1966) *Symp. Soc. Gen. Microbiol.* **16**, 281-293
GRANT, P. T. & BOWMAN, I. B. R. (1963) *Biochem. J.* **89**, 89P
GRANT, P. T. & FULTON, J. D. (1957) *Biochem. J.* **66**, 242-250
GRANT, P. T. & SARGENT, J. R. (1960) *Biochem. J.* **76**, 229-237
GRANT, P. T. & SARGENT, J. R. (1961) *Biochem. J.* **81**, 206-214
GRANT, P. T., SARGENT, J. R. & RYLEY, J. F. (1961) *Biochem. J.* **81**, 200-206
HALEVY, S. (1962) *Bull. Res. Counc. Isr.* **10E**, 65-68
HILL, G. C. (1972) in *Comparative Biochemistry of Parasites* (Van den Bossche, H., ed.), pp. 395-415, Academic Press, New York
HILL, G. C. & WHITE, D. C. (1968) *J. Bacteriol.* **95**, 2151-2157
HILL, G. C., CHAN, S. K. & SMITH, L. (1971a) *Biochim. Biophys. Acta* **253**, 78-87
HILL, G. C., GUTTERIDGE, W. E. & MATHEWSON, N. W. (1971b) *Biochim. Biophys. Acta* **243**, 225-229
KALLINIKOVA, V. D. (1968a) *Acta Protozool.* **5**, 395-403
KALLINIKOVA, V. D. (1968b) *Acta Protozool.* **6**, 87-96
KATZ, J. & WOOD, H. G. (1960) *J. Biol. Chem.* **235**, 2165-2177
KUSEL, J. P., SURIANO, J. R. & WEBER, M. M. (1969). *Arch. Biochem. Biophys.* **133**, 293-304
MANCILLA, R. & NAQUIRA, C. (1964) *J. Protozool.* **11**, 509-513
MÜHLPFORDT, H. & BAYER, M. (1961) *Z. Tropenmed. Parasitol.* **12**, 334-346
NEWTON, B. A. (1974) This symposium, pp. 285-301
PETTIGREW, G. W. (1972) *FEBS (Fed. Eur. Biochem. Soc.) Lett.* **22**, 64-66
RAW, I. (1959) *Rev. Inst. Med. Trop. São Paulo* **1**, 192-194
RAY, S. K. & CROSS, G. A. M. (1972) *Nature New Biol.* **237**, 174-175
RYLEY, J. F. (1956) *Biochem. J.* **62**, 215-222

RYLEY, J. F. (1962) *Biochem. J.* **85**, 211-223
SAGAN, L. (1967) *J. Theor. Biol.* **14**, 225-274
SANABRIA, A. (1963) *Exp. Parasitol.* **14**, 81-91
SANABRIA, A. (1966) *Exp. Parasitol.* **19**, 276-299
SEAMAN, G. R. (1953) *Exp. Parasitol.* **2**, 236-241
SHAW, J. J., VOLLER, A. & BRYANT, C. (1964) *Ann. Trop. Med. Parasitol.* **58**, 17-24
SINGER, T. P. (1965) in *Oxidases and Related Redox Systems* (King, T. E., Mason, H. S. & Morrison, M., eds.), vol. 1, pp. 448-481, Wiley, New York
SRIVASTAVA, H. K. (1971) *FEBS (Fed. Eur. Biochem. Soc.) Lett.* **16**, 189-191
SRIVASTAVA, H. K. & BOWMAN, I. B. R. (1971) *Comp. Biochem. Physiol.* **40B**, 973-981
THREFALL, D. R., WILLIAMS, B. L. & GOODWIN, T. W. (1965) *Prog. Protozool. Abstr. II Int. Conf. Protozool.*, ICS no. 91, p. 141, Excerpta Medica, Amsterdam
THURSTON, J. P. (1958) *Parasitology* **48**, 149-164
VICKERMAN, K. (1965) *Nature (Lond.)* **208**, 762-766
VICKERMAN, K. (1970) in *The African Trypanosomiases* (Mulligan, H. W., ed.), pp. 60-66, Allen & Unwin, London
VICKERMAN, K. (1974) This symposium, pp. 171-190
ZELEDÓN, R. (1960a) *Rev. Biol. Trop.* **8**, 25-33
ZELEDÓN, R. (1960b) *J. Parasitol.* **46**, 541-551

Discussion

Newton: Dr Bowman, you mentioned the use of acriflavin-induced mutants and concluded from experiments with such mutants that kinetoplast DNA might be involved in the synthesis of certain mitochondrial enzymes. I think this is a dangerous conclusion to draw at present because we don't know whether acriflavin acts only on kinetoplast DNA; it might interact with many other cell components.

Bowman: I agree. Acriflavin itself could directly affect enzymic activity rather than enzyme protein synthesis.

Zeledón: It is interesting that proline is quite well utilized by the culture forms of African trypanosomes which correspond to the dipteran forms. *T. rangeli* has a more intimate relationship with the *Rhodnius* vector than *T. cruzi*, since reproduction of the first takes place mainly in the haemolymph of the insect. Neither Mrs Monge, from my laboratory, nor I could find any glucose or trehalose in *Rhodnius prolixus* haemolymph. There is a high content of proline and some other amino acids and we showed that *T. rangeli* utilized these amino acids very well. This parallels what you said about the African forms, Dr Bowman.

Bowman: It seems to be a fair generalization to say that blood-feeding insects lack trehalose as their haemolymph sugar and seem to rely on proline as an energy source.

Njogu: Some years ago we tested cytochemically for the presence of oxidative enzymes, using tetrazolium salts. The amount of the deposit was significant when we used α-glycerophosphate as a substrate for this: the whole cell went black, indicating that there was a lot of α-glycerophosphate dehydrogenase.

We have also looked at the metabolism of trypanosomes in relation to the biosynthesis of antigens. We know that the antigens contain mannose, galactose and presumably amino acids. We have been measuring the incorporation of these metabolites into the cell using a system in which layers of various sucrose densities are put in a test tube with one layer, somewhere in the middle, containing the incubation medium which has labelled metabolites (Heinz *et al.* 1972). We then spin the trypanosomes through so that they have a very short time (six to nine seconds) in the incubation medium. Within that time the trypanosomes take into the metabolic pool about 70% of the total incorporated label of L-leucine, about 40% of D-mannose, and about 25% of D-galactose. A check of the possible intermediates for antigen (glycoprotein) biosynthesis has so far revealed the presence of three nucleotide sugars: uridine diphosphate (UDP) glucose, UDP-galactose and guanine diphosphate (GDP) mannose.

Vickerman: The α-glycerophosphate oxidase system is possibly located in the microbody-like structures (see p. 176). The evidence for its location in these microbodies is rather circumstantial. With light microscope-level cytochemistry Ryley (1966) found that using MTT-tetrazolium he could get quite good localization of the oxidase in bodies whose distribution corresponded to the microbodies one sees in electron micrographs. I have never succeeded in dehydrating and embedding similar cytochemical preparations in order to locate deposits in electron micrographs. The fact that no coupled phosphorylation is associated with this system is characteristic of microbody oxidase systems. You mentioned the iron components of the glycerophosphate oxidase system, Dr Bowman; is this component non-haem iron?

Bowman: I would like to think it is non-haem iron. I was very interested to read two reports that hydroxamates inhibit glycerophosphate oxidase activity, and hydroxamates are well known chelators of iron in particular. But the hydroxamate might be inhibiting somewhere further down the electron transfer chain. For example, with mung bean mitochondria, hydroxamates, far from abolishing the electron paramagnetic resonance signal, in fact potentiate it (Schonbaum *et al.* 1971). If there had been a direct chelation between hydroxamate and non-haem iron, the $g = 1.94$ signal should have been abolished, not potentiated.

Vickerman: Evans & Brown (1973) in my laboratory have found that about eight hydroxamic acids that they tested were specifically antagonistic to the α-glycerophosphate system in *T. brucei*.

Bowman: I would never advise anyone to use tetrazolium with whole cells or cell homogenates. The result is just a mess. One has to purify first. You fix your biological material in glutaraldehyde first, Dr Vickerman, so what you are left with is a vanishingly small percentage, I would guess, of the enzyme activity, since glutaraldehyde is a good protein cross-linking reagent.

Vickerman: For the MTT localization of the α-glycerophosphate oxidase, the cells were not fixed, which is why the localization of enzyme activity was not so satisfactory as with the NADH tetrazolium reductase reaction where one can use fixed cells.

Bowman: The choice is either to fix the material and beat down the enzyme activity, or to fractionate the enzyme activity so that one can be more specific in the use of tetrazolium.

Njogu: We tested quite a lot of metabolites for dehydrogenases, using not MTT but nitroblue tetrazolium, one of the new tetrazolium salts, after pre-fixing the cells by heat. Some of the substrates seem to have their enzymes localized; it is only α-glycerophosphate dehydrogenase that seems to be distributed all over the cell, according to the pattern of formazan deposit.

Trager: The iron metabolism of trypanosomes must be fundamental yet not much work has been done on it. Is cytochrome *o* the terminal oxidase in the culture forms of *T. brucei*?

Bowman: I think so.

Trager: This is not present in the blood forms, not even in the stumpy forms.

Bowman: No; we should have been able to pick this up. We have run a total pyridine haemochrome on freeze-dried short stumpy preparations, and we can get a vanishingly small signal.

Trager: Is there any cytochrome in the stumpy forms?

Bowman: I consider there is none. Any haemoprotein which is present could be due to contamination with haemoglobin being carried over in the purification of the trypanosomes. So although the blood form is surrounded by all this haem, it has no haem requirement. The fact that we get no pyridine haemo-chrome formation indicates that no haem is present in either the long slender or the short stumpy trypanosomes, the bloodstream forms.

Trager: So they have to synthesize all of this when they get into the tsetse fly?

Bowman: Yes, this is part of the transformation process.

Trager: The quickest way to do that is to use the haem that is already present in the nutrient medium—the blood meal or the culture medium. The haem requirement might be an adaptation for allowing rapid synthesis of cytochromes without going through all the business of δ-laevulinic acid and so on that the other cells do.

Newton: How long does it take for cytochromes to appear in culture forms after they have been transferred from the bloodstream to culture?

Bowman: We haven't done a time-course study of the cytochromes.

Vickerman: We have looked at the acquisition of mammalian cytochrome *c* reductase activities, for what they are worth. Succinate–cytochrome *c* reductase activity becomes maximal after 48 h *in vitro*. There is some discrepancy between Dr Bowman's results in the transformation process and ours, but we are using different media.

Bowman: If one assumes that the ability of transforming trypanosomes to oxidize succinate is linked to the cytochrome electron transport system, these cytochromes will be fully organized certainly within five days and will come near to the maximum within three days of exposure to culture conditions. Our time-scales differ. We would also like to follow the transformation process, not only by using marker substrates but by studying marker enzymes. Amino-laevulinate synthetase in the microsomal pathway for the synthesis of the haem ring system *de novo* could be quite an interesting marker for the transformation process. I don't know whether the haem is formed *de novo* or whether it is derived from the haemoglobin of the blood meal.

Trager: By analogy with the insect flagellates or with *Leishmania tarentolae*, I would expect trypanosomes not to be able to synthesize their own haem but to take it from the surrounding medium.

Bowman: That is a good working hypothesis, but the experiment has still to be done.

Vickerman: We find maximal activity of succinoxidase, proline oxidase and mammalian cytochrome *c* reductases within 48 h of putting *T. brucei* stumpy forms into the blood lysate broth medium of Pittam (1970), whereas Dr Bowman's group find maximal activity within five days in their cultures on the biphasic medium of Tobie *et al.* (1950).

Newton: How many cell divisions have taken place during those 48 h?

Vickerman: There is a tenfold increase in numbers while the trypanosomes are transforming, which is interesting in relation to the supposed mutual exclusion of division and differentiation that Dr Baker raised earlier. This time-scale corresponds, as far as we can see, to what is happening in the tsetse fly. The same strain within two days will transform to the procyclic form.

Bowman: Did you find transformation slower in Tobie's biphasic medium?

Vickerman: Yes, at first the numbers drop. They stay level for three days and then begin to go into logarithmic growth.

Bowman: Evans & Brown (1971) showed that within the two-day period, succinoxidase activity is cyanide-insensitive. I find that very difficult to account for.

Njogu: How do you get stumpy forms from the polymorphic population, Dr Vickerman?

Vickerman: We use rats which had been immunosuppressed by 600 rads of γ-radiation one day before infection. After one week we get a population of over 90% stumpy forms.

Newton: A most interesting feature of the metabolism of salivarian trypanosomes is their ability to switch from a cyanide-resistant to a cyanide-sensitive respiration; work now being done on branched electron transport chains may lead to a better understanding of this. The basic work has been done on *Crithidia* spp. and *T. mega* but G. A. M. Cross now has evidence for a branched electron transport chain in *T. brucei*.

Bowman: Are both oxidases present throughout the growth curve? Are they both present in log phase growth?

Newton: We don't know this yet for *T. brucei*.

Bowman: This was a striking finding with *Crithidia oncopelti* which has cytochrome *o* in log phase and both cytochromes a_3 and *o* in stationary phase (Srivastava 1971), and there are parallels in bacterial systems.

Vickerman: Why does the cyanide-insensitive succinoxidase puzzle you if you have the cytochrome *o* branch?

Bowman: The concentrations of cyanide which Evans & Brown (1971) used were quite high, up to 10 mM, which would inhibit cytochrome *o*.

Trager: The rate of transformation in different media is very interesting. Again, glucose may be one of the inhibiting materials, and I think Tobie's medium has glucose.

Bowman: Yes, there is glucose; of course there would be some glucose present in the blood as well.

Trager: A normal Hanks' solution has more glucose than the blood or the medium. There is some evidence that glucose itself inhibits transformation. What medium were you using, Dr Vickerman, when you got a more rapid change?

Vickerman: The monophasic medium of Pittam (1970); this medium is considerably hypertonic to Hanks' solution.

Baker: Does it have added glucose?

Vickerman: Yes.

Bowman: One can assume that within a few hours of the blood meal being taken, the blood glucose would have been exhausted in the tsetse fly.

Vickerman: Yes, the concentration of carbohydrates in the blood meal is very low (0.1%) and bloodstream trypanosomes would rapidly consume it.

Baker: When something is grown in culture, one is selecting maybe a minute proportion of what goes in, so what one actually examines in the culture may not bear very much relationship to the natural population of the organisms.

Vickerman: This is why it is very important to compare in detail the culture forms with forms from the vector, as far as one can physiologically, but certainly ultrastructurally and cytochemically.

Baker: When *Crithidia fasciculata* has been maintained in culture for generations, one wonders how much relationship it has to 'natural' *C. fasciculata*.

Vickerman: The *C. fasciculata* strain isolated in 1926 by Noguchi and Tildan will still infect mosquito larvae quite well and will multiply, attached to the gut linings (Brooker 1971).

Peters: That depends on which mosquito strain one uses.

Vickerman: Brooker used species A of the *Anopheles gambii* complex (Man/RR).

Bray: *L. tarentolae* will not infect lizards, and Dr Simpson told me he was unsuccessful in trying to recover a new strain from Algeria recently.

Trager: Simpson's efforts, whether to infect lizards or to recover a new strain, were very superficial, as I know because I was associated with them. Certainly we all have to keep in mind what Dr Baker said about cultures. Nevertheless we can also be encouraged, as Dr Newton just said, by the fact that the cytochrome *o* situation and the branched chain for the respiratory metabolism of the culture form of *T. rhodesiense* turn out to be the same as Hill (1972) found with *C. fasciculata*. Similarly, the interest in proline would indicate that Krassner's (1969) findings with *L. tarentolae*, which is admittedly a laboratory beast and not a natural animal at all, are of general significance. We can't say that what one finds with laboratory animals is applicable to the natural situation, but it might well be.

Newton: I believe work with *T. mega* isolated from the African toad, *Bufo regularis* (Boné & Steinert 1956), provided the first example of *in vitro* transformation of culture forms to bloodstream forms. *T. mega* also provides an example of the way organisms change when maintained in culture for long periods. In 1958 Steinert reported that 'transformation' of *T. mega* could be induced by the addition of urea to the culture medium; 50–60% of organisms in a culture would transform under optimal conditions. Dr S. K. Ray (unpublished observations) working in my laboratory in 1968 confirmed these findings with the same strain of *T. mega*. After a further year of subculturing only about 1–2% transformation could be obtained, and I believe Dr Steinert has had a similar experience.

Trager: Has anybody tried to isolate that strain from toads again to see whether it works?

Newton: Dr Baker has recently isolated several strains of trypanosomes from frogs and toads in Ethiopia but unfortunately the strains we have examined differ from Steinert's *T. mega* in their DNA base composition. We have not yet examined the effect of urea on their morphology.

Baker: An avian trypanosome being studied in our laboratory undergoes morphological transformation into what look like bloodstream trypomastigotes under certain conditions of culture (Shinondo 1972). But even when we maintained this strain by *in vitro* culture with occasional passage through a bird, it gradually lost the ability to transform. When we went back to a frozen stabilate near the original isolation, it then had the ability to transform. This rather shook me, because I thought that by passaging it every two or three months through a bird, it would maintain at least more of its natural characteristics, but it appeared not to do so.

Lumsden: The importance of early cryopreservation must also be emphasized. If we are looking for differences between organisms, we shouldn't subject them to the possibility of convergent selection by long maintenance in the laboratory before we start to deal with them. Our technique has always been to cryopreserve them at the earliest possible moment. Even though one transmits them cyclically in the laboratory, one is still doing something different from what happens in the field. The other advantage of cryopreservation is that one can put down a large number of samples of the suspension, and from successive samples of that material one can set up much more reproducible experimental situations than if one passages from an infected animal or from a culture in which there may be unmeasured changes in the infectivity of the organisms.

Newton: I agree entirely with what you say, Professor Lumsden, but unfortunately cryopreservation doesn't provide a complete answer to the biochemist's problems. It is generally necessary to passage newly isolated strains of trypanosomes many times before they will grow sufficiently well in laboratory rodents to provide enough material for biochemical studies.

Lumsden: Here again we need to do more work on how to get all our organisms quickly into a condition in which we may study them. The use of irradiated animals has been a great advance. But some work still has to be done to bring the difficult organisms into an amenable situation.

Bray: We probably ought to look more at freeze-drying. Russian workers (Serebryakov *et al.* 1967) have freeze-dried the promastigotes of *Leishmania* and I have heard that the Italians confirmed that work. That surprised me greatly, since leishmania are much more difficult to freeze for cryopreservation than the trypanosomes. Has anybody tried to freeze-dry trypanosomes?

Newton: Annear (1956) described a technique for 'snap freezing' *Crithidia oncopelti* on a 'peptone plug'. As far as I know this procedure has never been tried with trypanosomes.

Trager: Freeze-drying in particular might have considerable selective effect, whereas when one thaws a properly frozen suspension of some of these flagellates at least 95% of them are mobile, and one can hope that no selection has happened.

Bray: Motility is not really the point, particularly with promastigotes. They are frequently motile but will not divide.

Goble: Those of us who have irradiated trypanosomes know that motility is no indication of what they can do.

Lumsden: We need much more quantitative information about what comes back as compared to what goes in. Overdulve & Antonisse (1970a, b) showed that *Babesia rodhaini* lost about two logs, i.e. about 1% of the organisms survived. It is probably the same with *Trichomonas*, but again there is very little good quantitative information. One would expect to find much larger losses by lyophilization than by simple cryopreservation.

Njogu: When we freeze-dry the surface antigens, they don't behave properly on electrophoresis. It may be the technique, but I doubt it; I think freeze-drying has an effect on these proteins.

Vickerman: There was no proline among the amino acids you listed for Simpson's transformation, Professor Trager.

Trager: We didn't know then about the effects of proline on *L. tarentolae*. In the work on *L. donovani* proline certainly did not seem to play a specific role in transformation.

Vickerman: Yet the culture forms of *L. donovani* utilize proline.

Trager: Yes, they do. This all needs further investigation.

Vickerman: This might be relevant to a point I made elsewhere about replacing the glucose in Dr Bowman's biphasic medium with proline. When Dr D. A. Evans and I put stumpy *T. brucei* from irradiated rats into such modified biphasic medium, the trypanosomes stay as stumpy forms for three days in culture; they retain their surface coat and their stumpy form mitochondria; the only morphological change is the accumulation of microtubules close to the flagellar pocket. After three days they undergo normal transformation. Slender forms change to stumpy forms over three days in the same culture medium, then stay as stumpy forms for three days and eventually transform after a week in culture. So proline appears to be inhibiting the transformation, because in the presence of glucose the stumpy forms transform immediately they are put into culture. Have you any explanation for that?

Trager: No; all I can say is that we must do some more work.

Bowman: My simple-minded attitude here is that one shouldn't deprive the bloodstream trypanosomes too quickly of their glucose. They will need something to struggle by on while they develop their mitochondrial apparatus for the utilization of amino acids, proline in particular.

Vickerman: There is a very low level of proline oxidase activity in the stumpy bloodstream form. It seems as though one cannot accelerate the increase in this activity by putting proline in the transformation medium.

Trager: It might all depend on the microanatomy of the fly. When the fly takes its blood meal, at first there is some glucose helping these organisms along. In time they start transforming via their proline oxidase and by that time—two days—the blood meal has been digested. It may be that at that time they really are first ready to make use of the proline. Obviously they have a very active proline oxidase and proline may well play no role in the transformation but may play a role in the metabolism of insect forms.

Bowman: Have the authors of the branched electron transport chain in *T. mega* (Ray & Cross 1972) studied phosphorylation associated with re-oxidation?

Newton: Not in sufficient detail for me to comment on it.

Bowman: So we can't yet talk about energy efficiency in the culture forms.

Zeledón: Have any new efforts been made to culture *T. cruzi* on the same lines as has been done for *T. brucei*? A synthetic medium for *T. cruzi* would be extremely useful, and theoretically *T. cruzi* should be easier to culture than *T. brucei*.

Newton: I don't think much progress has been made since the early work of Citri & Grossowicz (1955). As I recall these workers did not obtain a fully defined medium; there was a requirement for a 'tomato juice factor'. We have never had any success with their medium, but we used Cambridge and not Israeli tomatoes!

Trager: S. M. Krassner (unpublished results) long ago tried the *L. tarentolae* medium for one strain of *T. cruzi* and one of *T. vespertilionis*. He supplemented the medium with stearate. The cultures went quite beautifully for three transfers but stopped on the fourth. This emphasizes the point previously raised about how many transfers one makes. Dr J. O'Daly is working on a defined medium for *T. cruzi*. He is using the *L. tarentolae* medium, but at a less alkaline initial pH, and he adds certain serum fractions to it. This systematic approach may give the desired results.

Lumsden: If the pH in the medium changes during the course of multi-plication, shouldn't one try to run these in continuous culture systems at the optimum pH all the time?

Newton: Dr R. A. Klein spent much of last year trying to do this at the Mol-teno Institute. Unfortunately it is much easier said than done. Introduction of electrodes into cultures of such fragile organisms as trypanosomes creates all sorts of problems. However, I think he now has a system in which the pH can be continually and adequately controlled for the growth of *T. mega*. This has

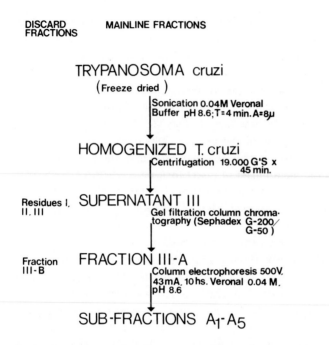

FIG. 1 (Pulido). Purification of soluble fractions from *T. cruzi*.

not yet been achieved for *T. brucei*. It appears from G. A. M. Cross's work that in a defined or semi-defined medium lacking crude blood constituents it may be necessary to control pH to within 0.1 of a pH unit to maintain growth of *T. brucei*.

Pulido: Dr Vickerman spoke about the importance of working with special selected forms of *T. cruzi*. This also applies to other problems bearing on diagnosis, as indicated by preliminary work (D. Lares, L. Ulpino) with Dr Maekelt. In these studies with *T. cruzi*, our main objective was to fractionate the soluble proteins present in the parasite. Lyophilized *T. cruzi* was resuspended in buffer and ultrasonicated. We then put the homogenate through the centrifuge at 19 000–20 000 g and obtained a supernatant containing roughly 70–80% of the proteins initially present in the parasite (Fig. 1). We submitted this material to column chromatography on Sephadex G-200 or G-50 and then to another purification step consisting essentially of preparative column electrophoresis, after which we obtained several subfractions (Fig. 2). The main objective was to prepare the protein subfractions of the whole antigen as usually used in the complement fixation test. From the first separation we obtained two quite different fractions of different molecular weights. Our

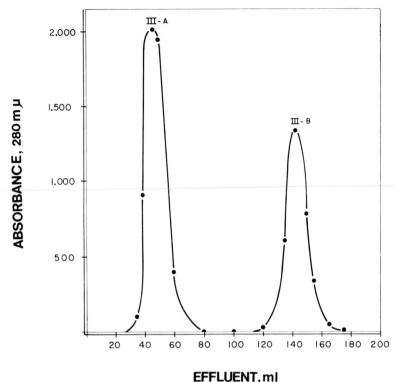

Fig. 2 (Pulido). Gel filtration chromatography of supernatant III from *T. cruzi* (Sephadex G-200, 0.005 M-Tris-HCl, pH 8.6, Vt 140 ml).

findings support what has been said about the heterogeneity of the protein fractions. We tested the first macromolecule, fraction III-A, to see how it behaved antigenically in the complement fixation test (Fig. 3). We compared the initial material, the sonicated trypanosomes (*T. cruzi*), with fraction III-A, and then with the III-B fraction which has a low molecular weight. The low molecular weight protein has no antigenic capacity but fraction III-A and the initial material behave essentially similarly. Similar results were obtained in a double diffusion experiment (Fig. 4). Although the antigen concentration was not optimal in this experiment, there was some precipitation against the initial material and with fraction III-A but none whatsoever in fraction III-B. The antiserum used was obtained from rabbits previously sensitized by successive injections of the whole parasite.

We are now working on the purification of the several different protein fractions and on studying the chemical composition and perhaps the antigenic

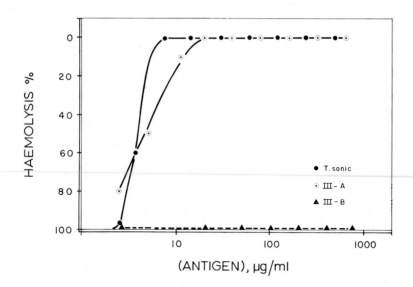

Fɪɢ. 3 (Pulido). Purified protein fractions from *T. cruzi*: antigenic behaviour in the complement-fixation test.

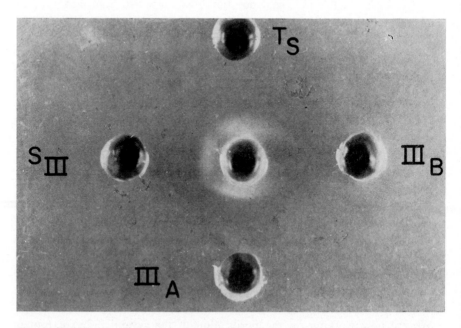

Fɪɢ. 4 (Pulido). Purified protein fractions from *T. cruzi*: behaviour in double diffusion experiment.

behaviour of each fraction. This cannot be done with the whole population of trypanosomes that we are getting in culture. Dr O'Daly is starting to produce well-selected populations of each form.

O'Daly: We started by looking for a defined medium for growing *T. cruzi.* Modified Eagle's medium, a synthetic medium with no protein at all, can support growth of trypanosomes at room temperature (22°C) for at least five days. The trypanosomes can incorporate amino acids into protein and they can synthesize DNA, but at a very low rate. By adding fetal calf serum, we can increase the rate of multiplication of the trypanosomes by six to eight times, and serial passaging of the *T. cruzi* has now been going on for two months, with a doubling of the population every 10 to 12 hours, as measured with tritiated thymidine. When trypanosomes are transferred from 22°C to 37°C they change their appearance, as judged from cytocentrifuge preparations, stained with May-Grünwald Giemsa. Twenty-four hours of incubation at 37°C gives: 27% amastigotes; 1.8% sphaeromastigotes; 70.6% promastigotes and 0.8% epimastigotes. The peak numbers of amastigotes were observed at the fifth day, with 56% of this form, 7.3% of sphaeromastigotes, 36.1% of promastigotes and 0.5% epimastigotes. A few trypomastigotes were observed, in numbers similar to the epimastigotes. The key to stabilizing pH to allow the growth of *T. cruzi* was the use of piperazine derivatives ('PIPES', 'BES' and 'HEPES'). The defined medium contains amino acids, vitamins, nucleotides and piperazine derivatives to stabilize the pH. We are also using serum factors purified by chromatography as substitutes for the fetal calf serum, with some success. A complete account of this work will be published shortly.

Goodwin: Professor Trager, you mentioned that folate was necessary for nucleoprotein synthesis. Can the organisms make do with *p*-aminobenzoate?

Trager: No. My original *L. tarentolae* medium contained PABA. There was no indication that it was doing anything but it was there, and it is very easy with the PABA present to show the folate requirement.

Goodwin: That means there is a very good reason why sulphonamides and substances like pyrimethamine don't work on trypanosomes.

Newton: Dr Bowman suggested that *T. cruzi* is perhaps more primitive and more closely resembles its host than do the African trypanosomes and that this is why it has been so difficult to find an effective chemotherapeutic agent, but surely the important fact is that *T. cruzi* undergoes intracellular development. There are drugs which are active against bloodstream forms of *T. cruzi* but none which can clear intracellular forms in chronic infections.

References

ANNEAR, D. I. (1956) Preservation of *Strigomonas oncopelti* in the dried state. *Nature (Lond.)* **178**, 413

BONÉ, G. J. & STEINERT, M. (1956) Isotopes incorporated in the nucleic acids of *Trypanosoma mega*. *Nature (Lond.)* **178**, 308-309

BROOKER, B. E. (1971) Flagellar attachment and detachment of *Crithidia fasciculata* to the gut wall of *Anopheles gambiae*. *Protoplasma* **73**, 191-202

CITRI, N. & GROSSOWICZ, N. (1955) A partially defined culture medium for *Trypanosoma cruzi* and some other haemoflagellates. *J. Gen. Microbiol.* **13**, 273-278

EVANS, D. A. & BROWN, R. C. (1971) Cyanide insensitive culture form of *Trypanosoma brucei*. *Nature (Lond.)* **230**, 251-252

EVANS, D. A. & BROWN, R. C. (1973) *m*-Chlorobenzhydroxamic acid – an inhibitor of cyanide insensitive respiration in *Trypanosoma brucei*. *J. Protozool.* **20**, 157-160

HEINZ, E., RING, K. & GECK, P. (1972) Amino acid transport in animal and bacteria cells, in *Laboratory Instruction* (International Cell Research Organization [ICRO] – European Molecular Biology Organization [EMBO] Training Course on Membrane Physics), University of Berne

HILL, G. C. (1972) Recent studies on the characterization of the cytochrome system in Kinetoplastidae, in *Comparative Biochemistry of Parasites* (Van den Bossche, H., ed.) pp. 395-415, Academic Press, New York & London

KRASSNER, S. M. (1969) Proline metabolism in *Leishmania tarentolae*. *Exp. Parasitol.* **24**, 348-363

OVERDULVE, J. P. & ANTONISSE, H. W. (1970a) Measurement of the effect of low temperature on protozoa by titration. I. A mathematical model for titration using the prepatent period or survival time; with discussion of the method of the ID_{63}. *Exp. Parasitol.* **27**, 310-322

OVERDULVE, J. P. & ANTONISSE, H. W. (1970b) Measurement of the effect of low temperature on protozoa by titration. II. Titration of *Babesia rodhaini* using prepatent period and survival time before and after storage at $-76\,°C$. *Exp. Parasitol.* **27**, 323-341

PITTAM, M. D. (1970) Medium for *in vitro* cultivation of *Trypanosoma rhodesiense* and *T. brucei*. *Comp. Biochem. Physiol.* **33**, 127-128

RAY, S. K. & CROSS, G. A. M. (1972) Branched electron transport chain in *Trypanosoma mega*. *Nature New Biol.* **237**, 174-175

RYLEY, J. F. (1966) Histochemical studies on blood and culture forms of *Trypanosoma rhodesiense*. *Proc. I Int. Congr. Parasitol.* **1**, 41-42, Pergamon, Oxford

SCHONBAUM, G. R., BONNER, W. D., STOREY, B. T. & BAHR, J. T. (1971) Specific inhibition of the cyanide-insensitive respiratory pathway in plant mitochondria by hydroxamic acids. *Plant Physiol.* **47**, 124-128

SEREBRYAKOV, V. A., YUSUPOV, K. A., NI, G. V. & SHISHLYAEVA-MATOVA, Z. S. (1967) Experiments on lyophilisation of *Leishmania tropica major* culture [in Russian]. *Med. Parazitol. Parazit. Bolezn.* **36**, 267-269

SHINONDO, C. J. (1972) Transformation in vitro of *Trypanosoma avium* from epimastigote to bloodstream trypomastigote. *J. Protozool.* **19** (suppl.), 52

SRIVASTAVA, H. K. (1971) Carbon monoxide-reactive hemoproteins in parasitic flagellate *Crithidia oncopelti*. *FEBS (Fed. Eur. Biochem. Soc.) Lett.* **16**, 189-191

STEINERT, M. (1958) Etudes sur le déterminisme de la morphogenèse d'un trypanosome. *Exp. Cell Res.* **15**, 560-569

TOBIE, E. J., BRAND, T. VON & MEHLMAN, B. (1950) Cultural and physiological observations on *Trypanosoma rhodesiense* and *Trypanosoma gambiense*. *J. Parasitol.* **36**, 48-54

The chemotherapy of trypanosomiasis and leishmaniasis: towards a more rational approach

B. A. N EWTON

Medical Research Council Biochemical Parasitology Unit, Molteno Institute, University of Cambridge

Abstract There is no effective drug treatment for Chagas' disease and an outstanding characteristic of the causative organism, *Trypanosoma (Schizotrypanum) cruzi*, is its resistance to drugs used against African trypanosomiasis and some forms of leishmaniasis. Chemotherapy of the two latter diseases at present depends on a relatively small number of synthetic drugs and resistance has been reported to occur against most of these; no effective new drugs have been introduced in recent years. These facts emphasize how narrow is the margin of security in the treatment of African trypanosomiasis in man and domestic animals and how urgent is the need for a new lead on which to base the development of future trypanocides and leishmanicides. Such a lead could come from a detailed knowledge of the biochemistry of trypanosomes and leishmania, together with an understanding of the mechanism of action of existing drugs. The mechanism of action of trypanocidal drugs is discussed in relation to aspects of parasite physiology which seem to offer the greatest promise to those who seek a more rational approach to chemotherapy. Qualitative and quantitative differences between parasites and hosts which may provide targets for chemotherapeutic attack are emphasized.

The need for new trypanocides and leishmanicides cannot be overemphasized.

At present chemotherapy of African trypanosomiasis is dependent on a relatively small number of synthetic drugs. Suramin (I) and pentamidine (II) are used for prophylaxis and treatment of early stages of the disease in man; organic arsenicals such as tryparsamide (III) and melaminyl compounds (IV) for advanced cases, when trypanosomes have invaded the central nervous system. The disease in cattle and other domestic animals is controlled by quaternary ammonium trypanocides (Antrycide [V], Ethidium [VI], Prothidium [VII] and related drugs) and by the aromatic diamidine, Berenil (VIII). Resistance has been reported to occur against all these drugs and development of resistance to one compound is often accompanied by cross-resistance to others.

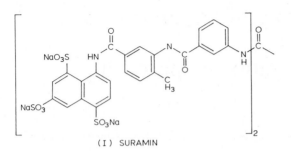

(I) SURAMIN

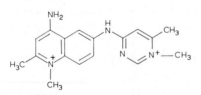

(II) PENTAMIDINE

MELARSEN
OXIDE

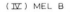

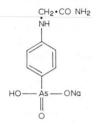

(III) TRYPARSAMIDE

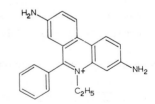

(IV) MEL B

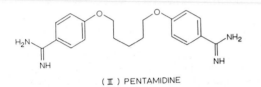

(V) ANTRYCIDE

(VI) ETHIDIUM

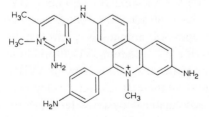

(VII) PROTHIDIUM

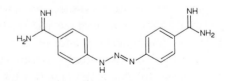

(VIII) BERENIL

A similar picture emerges when we consider present-day chemotherapy of visceral and cutaneous leishmaniasis; the choice of drugs is mainly limited to pentavalent antimony compounds and aromatic diamidines such as pentamidine. There are numerous reports in the literature of other compounds being used successfully for the treatment of cutaneous leishmaniasis but the success of a particular drug appears to vary from locality to locality, presumably due to strain differences in *Leishmania* sp. An additional difficulty in evaluating the success of chemotherapy against this form of leishmaniasis is the assessment of the contribution of spontaneous healing to the cure (Bray 1972).

Trypanosoma cruzi infections are characterized by their resistance to all drugs in general use for the treatment of African trypanosomiasis and leishmaniasis. This fact first emerged from the work of Mayer & Rocha Lima in 1912 and in spite of 60 years' research effort there is still no effective treatment for Chagas' disease. Recent studies on a nitrofuran derivative (IX) (Bayer

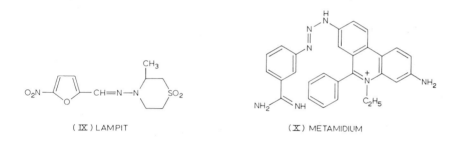

(IX) LAMPIT   (X) METAMIDIUM

2502: Lampit) appear encouraging (Haberkorn *et al.* 1970) but it is still too early to assess the value of this compound for the control of South American trypanosomiasis. Nitrofurans in general are broad-spectrum inhibitors and their usefulness in the treatment of systemic infections is limited by their toxicity. Preliminary clinical trials suggest that Lampit may suffer from this disadvantage.

These facts stress the urgency of the requirement for new prophylactic and curative drugs to combat all forms of trypanosomiasis and leishmaniasis.

Without exception the drugs used at present result from the empirical approach of the chemist to the problem of selective toxicity, and it has to be recognized that this approach has yielded more useful drugs than any other. However, no effective new compounds have been introduced recently and many of the drugs developed in the last 20 years were produced by combining portions of known trypanocides (a procedure termed 'hybrid synthesis' by Williamson 1962); for example, Metamidium (X) contains a portion of the Berenil molecule linked to Ethidium and Prothidium contains the pyrimidyl moiety of Antrycide linked to a phenanthridine closely related to dimidium. Although these compounds have some virtues as trypanocides, Whiteside's (1962) observation that development of resistance to quaternary ammonium drugs is frequently accompanied by cross-resistance to structurally related substances demonstrates the danger of continuing to produce new drugs by 'hybrid synthesis': the need for a new approach is clear. The chemist's achievement has been greatly limited by his lack of information about the nature of primary drug-binding sites in sensitive cells and about the essential reactions he should aim to block: he has been working blind.

In this paper I shall attempt to assess some of the immediate problems delaying development of a more rational approach to chemotherapy of trypanosomiasis and leishmaniasis and then try to define possible lines for future research by reviewing advances in our understanding of trypanocide action in relation to knowledge of parasite physiology.

First it may be helpful to consider what is known about the basis of the selective toxicity of other types of antimicrobial agents. In the last decade there have been major advances in knowledge of the mechanism of action of antibacterial agents, particularly antibiotics, so that we are now in a position to make some generalizations. An antimicrobial agent may be selective because it acts in one or more of the following ways:

(1) It may inhibit the synthesis or cause disorganization of some cell constituent of the parasite which is either not present in the host or not essential to the host (e.g. penicillin inhibits the synthesis of components unique to the cell wall of certain bacteria).

(2) It may block a metabolic pathway vital to the parasite but relatively unimportant or absent in the host. It may achieve this by inhibiting an enzyme or by acting as a metabolite analogue (e.g. the action of sulphonamides on folic acid synthesis).

(3) It may inhibit a biosynthetic process which occurs in both parasite and host but which involves enzymes or other cell constituents that in the parasite have a higher affinity for the drug than those in the host (e.g. isoenzymes are known to have different drug affinities; phosphofructo-kinase from *Schistosoma mansoni* is more sensitive to organic antimonials than the mammalian enzyme; chloramphenicol selectively inhibits protein synthesis in bacteria because it binds to and inactivates 70S ribosomes but does not inactivate the 80S ribosomes of eukaryotic cells).

(4) It may penetrate cells of the parasite more readily than host cells.

These conclusions indicate an obvious approach to the problem of developing new chemotheropeutic agents: detailed comparisons of homologous enzymes in host and parasite must be made, unique cell components or metabolic pathways in parasites must be sought and the basis of the selective toxicity of known drugs must be elucidated. These ideas have been stated often—they are little more than extensions of Paul Ehrlich's thoughts on chemotherapy— and a great deal of effort has already gone into developing them, but so far with little or no tangible success in terms of new drugs. The reasons for this failure are many, but in the particular case of chemotherapy of trypanosomiasis and leishmaniasis, the main bottleneck delaying research has been the difficulty of obtaining parasite material in the quantities required for biochemical research.

Salivarian species of *Trypanosoma* can only be grown continuously *in vitro* in a form which resembles the initial developmental phase of the invertebrate cycle. The medium generally used is complex and contains blood constituents; however some progress towards a completely defined medium for the growth of *T. brucei* has recently been made (Cross 1973a). Bloodstream (haematozoic) forms of salivarian trypanosomes cannot be cultured *in vitro*: the best that has been achieved is an increase in cell numbers of eight to tenfold in the presence of L cells maintained in a tissue culture medium (Le Page 1967). Intracellular developmental forms in the vertebrate cycle of *T. cruzi* and *Leishmania* spp. have proved even more difficult to culture. Very limited success has been achieved in growing amastigotes of these species in non-cellular media (Trager 1953; Lemma & Schiller 1964; Pan 1971). They can be grown in tissue culture (Pipkin 1960; Zuckerman 1966), but such systems are almost as complex as those using a living vertebrate.

These difficulties have restricted our knowledge of the biochemistry of these parasites to a relatively superficial level compared to that of many other micro-organisms and have imposed severe limitations on studies of drug action. However, in the absence of cultures of trypomastigote and amastigote forms the effects of drugs have been studied on a number of systems, including non-pathogenic flagellates which can be readily grown on defined media, culture forms of laboratory strains of pathogens, bloodstream forms either *in vivo* or *in vitro* as washed suspensions of non-dividing cells, and enzymes and other cell constituents isolated from parasites. Each of these experimental systems has its limitations but all are capable of providing calculable information about mechanisms of drug action and some important facts, which provide pointers to further lines of research, are now emerging.

MECHANISMS OF ACTION OF TRYPANOCIDES AND LEISHMANICIDES:
CURRENT HYPOTHESES

In summarizing current ideas it will be most convenient to divide the drugs
into three groups (Table 1) on the basis of their metal content and ionic nature
at a physiological pH (Williamson & Rollo 1959).

TABLE 1

Drugs in current use for treatment of trypanosomiasis and leishmaniasis

Drug group	Drug	Ionization at blood pH	African trypanosomiasis		Leishmaniasis
			In man	In animals	
Neutral aromatic arsenicals	Tryparsamide	Weak	+		
Melaminyl arsenicals and antimonials	Melarsen Mel B Stibenyl Neostibosan		+ +		+
Diamidines	Pentamidine (P) Berenil	Cationic	+ (+ ?)	+	+
Phenanthridines	Ethidium Prothidium (P) Metamidium (P)			+ + +	
Aminoquinaldines	Antrycide (P)			+	
Sulphated naphthylamine	Suramin	Anionic	+	+	

(P = prophylactic activity)

(1) *Organometallic drugs*

The cytotoxicity of aromatic arsenicals is undoubtedly due to inactivation of
metabolically active thiol groups by trivalent arsenic (Johnstone 1963) but this
well-established inhibitory action does not explain the selective activity of these
trypanocides and there is good evidence (reviewed by Williamson 1970) that
the specificity of these drugs is controlled by the non-metallic portion of the
molecules. Changes in the substituent groups of organic arsenicals may alter
the affinity of compounds for binding sites on enzymes or their ability to penetrate cell permeability barriers, or both. It seems likely that the arsenic
sensitivities of enzymes catalysing phosphorylation reactions (e.g. adenosine
triphosphatase and hexokinase) and involved in the cyanide-resistant terminal

respiration system of bloodstream forms of *T. brucei* spp. (Grant & Sargent 1960; Bowman, this symposium) are of importance in the trypanocidal activity of these drugs.

Goodwin (1964) listed over thirty enzymes known to be inhibited by arsenicals and antimonials; subsequent investigations have shown that trypanosomal kinases are particularly sensitive to Melarsen oxide (Grant 1966) and Flynn & Bowman reported (1970) that pyruvate kinase, the terminal glycolytic enzyme in *T. brucei* spp. is selectively inhibited *in vitro* by this drug. A study of the kinetics of inhibition of Melarsen oxide-sensitive trypanosomal enzymes suggests that pyruvate kinase is the most likely site of action of trivalent arsenical drugs in long slender trypomastigote forms of *T. rhodesiense* (Bowman *et al.* 1970). The comparable host enzyme was found to be less sensitive to Melarsen oxide whereas host and parasite enzymes were equally sensitive to non-selective thiol inhibitors. A similar differential sensitivity of host and schistosome phosphofructokinase to trivalent antimonials was demonstrated nearly twenty years ago by Mansour & Bueding (1954).

Aromatic arsenicals and antimonials are well known to be active against *T. brucei* spp. but inactive against the *T. congolense–T. vivax* group, although both groups of parasites have an active pathway of aerobic glycolysis. Whether this selectivity reflects differences in the enzyme proteins in the region of active thiol groups or differences in cell permeability barriers is not known.

(2) *Non-metallic cationic trypanocides*

Some of the most widely used trypanocides for the control of African trypanosomiasis in man and domestic animals are included in this category and the mechanism of action of a number of them has been studied intensively. The most striking fact to emerge from these investigations is that several of these drugs are selective inhibitors of DNA synthesis. The compound which has received the greatest attention from biochemists and molecular biologists in recent years is the phenanthridinium trypanocide, Ethidium bromide. The first evidence that this drug is a potent and selective inhibitor of DNA synthesis was obtained using a non-pathogenic flagellate, *Crithidia oncopelti*, as a test organism (Newton 1957). Ethidium bromide inhibited the growth of this organism after an approximate doubling in cell numbers had occurred; at the time of growth inhibition the DNA content of cells was half the normal value. Further studies with washed cell suspensions showed that the drug rapidly inhibits DNA synthesis but permits RNA and protein synthesis to continue for a limited period. These findings led to studies on the effect of Ethidium on cell-free enzyme systems which will synthesize DNA from deoxyribonucleoside triphosphates in the presence of a DNA 'primer'. Elliott (1963) showed that Ethidium inhibits such an *in vitro* system and that the inhibition produced by a given concentration of drug is related to the amount of DNA primer present. This observation suggested that the drug inactivates the 'primer' molecule rather than the DNA polymerase and further work established that the drug formed a complex with DNA. A similar interaction was known to occur between proflavin and DNA and detailed study of these DNA–drug complexes (Lerman 1964; Waring 1965a) has shown that both acridines and phenanthridines combine with DNA by the heterocyclic chromophore of the drug molecules becoming inserted, or intercalated, between the adjacent base pairs in the double-stranded helix of DNA. Such intercalation is achieved by a partial uncoiling of the DNA helix, which results in the base pairs above and below the bound drug molecule becoming separated by twice their normal distance. Substituents of the chromophore project out into one of the grooves of the DNA helix where they may contribute to the stabilization of the DNA–drug complex by interacting with oppositely charged groups. The distortion of the DNA molecule which results from this interaction is sufficient to prevent its replication and to prevent the DNA from acting as a template for RNA synthesis.

More recent work (Radloff *et al.* 1967; Crawford & Waring 1967) has shown that phenanthridines also bind to supercoiled circular DNA of the type found in certain tumour viruses, mitochondria of many cell types and kinetoplasts of trypanosomes. There is evidence that these drugs bind preferentially to such DNA *in vivo* and give rise to dyskinetoplastic trypanosomes (Steinert 1969) and 'petite mutants' of yeast (Slonimsky *et al.* 1968). The molecular basis of this preferential binding is not yet fully understood. Covalently closed circular DNA molecules may have a higher affinity for the drugs than linear DNA molecules, but other factors such as the apparent lack of histone in kinetoplasts (Steinert 1965) and differences in the permeability of kinetoplast, mitochondrial and nuclear membranes may also contribute (Newton 1970). These findings can adequately explain the growth inhibitory activity of phenanthridine drugs but it remains to be established whether their primary action on bloodstream forms of trypanosomes is to inhibit DNA synthesis. Other possibilities exist; for example Williamson (1965) has reported that Ethidium may also interact with lysosome membranes and prevent the reorganization of these structures which is associated with normal cell division.

Aromatic diamidines form a second important group of widely used cationic trypanocides but we do not have as much information about their mechanism of action as we do about the phenanthridines. However, recent work (Newton

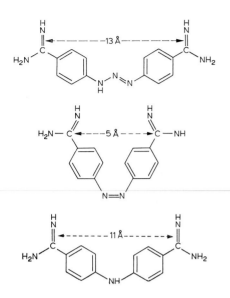

FIG. 1. Spacing of amidino groups in Berenil and derivatives. Top: maximum distance between groups; middle: after removal of one nitrogen atom from the triazine bridge; bottom: after removal of two nitrogen atoms.

1967; Brack *et al.* 1972*b*) has shown that under certain conditions they too interact with DNA and can selectively block kinetoplast replication.

The earliest observed effect of the diamidine Berenil is localization in the kinetoplast of *T. brucei*. This can be detected by ultraviolet microscopy within an hour of a curative dose being injected intraperitoneally into infected mice (Newton & Le Page 1967) and within seconds of the drug being added to an *in vitro* suspension of trypanosomes. Further work (Newton 1967, 1972) has shown that Berenil can form complexes with purified DNA but, in contrast to the phenanthridines, there is good evidence (Waring 1970) that the complexes are not formed by intercalation. Drug-DNA binding studies (Newton 1972 and unpublished observations) suggest that spacing of the amidino groups of Berenil may be critical for the formation of a complex between this drug and DNA. The maximum distance between these groups in Berenil is 1.3 nm (13 Å); in a compound in which one nitrogen has been removed from the triazine bridge (Fig. 1) this distance may be reduced to 0.5 nm, with a resultant loss of growth inhibitory activity and ability to bind to kinetoplast and nuclear DNA *in vivo*; removal of a second nitrogen atom means that the molecule opens out again, increasing the distance between amidino groups to 1.1 nm, and restoring growth inhibitory activity and the ability to combine with intracellular DNA.

Further evidence that Berenil binds to critically spaced groups in DNA molecules comes from the observation that extension and untwisting of DNA by combination with compounds which intercalate prevents normal binding of Berenil.

Electron microscopy of trypanosomes treated with Berenil, pentamidine and hydroxystilbamidine *in vitro* (Delain *et al.* 1971) and *in vivo* (Macadam & Williamson 1972) supports the view that a very early effect of all three compounds is to disorganize kinetoplast DNA in *T. rhodesiense* and *T. cruzi*. A detailed examination of kinetoplast DNA isolated from Berenil-treated *T. cruzi* (Brack *et al.* 1972a) has shown that many of the small circular DNA molecules appear as branched structures; these forms, which are thought to be replicating molecules, are rarely seen in control preparations, suggesting that Berenil does not block the replication of kinetoplast DNA at initiation but binds preferentially to certain specific points in the circular DNA molecule. Later effects of diamidines detected by electron microscopy include aggregation and loss of ribosomes, nucleolar dispersion, and modification of cytoplasmic membranes and lysosomes. As for the phenanthridines, we are not yet able to say which, if any, of these effects is of primary importance in the trypanocidal action of diamidines and certainly many other effects on trypanosome metabolism have been reported. Studies of pentamidine action on *Crithidia fasciculata* (Gutteridge 1966, 1967) showed that transport of basic amino acids and biosynthetic processes in general were more sensitive to growth inhibitory concentrations of the drug than was respiration. Pentamidine and the closely related drugs, stilbamidine and propamidine, have all been shown to interact with ribosomes *in vitro* and to displace magnesium ions and polyamines from the particles (Wallis 1966). Pentamidine has also been reported to inhibit phospholipid synthesis in *Crithidia* (Gutteridge 1969) and bacteria (Gale & Folkes 1967).

A third type of cationic trypanocide is represented by Antrycide, an aminoquinaldine. There is evidence that this drug reduces the growth rate of *Crithidia* species *in vitro* by inactivating cytoplasmic ribosomes (Newton 1966); basophilic granules, formed from aggregations of ribosomes and bound drug, appear in the cytoplasm of organisms after a period of growth in the presence of the drug. Similar basophilic granules have been observed in trypanosomes isolated from infected animals treated with Antrycide (Ormerod 1951a). Suspensions of isolated ribosomes are also aggregated by the drug and it has been shown that magnesium ions and polyamines are displaced from the particles of Antrycide (Newton 1963).

Antrycide does not immediately inhibit the growth of trypanosomes in rats or mice (Ormerod 1951b; Hawking & Sen 1960); and Sen *et al.* (1955) have reported that splenectomy prevents this drug from curing an experimental infection in mice, which suggests that host defence mechanisms play an important role in the action of Antrycide *in vivo*. These findings are in keeping with the results obtained with the *Crithidia* test system (Newton 1966) and are consistent with the hypothesis that Antrycide is not trypanocidal but reduces growth rate to a level at which host defence mechanisms can control, and eventually overcome, the infection.

An additional effect of Antrycide (at a concentration of 10^{-5}M) on *Crithidia oncopelti* is that it rapidly inhibits incorporation of [^{14}C]adenine into ribosomal RNA. Incorporation of this precursor into transfer RNA and DNA is either unaffected or slightly stimulated by a similar concentration of drug, and RNA synthesis from purines synthesized *de novo* is unaffected (Newton 1961). These findings raise a number of interesting questions about compartmentalization of nucleotide pools in *Crithidia oncopelti* which are not relevant to the present discussion, although the observed sensitivity of enzymes involved in the utilization of preformed purines may be of importance when the action of Antrycide on pathogenic trypanosomes is being considered, as it appears that most species of trypanosome are unable to synthesize the purine ring. However, further examination of this effect must await the development of an *in vitro* system which will support the growth of bloodstream forms of these organisms.

(3) *Anionic drugs*

The only widely used compound of this type is Suramin. It has been in use for over half a century and many workers have studied its mechanism of action without success. *In vitro* exposure of trypanosomes to Suramin at concentrations as low as 10^{-5}M is known to reduce their infectivity whereas concentrations as high as 10^{-2}M do not affect the motility or respiration of cells. As would be expected from its structure, the drug binds avidly to basic proteins and is known to inhibit many isolated enzymes (see Newton 1963; Williamson 1970), possibly by binding free cationic amino acid residues in the vicinity of the active centre. In the case of RNA polymerase it seems possible that Suramin may compete with DNA for attachment sites on the enzymes (Waring 1965b). The ready adsorption of this drug by plasma proteins may well account for the long retention time of the compound in man and animals and contribute to its value as a prophylactic agent. The question of how a molecule as large as Suramin enters trypanosomes is an interesting one and it seems possible that, when protein-bound, the drug actively stimulates pinocytosis. There is evidence that Suramin, like a number of other trypanocides, becomes localized in lysosomes but whether this is important to the trypanocidal action of the drug or whether it is a secondary phenomenon is unknown.

SPECULATIONS ON THE BASIS OF SELECTIVE TOXICITY OF TRYPANOCIDES AND LEISHMANICIDES

Perhaps the most surprising, and most disappointing, fact to emerge from all the available information about the mechanism of action of trypanocides and leishmanicides is that none of the drugs in current use appears to inhibit a metabolic process which is unique to these parasites. The drugs which have been discussed appear to block such universal processes as carbohydrate catabolism or nucleic acid or protein synthesis. It may be that this situation merely reflects our lack of knowledge of the biochemistry of trypanosomes and leishmania. It is important to stress that knowledge of the mechanism of action of a drug can never be in advance of knowledge of the biochemistry of the cell, and certainly our knowledge of the biochemistry of these flagellates lags far behind that of many bacteria and other microorganisms. However, there is no evidence from studies of cell-free systems that the specificity of the drugs discussed (with the possible exception of Melarsen oxide) lies at the site of drug action. If we assume that the primary action of Ethidium in a susceptible trypanosome is to combine with kinetoplast DNA, so blocking its replication and function, and that later, when available drug-binding sites on this DNA are saturated, it combines with and inhibits the replication of nuclear DNA, how can we explain the success of this drug as a trypanocide? DNA's isolated from plant, mammalian, protozoal and bacterial cells all appear to have the same affinity for Ethidium. This finding directs our attention to the possibility of differences in the permeability of membranes of host and parasite. Similarly the binding of diamidines to DNA and Antrycide to ribosomes displays no species-specificity, again indicating the importance of making comparative studies of the osmotic barriers of host and parasite if we seek to understand the basis for the selective activity of these drugs.

Recent studies (Hollingshead *et al.* 1963; Vickerman 1969; Wright & Hales 1970) are beginning to yield some information about the surface structure of trypanosomes. It is particularly interesting that bloodstream forms of *T. rhodesiense* differ from other freely circulating cells in the bloodstream in that they either have no net charge or are slightly positively charged at a physiological pH: lymphocytes and red blood corpuscles carry a net negative charge. Electron microscopy (Godfrey & Taylor 1969; Vickerman 1969 and this

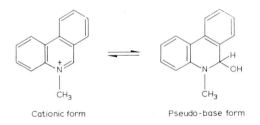

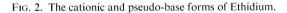

Cationic form   Pseudo-base form

FIG. 2. The cationic and pseudo-base forms of Ethidium.

symposium) has shown that bloodstream forms of African trypanosomes have a layer of moderately electron-dense material (12–15 nm thick) outside the plasma membrane. This 'coat' layer is absent in 'culture' and 'midgut' forms of these trypanosomes; such forms have a net negative charge and thus will have a quite different affinity for charged drug molecules. The neutral or slightly positive charge of bloodstream forms at physiological pH will undoubtedly affect the nature of the primary interaction of these organisms with drug molecules carrying a positive charge at this pH. Watkins (1952) suggested that Ethidium may enter trypanosomes in the form of a neutral pseudo-base (Fig. 2) rather than as a charged cation; the pseudo-base is more soluble in lipids than the charged molecule. Ethidium is known to be a more effective trypanocide than the methyl quaternary homologue (dimidium); perhaps this is due to the fact that Ethidium forms twice as much pseudo-base as dimidium at a physiological pH. In view of this difference it is interesting to note that Ethidium and dimidium show the same affinity for DNA *in vitro* (B. A. Newton, unpublished observations). Clearly we need to know much more about the interaction of trypanocidal drugs with lipoprotein structures of cell surfaces and about the factors which influence the penetration of drug molecules through such structures under physiological conditions if we are to understand the basis of their selective toxicity. Unfortunately such investigations are proving extremely difficult in the absence of radioactively labelled drugs of high specific activity. The availability of such labelled trypanocides would also open up new approaches to the problem of drug resistance (see Peters, this symposium), and in my opinion their synthesis should be a top priority in future research programmes on the chemotherapy of leishmaniasis and trypanosomiasis.

PROSPECTS

Other contributors to this symposium (Vickerman, Trager and Bowman) have discussed recent advances in knowledge of the ultrastructure, nutrition and metabolism of pathogenic flagellates. The work they have described provides some evidence of differences between parasites and their hosts which might be exploited in the future development of drugs. The L-glycerophosphate reductase system of *T. brucei* group trypanosomes appears to be unique; isoenzymes with differing drug sensitivities are now being found in parasites and mammalian cells. Nutritional studies are beginning to reveal metabolic deficiencies in trypanosomes (such as their inability to synthesize the purine ring); greater knowledge of such deficiencies may lead to the development of new metabolite analogues. The kinetoplast of trypanosomes is now regarded as a specialized area of a unique type of mitochondrion which plays a vital role in the developmental cycle of both trypanosomes and leishmania; in the *T. brucei* group the presence of kinetoplast DNA appears to be mandatory for the development of the parasite in culture and in its insect vector. Inhibition of the synthesis of kinetoplast DNA by acridines, phenanthridines and diamidines gives rise to 'dyskinetoplastic' organisms which are unable to infect the insect vector. Compounds that act in this way have long been known, but their ability to block the natural developmental cycle of trypanosomes has not been fully exploited (Newton 1966); they may prove valuable in controlling the spread of drug-resistant strains, if used in conjunction with other drugs.

Another well established characteristic of the *T. brucei* group is their ability to undergo antigenic variation in the mammalian host (de Raadt, this symposium). Successful immunization against African trypanosomiasis has been impossible because of the apparently unlimited capacity of these trypanosomes for changing their antigenic character (Gray 1965). Such an ability suggests the operation of an unusual system for the control of antigen synthesis; detailed knowledge of the chemical structure of these antigens and of factors controlling their synthesis may reveal biochemical mechanisms sufficiently different to those functioning in host cells for them to become targets for chemotherapeutic attack. Restriction of antigenic variation would give host defence mechanisms a better chance of controlling infections and would possibly permit the development of a technique of immunization. Methods recently described by Cross (1973b) for the isolation of highly purified surface proteins of *T. brucei* are perhaps the first step towards this goal.

Other biochemical peculiarities of African trypanosomes which, on further investigation, may provide sites for the action of selective inhibitors include the branched electron transport pathway (Hill 1972; Ray & Cross 1972) and the biosynthetic and biodegradative reactions involved in the changes in lipid and sterol composition of trypanosomes during their developmental cycle (Newton *et al.* 1973).

The promastigote to amastigote change in leishmania and the trypomastigote–promastigote–amastigote cycle in *T. cruzi* also involve considerable changes in cell structure and function. In contrast to African trypanosomes it seems that some of the changes which occur during the developmental cycle of *T. cruzi*, such as the activity of tricarboxylic acid cycle enzymes and cytochromes, may only be quantitative changes; however, it seems not unreasonable to predict that further studies will ultimately reveal reactions unique to these parasites. A vital step in the life cycle of both *Leishmania* and *T. cruzi* is the penetration of host cells. What factors stimulate these parasites to leave the bloodstream and, in the case of *T. cruzi*, how do they select and penetrate muscle and glial cells? *T. cruzi* is known to penetrate host cells posterior end first; electron microscopy has shown the presence of a vesicle at the posterior end of the flagellates and it has been suggested (Meyer *et al.* 1958) that this may contain enzymes used in the penetration process; we still have no information about these. Once it is established at an intracellular site, *T. cruzi* resists all known chemotherapeutic agents; knowledge of factors controlling cell penetration may aid the development of compounds which could restrict *T. cruzi* to the bloodstream.

An outstanding characteristic of all pathogenic flagellates is the complexity of their life cycles. The changes which occur during their development must all result, directly or indirectly, from changes in gene activity but, as in other differentiating systems, we know nothing of the mechanisms of gene repression and derepression which give rise to parasites able to respond to changing environmental stimuli. Such knowledge should be the goal of future research; it may well provide the basis for a more rational approach to chemotherapy.

References

BOWMAN, I. B. R. (1974) This volume, pp. 255-271
BOWMAN, I. B. R., FLYNN, I. W. & FAIRLAMB, A. H. (1970) *J. Parasitol.* **56**, 402
BRACK, C. H., DELAIN, E. & RIOU, G. (1972a) *Proc. Natl. Acad. Sci. U.S.A.* **69**, 1642-1646
BRACK, C. H., DELAIN, E., RIOU, G. & FESTY, B. (1972b) *J. Ultrastruct. Res.* **39**, 568-579
BRAY, R. S. (1972) *Br. Med. Bull.*, **28**, 39-43
CRAWFORD, L. V. & WARING, M. J. (1967) *J. Mol. Biol.* **25**, 23-30
CROSS, G. A. M. (1973a) *Trans. R. Soc. Trop. Med. Hyg.* **67**, 255-256
CROSS, G. A. M. (1973b) *Trans. R. Soc. Trop. Med. Hyg.* **67**, 261
DELAIN, E., BRACK, C. H., RIOU, G. & FESTY, B. (1971) *J. Ultrastruct. Res.* **37**, 200-218
ELLIOTT, W. H. (1963) *Biochem. J.* **86**, 562-567
FLYNN, I. W. & BOWMAN, I. B. R. (1970) *Trans. R. Soc. Trop. Med. Hyg.* **64**, 175-176
GALE, E. F. & FOLKES, J. P. (1967) *Biochim. Biophys. Acta* **144**, 467-469
GODFREY, D. G. & TAYLOR, A. E. R. (1969) *Trans. R. Soc. Trop. Med. Hyg.* **63**, 115-116
GOODWIN, L. G. (1964) in *Biochemistry and Physiology of Protozoa III* (Hutner, S. H., ed.), pp. 495-524, Academic Press, New York

GRANT, P. T. (1966) in *Biochemical Studies of Antimicrobial Drugs*. (Newton, B. A. & Reynolds P. E., eds.), pp. 281-293, Cambridge University Press, London
GRANT, P. T. & SARGENT, J. R. (1960) *Biochem. J.* **76**, 229-237
GRAY, A. R. (1965) *J. Gen. Microbiol.* **41**, 195-214
GUTTERIDGE, W. E. (1966) *Trans. R. Soc. Trop. Med. Hyg.* **60**, 120
GUTTERIDGE, W. E. (1967) *Trans. R. Soc. Trop. Med. Hyg.* **61**, 136
GUTTERIDGE, W. E. (1969) *J. Protozool.* **16**, 306-311
HABERKORN, A., BOCK, M. & GONNERT, R. (1970) *Proc. II Int. Congr. Parasitol., Washington*, Part 4, p. 15, abstr. no. 895
HAWKING, F. & SEN, B. S. (1960) *Br. J. Pharmacol.* **15**, 567-570
HILL, G. C. (1972) in *Comparative Biochemistry of Parasites* (Van den Bossche, H., ed.), pp. 395-416, Academic Press, New York
HOLLINGSHEAD, S., PETHICA, B. A. & RYLEY, J. F. (1963) *Biochem. J.* **89**, 123-127
JOHNSTONE, R. M. (1963) in *Metabolic Inhibitors* (Hochester, R. M. & Quastel, J. H., eds.), vol. 2, pp. 99-118, Academic Press, New York
LEMMA, A. & SCHILLER, E. L. (1964) *Exp. Parasitol.* **15**, 503-513
LE PAGE, R. W. F. (1967) *Nature (Lond.)* **216**, 1141-1142
LERMAN, L. S. (1964) *J. Cell. Comp. Physiol.* **64** (Suppl. 1), 1-18
MACADAM, R. F. & WILLIAMSON, J. (1972) *Trans. R. Soc. Trop. Med. Hyg.* **66**, 897-904
MANSOUR, T. E. & BUEDING, E. (1954) *Br. J. Pharmacol.* **9**, 459-462
MAYER, M. & ROCHA LIMA, H. DA (1912) *Arch. Schiffs- & Tropenhyg.* **16**, 90-94
MEYER, H. M., MUSACCHIO, M. DE O., & MENDONCA, I. DE A. (1958) *Parasitology*, **48**, 1-8
NEWTON, B. A. (1957) *J. Gen. Microbiol.* **17**, 718-730
NEWTON, B. A. (1961) *Prog. Protozool. (Proc. I Int. Congr. Protozool.)*, pp. 170-172, Pergamon, Oxford
NEWTON, B. A. (1963) in *Metabolic Inhibitors* (Hochester, R. M. & Quastel, J. H., eds.), pp. 385-310, Academic Press, New York
NEWTON, B. A. (1966) in *Biochemical Studies of Antimicrobial drugs* (Newton, B. A. & Reynolds, P. E., eds.), pp. 213-234, Cambridge University Press, London
NEWTON, B. A. (1967) *Biochem. J.* **150**, 50p.
NEWTON, B. A. (1970) *Adv. Pharmacol. Chemother.* **8**, 149-184
NEWTON, B. A. (1972) in *Comparative Biochemistry of Parasites* (Van den Bossche, H. ed.), pp. 127-138, Academic Press, New York
NEWTON, B. A. & LE PAGE, R. W. F. (1967) *Biochem. J.* **105**, 50p
NEWTON, B. A., CROSS, G. A. M. & BAKER, J. R. (1973) in *Microbial Differentiation* (Ashworth, J. M. and Smith, J. E., eds.), pp. 339-374, Cambridge University Press, London
ORMEROD, W. E. (1951a) *Br. J. Pharmacol.* **6**, 334-341
ORMEROD, W. E. (1951b) *Br. J. Pharmacol.* **6**, 325-333
PAN, C. T. (1971) *J. Protozool.* **18**, 556-560
PETERS, W. (1974) This volume, pp. 309-326
PIPKIN, A. C. (1960) *Exp. Parasitol.* **9**, 167-203
RAADT, P. DE (1974) This volume, pp. 199-216
RADLOFF, R., BAUER, W. & VINOGRAD, J. (1967) *Proc. Natl Acad. Sci. U.S.A.* **57**, 1514-1521
RAY, S. K. & CROSS, G. A. M. (1972) *Nature (Lond.)* **237**, 174-175
SEN, H. G., DUTTA, B. N. & RAY, H. N. (1955) *Nature (Lond.)* **175**, 778-779
SLONIMSKY, P. P., PERRODIN, G. & CROFT, J. H. (1968) *Biochem. Biophys. Res. Commun.* **30**, 232-239
STEINERT, M. (1965) *Prog. Protozool. (Abstr. II Int. Conf. Protozool.)*, pp. 40-41, ICS no. 91, Excerpta Medica, Amsterdam
STEINERT, M. (1969) *Exp. Cell Res.* **55**, 248-252
TRAGER, W. (1953) *J. Exp. Med.* **97**, 177-188
TRAGER, W. (1974) This volume, pp. 225-245
VICKERMAN, K. (1969) *J. Cell Sci.* **5**, 163-193

VICKERMAN, K. (1974) This volume, pp. 171-190
WALLIS, O. C. (1966) *J. Protozool.* **13**, 234-238
WARING, M. J. (1965*a*) *J. Mol. Biol.* **13**, 269-282
WARING, M. J. (1965*b*) *Mol. Pharmacol.* **1**, 1-13
WARING, M. J. (1970) *J. Mol. Biol.* **54**, 247-279
WATKINS, T. I. (1952) *J. Chem. Soc. (Lond.),* p. 3059-3064
WHITESIDE, E. F. (1962) in *Drugs, Parasites and Hosts* (Goodwin, L. G. & Nimmo-Smith, R. H., eds.), pp. 116-141, Churchill, London
WILLIAMSON, J. (1962) *Exp. Parasitol.* **12**, 274-367
WILLIAMSON, J. (1965) *Prog. Protozool. (Abstr. II Int. Conf. Protozool.),* pp. 81-82, ICS no. 91, Excerpta Medica, Amsterdam
WILLIAMSON, J. (1970) in *The African Trypanosomiases* (Mulligan, H. W., ed.), pp. 125-221, Allen & Unwin, London
WILLIAMSON, J. & ROLLO, I. M. (1959) *Br. J. Pharmacol.* **14**, 423-430
WRIGHT, K. A. & HALES, H. (1970) *J. Parasitol.* **56**, 671-683
ZUCKERMAN, A. (1966) *Ann. N.Y. Acad. Sci.* **139**, 24-38

Discussion

Baker: You told us that things like Berenil bind to the kinetoplast DNA of *T. cruzi* and I take it this applies to the bloodstream forms, Dr Newton. Presumably, therefore, although such drugs could be used to prevent onward transmission from man, there are so many non-human mammalian reservoirs this would be quite pointless.

Newton: It would be useful to have compounds that could selectively block kinetoplast replication even if they did not kill trypanosomes, because they might be useful in stemming the spread of drug resistance. They would stop a drug-resistant parasite being carried on to an insect vector. In African trypanosomes, at least, this is a possibility, and it might be valuable to use such a compound in conjunction with another drug.

Bowman: I think one would tend to get a long slender population rather than a pleomorphic population. The long slender trypanosomes seem to kill rats much quicker than the pleomorphic forms.

Newton: Yes, but the long slender forms won't go into the insect vectors, so they won't be spread around.

Bowman: They won't be spread around but it is no further help to kill the host quicker.

Newton: One would use a drug cocktail.

Bowman: If you are going to use this chronically, what happens to the host mitochondrial DNA? In long-term treatment won't oxidative deficiency occur in host cells through mitochondrial damage?

Newton: I don't know of any evidence that drugs known to be highly selective for the mitochondrial DNA of trypanosomes produce mitochondrial damage in the host.

Bowman: Kroon seemed to consider that chronic treatment with chloramphenicol was not a good idea (Kroon & Jansen 1968).

Newton: But chloramphenicol is not a selective inhibitor of mitochondrial DNA replication. Its action is on ribosomes.

Baker: Is there any epidemiological situation in which it might be of value to block onward transmission of *T. cruzi* from the human host only?

Goodwin: People thought that pamaquin would help in this way in malaria but it never did.

Vickerman: Is Ethidium bromide useful in the chemotherapy of dyskinetoplastic trypanosome infections?

Newton: The drug is certainly active against dyskinetoplastic strains. This of course supports my view that the trypanocidal action of Ethidium cannot be explained in terms of selective binding to kinetoplast DNA. In strains containing a kinetoplast this organelle appears to be the primary binding site for the drug (that is as far as we can judge by available techniques). Once the binding sites on kinetoplast DNA have been saturated, Ethidium certainly binds to nuclear DNA, ribosomes and probably many other cell constituents. I think it is much more likely that the trypanocidal activity of Ethidium results from such secondary binding to as yet unidentified cell components than from selective inhibition of kinetoplast DNA replication.

Peters: Chloroquine and similar drugs can be shown to bind to the DNA from a malaria parasite, but much evidence suggests that the way in which chloroquine kills the malaria parasite bears little if any relation to the DNA. Binding may happen as a terminal event but it certainly is not the way the drug cuts the parasite down in the first place. Some trypanocidal drugs have many actions on different enzymes, for example, about which we know nothing. Work on extracted enzymes would be useful, although it is very difficult to interpret.

Goodwin: Some old evidence on what phenanthridinium compounds do to trypanosomes suggests that something other than the DNA may be involved. If an animal with a blood infection is given a very small dose of dimidium, then although the trypanosomes swim around for 48 hours before they disappear, within half an hour of exposure to the drug they are quite incapable of multiplying in another host (Lock 1950).

Newton: That would agree with my findings. One can do the same type of experiment with *in vitro* cultures. The binding of Ethidium to DNA can be readily reversed but the effect on cells which have been grown in the presence of the drug for one generation time cannot (Newton 1957).

Goodwin: Have you any evidence that the cells of the host are more resistant than trypanosomes to penetration of the drug?

Newton: No; all I can say is that Ethidium gets into tissue culture cells (HeLa) at about the same rate as it penetrates trypanosomes.

Goodwin: If there is no difference in the rate at which it goes in, then it must be able to come out more easily.

Newton: That is one possibility, but if Ethidium penetrates into a cell I would be very surprised if it did not bind to DNA in that cell. I agree that we need to know much more about factors affecting the permeability of host and parasite cells to drugs like Ethidium.

Trager: Phyllis Strauss (1972) has used tritiated acriflavin in *Leishmania tarentolae*. By light microscopy and fluorescence it certainly looked as if acriflavin localized preferentially in the kinetoplast of this haemoflagellate, but when she did this with the tritiated compound and used electron microscope autoradiography, there was not nearly such a clear-cut localization. Acriflavin was in the whole mitochondrion as well as in the kinetoplast, and perhaps there was more acriflavin in some of the lipid bodies.

Newton: I am sure you are right. What we can observe at present is limited by the sensitivity of our techniques. Williamson (1965) also found that a number of quaternary ammonium drugs become localized in lysosomal membranes and suggested that the inhibition of cell division by these compounds might be due to a stabilizing effect on lysosomal membranes. Certainly many of these drugs have a high affinity for lipoprotein structures in cells.

Goodwin: Is there any chance that anyone will provide radioactively labelled forms of trypanocidal drugs?

Newton: Some of the pharmaceutical firms have been very helpful and have produced small amounts of radioactive trypanocides, but unfortunately these have generally been of such low specific activity that they have not been suitable for studying drug uptake and localization in trypanosomes. It is of course an expensive exercise to make drugs of high specific activity with the label (preferably ^{14}C) in a position in the molecule from which it cannot be readily removed by normal cell metabolism or by exchange.

Njogu: We sometimes carry out field trials of new drugs but we have only had one new drug in the last eight years. We can carry on with our inhibitor studies, but we are only playing with a familiar part of an old sequence.

Goodwin: It is not a financially attractive proposition for a drug firm to go into the long and difficult problems involved in synthesizing and testing new chemotherapeutic substances for a disease of importance to a relatively small number of poor people and their domestic stock. But it should be done, even though it is more profitable to sell new cough medicines to more wealthy people.

Peters: Could you say more about the possibility of using drug combinations to prevent the emergence of drug resistance rather than trying to produce individual compounds, each with a better action *per se*?

Newton: I have always been surprised that this approach has not been used more frequently in the treatment of trypanosomiasis. In bacterial chemotherapy a 'cocktail' of antibiotics is frequently used. Whiteside (1962) studied a number of drug combinations in the treatment of cattle trypanosomiasis. Williamson & Desowitz (1956) showed that Suramin and Ethidium could be used together with advantage as they formed a relatively insoluble complex which formed a depot at the site of injection and so was retained longer and provided increased prophylaxis. But it seems that combinations of drugs are not routinely used. Clearly if this approach is to be effective in reducing drug resistance it is essential to select pairs of drugs which act on different metabolic pathways.

Peters: Two drugs which act at two different points on the same general pathway would be more effective.

Newton: Possibly, but the important point is that they must act in different ways and not compete for the same binding sites.

Peters: In malaria another approach to the question of drug combinations is to use a rather specific antimalarial together with another drug which slows down the rate at which resistant parasites emerge. We found that a combination of a sulphonamide with mepacrine slows down the rate at which resistance develops to the sulphonamide (Peters 1969). Has any work of that type been done in trypanosomiasis? It seems a very rational approach to take. It is surprising how many avenues are unexplored in this field.

Goodwin: Because of the follow-up problem it is very difficult to organize this kind of work in tropical Africa, and I should imagine it is equally difficult in tropical America. Even with cattle, fairly large numbers are needed under control for a fairly long time. Whiteside (1962) had a splendid system of preventing the development of drug resistance in Kenya by changing the drug issued by the Veterinary Department. The veterinary officer just had to sit in his office in Nairobi and get records of the number of positive cases of trypanosomiasis. As soon as they started to rise in a particular area, he banned Berenil and sent out isometamidium; then he waited until the number of cases started to rise again a year or two later, when he banned isometamidium and sent out Berenil; and so on. This worked extremely well and it is very simple and straightforward. Of course it depends on the fact that every two years, or even less, most of the cattle are slaughtered and eaten, so there is no continuing source of infection as there is in man.

Bray: Even that won't work with people like the Borana or the Masai, who have no intention of slaughtering their animals at all.

Goodwin: That is right; it was used only on farms in Kenya, where the animals are killed.

Baker: Why don't antileishmanial drugs work on *T. cruzi* amastigotes? Is it parasite specificity or is it a difference in host cells and their permeability?

Newton: I don't know. Perhaps they don't get into the amastigotes.

Baker: But why not, if they do get at *Leishmania*?

Peters: I have those questions in my paper but not the answers.

Newton: Perhaps in talking about future developments in chemotherapy I overstressed the need to look for *major* differences between host and parasite. There are now a number of well established examples of isoenzymes from microbial and mammalian cells which differ significantly in sensitivity to certain drugs. This emphasizes the importance of detailed comparisons of enzymes common to both parasite and host. Dr Bowman's work on arsenical drugs illustrates this point.

Bowman: We thought that if a fast-acting drug such as a trivalent arsenical was going to act on an energy-producing pathway the ideal target site would be glycerophosphate oxidase, which is perfectly suited for selective action, being present in the parasite and not in the host. However, Melarsen oxide didn't inhibit the glycerophosphate oxidase at all. We then examined most of the enzymes in the glycolytic sequence and found only one, pyruvate kinase, was affected by this trivalent arsenical. Here we began to realize the subtlety of arsenical action. This is an isofunctional enzyme. Pyruvate kinase is present, of course, in the host tissues. We were next delighted to find that pyruvate kinase in mammalian muscle was not inhibited by the trivalent arsenical. Nevertheless the arsenical is toxic to the host. This could of course be due to the trivalent arsenical reacting with dihydrolipoate dehydrogenase enzymes such as the α-oxo-acid decarboxylases, which are the two further enzyme complexes which I said had developed in the short stumpy forms and are also present in the host. We then began to look at other tissue pyruvate kinases, especially in the liver. There are two isoenzymes in the liver. One, called M because it looks a bit like the muscle enzyme, was not inhibited to any marked extent by Melarsen oxide. But the other, inducible, form of pyruvate kinase (L form) turned out to be well inhibited by melarsen oxide. This may be a further reason for the toxicity of Melarsen oxide to the host, since it affects not only the lipoamide enzymes and the coenzymes of the α-oxo-acid decarboxylases but also this form of pyruvate kinase in the liver.

In a curve of velocity versus substrate concentration, if the enzyme is allosteric we get a sigmoid profile; if it is not an allosteric enzyme, a hyperbolic profile will be obtained. The trypanosome enzyme is allosteric and is activated by fructose-1,6-diphosphate (FDP), while the muscle enzyme is not, and the liver L form is allosteric and is activated by FDP. It seems to be the allosteric property which is affected and inhibited by the Melarsen oxide. The concentration required to inhibit the trypanosome pyruvate kinase is 10^{-5}M and 10^{-6}M in the liver L form. If we dissect the molecule of Melarsen oxide, it can be shown that arsenite, the basic reactive constituent, has no effect at all on the trypanosome pyruvate kinase. If a benzene ring is substrated onto arsenite, forming phenylarsenoxide, it is then a good inhibitor of the trypanosome enzyme. If an amino group is put in the *para* position, it is still a good inhibitor of the parasite enzyme. The melamine molecule has no effect on pyruvate kinase but the substitution of the *p*-amino group by this melamine ring system making Melarsen oxide, improves the efficacy of the drug. What do we mean by improved efficacy? In fact, the ID_{50} of the *p*-aminophenylarsenoxide is not so different from Melarsen oxide.

What we think this residue is doing is to facilitate the uptake of the drug into the trypanosome or to obstruct the uptake of the drug into the mammalian cell. Or the presence of the positively charged melamine ring may make the drug less toxic to the mammalian enzymes, which may have adjacent positive charges, so that the charges are repelled. But that is all hypothesis.

Maekelt: In 1967 we started to evaluate the new Bayer compound, Bayer 2502 or Lampit, in cases of chronic Chagas' disease, using immunoserological procedures. Preliminary results were reported at the Chagas' Symposium held in Santiago de Chile in 1968 (Maekelt 1969). Since we observed no changes in serum antibody titres in patients during and after treatment with increasing doses (5 to 25 mg/kg body weight daily for 120 days), we concluded that the effectiveness of this chemotherapeutic agent was not measurable by serological procedures (G. A. Maekelt 1969, unpublished).

Schenone *et al.* (1969) were the first to report parasitological cure in adult hospitalized patients with chronic Chagas' disease treated with this drug. Xenodiagnosis in ten patients receiving Lampit became consistently negative after the first month of treatment and remained negative during a follow-up study of 13 months after treatment. In their control group of six patients given placebos, the follow-up study with xenodiagnosis showed that two-thirds of the tests on average were positive. A similar evaluation of 28 hospitalized psychiatric patients given Lampit in daily doses of 15 mg/kg and of nine control patients, was done by Rabinovich in Buenos Aires (see Cerisola *et al.* 1972). His parasitological follow-up, with xenodiagnosis of the treated patients for 24 months after chemotherapy, using 80 reduviid bugs per xenodiagnosis, gave consistently negative results. In the placebo group, xenodiagnosis remained positive in 65.1 % of tests.

We repeated this drug evaluation study on ten control patients and 18 others who received an average of 8.87 mg Lampit/kg daily for 114.6 days, and we used xenodiagnosis for the parasitological follow-up study (28 reduviid bugs per test). In the control group, xenodiagnosis remained positive in 47.2% of tests during 20 months of observation. In a 24-month follow-up study only one of the 18 patients still had a positive xenodiagnosis. This patient was the only one who had not lost weight during treatment.

From these results we may conclude that treatment of patients with chronic Chagas' disease with Lampit for 120 days brought about a parasitological cure in most cases, as measured by xenodiagnosis in a 24-month post-treatment follow-up study (Maekelt 1972).

References

CERISOLA, J. A., LUGONES, H. & RABINOVICH, L. B. (1972) *Tratamiento de la Enfermedad de Chagas*, p. 7, Fundación Rizzuto, Buenos Aires

KROON, A. M. & JANSEN, R. J. (1968) The effect of low concentrations of chloramphenicol on beating rat-heart cells in tissue culture. *Biochim. Biophys. Acta* **155**, 629-631

LOCK, J. A. (1950) The chemotherapeutic action of phenanthridine compounds. Part IV: Activity *in vitro. Br. J. Pharmacol.* **5**, 398

MAEKELT, G. A. (1969) *Bol. Chil. Parasitol.* **24**, (1/2), 95

MAEKELT, G. A. (1972) in *Symposium Internacional sobre la Enfermedad de Chagas*, Sociedad Argentina de Parasitologia, Buenos Aires, in preparation

NEWTON, B. A. (1957) The mode of action of phenanthridines: the effect of ethidium bromide on cell division and nucleic acid synthesis. *J. Gen. Microbiol.* **17**, 718-730

PETERS, W. (1969) Partial inhibition by mepacrine of the development of sulphonamide resistance in *Plasmodium berghei. Nature (Lond.)* **223**, 858-859

SCHENONE, H., CONCHA, L., ARANDA, R., ROJAS, A. & ALFARO, E. (1969) Experiencia terapeutica con el Bay 2502 en la infeccion chagasica cronica del adulto. Importancia del uso adecuado del xenodiagnostico. *Bol. Chil. Parasitol.* **24** (1/2), 66

STRAUSS, P. R. (1972) Acriflavin resistance in the hemoflagellate, *Leishmania tarentolae. J. Cell Biol.* **53**, 312-334

WHITESIDE, E. F. (1962) Interactions between drugs, trypanosomes and cattle in the field, in *Drugs, Parasites and Hosts* (Goodwin, L. G. & Nimmo-Smith, R. H., eds.), p. 116-141, Churchill, London

WILLIAMSON, J. (1965) New aspects of trypanocidal drug action. *Prog. Protozool. (Abstr. II Int. Conf. Protozool.)*, pp. 81-82, ICS No. 91, Excerpta Medica, Amsterdam

WILLIAMSON, J. & DESOWITZ, R. S. (1956) Prophylactic activity of suramin complexes in animal trypanosomiasis. *Nature (Lond.)* **177**, 1074-1075

Drug resistance in trypanosomiasis and leishmaniasis

W. PETERS

Department of Parasitology, Liverpool School of Tropical Medicine

Abstract Although the problem of drug resistance in the African trypanosomes has received considerable attention, it is only recently that we have begun to understand the molecular basis of the action of the numerous potent trypanocides that are available and the significance of the interaction between drug, parasite and host. The situation is quite different in *Trypanosoma (Schizotrypanum) cruzi*, since few drugs have any significant action against their tissue-dwelling amastigotes. The problem of drug resistance as such has therefore aroused little interest in relation to this parasite.

On the other hand, drug resistance has proved to be a matter of practical concern in the treatment of the leishmaniases. Little is known of the interaction of drug, parasite and host immunity when drugs are employed against the amastigotes of either *T. cruzi* or the *Leishmania* species. In order to study this problem we are examining a wide spectrum of chemical structures in tissue culture and *in vivo*.

The pentavalent and trivalent organic antimonials that are classically employed as leishmanicides and against which resistance is known to develop display no selective toxicity against intracellular *Leishmania* amastigotes in tissue culture, although some affect extracellular organisms. Primaquine, pentamidine and amphotericin B inhibit the growth of the intracellular amastigotes. A comparison is being made of the activity of antileishmanial compounds in intact and in immunosuppressed hosts. Antigenic variation, which is associated with drug resistance in some salivarian trypanosome infections, may be of significance too in the leishmaniases. The immunosuppressive action of the infections themselves may also play a role in some individuals in the emergence of drug resistance.

Although the problem of drug resistance in the African trypanosomes has received considerable attention, it is only recently that we have begun to understand the molecular basis of the action of the numerous potent trypanocides that are available, and the significance of the interaction between drug, parasite and host. The situation is quite different in *Trypanosoma (Schizotrypanum) cruzi*, since few drugs have any significant action against its tissue-dwelling amastigotes. The problem of drug resistance as such has therefore aroused little interest in relation to this parasite.

On the other hand, drug resistance has proved to be a matter of practical concern in the treatment of the leishmaniases. Little is known of the inter-action of drug, parasite and host immunity when drugs are employed against the amastigotes of either *T. cruzi* or the *Leishmania* species. In order to study this problem we are examining a wide spectrum of chemical structures in tissue culture and *in vivo*. Our preliminary observations and data published by other workers indicate that the main obstacle to chemotherapy of infection with these organisms is, in fact, 'resistance to therapy' rather than 'drug resistance'.

THE PROBLEM DEFINED

The African trypanosomiases

Trypanosomiasis of man and, even more, of his domestic animals is re-cognized to be a major scourge, and a barrier to economic and agricultural development in large areas of tropical Africa. In the practical control of trypano-somiasis of livestock, chemotherapy plays a major role. The use of chemo-prophylaxis however is viewed with considerable caution because of the frequency with which the use of trypanocidal agents for this purpose has culminated in the rapid and widespread dissemination of drug resistance. Even the most promising drugs, such as diminazene aceturate, have failed to sustain their early promise and, for example, strains of both *Trypanosoma congolense* and *T. vivax* have been reported in Nigeria to be resistant to this compound (Maclennan 1970). Gray & Roberts (1971) have demonstrated that the resistance to diminazene aceturate, to homidium bromide (Ethidium bromide), quinapyramine sulphate and isometamidium chloride, remains un-changed after several cyclical passsages through *Glossina*.

The application of drugs for chemoprophylaxis has, on the other hand, contributed significantly to the reduction of the reservoir of human infection in West and Central Africa, and possibly to some degree to the protection of individuals exposed to infection by *T. rhodesiense* further East (Waddy 1970). The problem of drug resistance has become of less importance since the discontinuation of tryparsamide for the treatment of established cases, and its replacement by melaminyl derivatives of arsenic such as melarsoprol and melarsonyl potassium.

Overall, then, the problem of drug resistance has been of sufficient practical importance to attract the attention of numerous research workers, and indeed provided one of the first targets for Ehrlich's search for a 'Chemotherapia specifica'. The field has been reviewed recently in a masterly paper by Williamson (1970) and will therefore not be discussed further here.

Chagas' disease and leishmaniasis

Quite a different situation exists, however, in relation to Chagas' disease caused by the New World trypanosome, *Trypanosoma (Schizotrypanum) cruzi*, and to the complex of diseases known under the generic term of 'leishmaniasis'. In the first place, the existing battery of drugs available for their treatment is extremely limited both in number and efficacy. In the second place, drug resistance undoubtedly occurs in some types of leishmanial infection. Finally, neither Chagas' disease nor leishmaniasis are considered by most controllers of research funds to be of sufficient economic or public health importance to merit devoting to them the intensive multidisciplinary effort that is needed to overcome them.

In its way Chagas' disease presents the more acute problem since no completely safe and effective drug is available, even today, that will guarantee a radical cure, and yet probably at least seven million people are infected with *T. cruzi*. Both animal and clinical studies indicate that there are great variations in the response of *T. cruzi* to drugs, but this cannot be considered as drug resistance. There are many strains of this organism in different parts of its geographical range. They induce a wide variety of changes in the mammalian host. Köberle (1968) has drawn attention to the marked regional variations in the pathological manifestations in man, adding that he is unable to account for this phenomenon. I believe that this is readily understood if one considers *T. cruzi* as a complex of morphologically similar (Brener 1965) but physiologically and antigenically (González Cappa & Kagan 1969) distinct organisms, rather than as a single taxon. It is well established that different strains show divergent responses to drugs (Brener & Chiari 1967; Wilson 1972), and different degrees of infectivity to both invertebrate and vertebrate hosts (animal and human) as well as of cardiotropism or neurotropism. Clinical responses to one of the latest trypanocides, nifurtimox (Bayer 2502, Lampit), although of course the parameters of cure differ, vary from excellent in parts of Argentina to virtual failure in some Brazilian centres.

The leishmaniases present an interesting parallel in certain respects. Morphologically the several 'species' of *Leishmania* that affect mammals, including man, are for all practical purposes indistinguishable. Unlike '*T. cruzi*' they are named firstly on the basis of the clinicopathological picture they induce in the human host, secondly on characteristics of the culture forms, thirdly on certain immunological criteria and, more recently, on the basis of biochemical characteristics. Even such recent classifications as that of Lainson & Shaw (1972) are open to controversy. It is quite clear that the responses of the different clinical syndromes, kala azar, Oriental sore, espundia etc., to given therapeutic regimens are very different, and frequently quite unpredictable. Whereas very few reports have appeared on the subject of drug resistance in *T. cruzi*, for the simple reason that almost no drug destroys this organism *in vivo*, several workers have investigated and demonstrated resistance to various drugs in leishmaniasis, both in the clinic and in animal models.

In her review, Beveridge (1963) stressed that, although there was a great variation in the response to antimonials in different geographical areas, isolates from 'antimony-resistant' cases of *L. donovani* had shown a normal response to these drugs in hamsters. Moreover, such cases responded well to therapy with diamidines, although those with post-kala azar dermal leishmanoid may prove very refractory to such treatment (Sen Gupta 1968). Most simple cutaneous types of leishmaniasis due to *L. tropica* and the *L. mexicana* complex appear to respond well to therapy with antimonials, to cycloguanil embonate and to other drugs, and may even heal spontaneously. The *L. braziliensis* complex however produces cutaneous lesions that, while they regress and may appear to heal, often relapse after some time in the form of metastatic lesions, commonly involving mucocutaneous areas of the nose, palate and mouth. Against the late manifestations of this disease most drugs currently available offer at the best a poor means of treatment, although healing may eventually occur.

The most refractory type of leishmaniasis is disseminated cutaneous leishmaniasis, which has now been identified in Venezuela, Bolivia and Brazil, Ethiopia, Haute Volta and Nigeria. This condition, which is associated with a complete failure of cell-mediated immunity on the part of the patient, is caused by infection not with *L. braziliensis* but, as far as we know, with organisms of the *L. mexicana* and *L. tropica* complexes. The organisms in these patients rapidly develop a solid resistance to all forms of chemotherapy. Ercoli (1966) showed that '*L. pifanoi*' isolated from a patient with untreated diffuse cutaneous leishmaniasis responded well to Glucantime in mice, whereas another isolate made from a long-treated patient with this type of infection was resistant to this antimonial on passage to mice. The importance of the host immune response in chemotherapy cannot be too strongly stressed. Conversely, the ease with which a failure of this response may lead to the emergence of drug resistance is well exemplified in this disease.

Recently Walton (1970) has demonstrated, using serial titration of anti-leishmanial antibodies with an indirect fluorescent antibody test, that infection persists in many patients whose primary ulcers have apparently healed on treatment with cycloguanil embonate. Biopsy and skin culture in individuals who have been infected with Panamanian strains of the *L. braziliensis* complex, and have been found to have a constant antibody titre in spite of apparent healing of their lesions, have revealed the survival of living *Leishmania*. Treatment of some of these individuals with stibophen has resulted in a fall of the antibody titre to zero, and parasitological cure.

RECENT STUDIES OF DRUG ACTION IN TISSUE CULTURE

In this confusion of '*T. cruzi*' and *Leishmania* species and strains, not to mention host variation, what part does the actual drug sensitivity of the parasite play in the clinical response, what indeed is the baseline sensitivity of any given parasite isolate, to what degree is drug resistance a factor in treatment failure, how do the drugs act, and how, if at all, do the parasites become resistant to them? Existing models for the study of drug response in leishmaniasis are not adequate to resolve these questions. Liquid cultures of promastigotes present an entirely false picture since the metabolism of the organisms differs in important ways from that of the amastigote stages that infect the vertebrate. None of the usual *in vivo* models (*L. enriettii* in the guinea pig, *L. tropica* in the mouse, *L. donovani* in the hamster) provide data that have proved consistently referable to the human situation.

T. cruzi

Similarly, no truly satisfactory animal model has so far been reported for *T. cruzi*. Several investigators have resorted to the use of tissue culture for the maintenance of *T. cruzi* and the study of drug action on these organisms (Brener 1968), but very little work has been done with tissue culture models for the study of leishmanicides because of the relative difficulty of growing *Leishmania* organisms in this way. The use of tissue culture offers the advantage of a parasite–host system which, for both *T. cruzi* and *Leishmania* infection, eliminates the intervention of almost all host immunity (except possible effects of parasite-induced interferon). It also has the advantage of allowing one to observe the effect of the drugs on the intracellular amastigote forms of these parasites, the forms that are most inaccessible to exogenous substances and hence the most difficult to eliminate by the selective toxicity of chemotherapeutic agents.

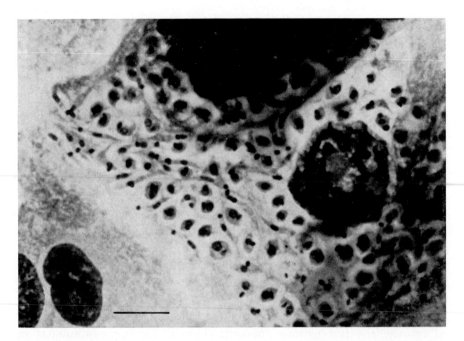

FIG. 1. An 8-day culture of *T. cruzi* in human amnion cells (KAM) grown at 35 °C. The cytoplasm of the host cell is filled with amastigotes and a number of trypomastigotes that are ready to erupt into the culture medium. Bar = 10 μm. (Original micrograph by Miss N. Mattock; Giemsa stain.)

We began our studies by establishing a strain of *T. cruzi* (Petana's strain from British Honduras) in a human amnion (KAM) cell line (Mattock & Peters 1972) and graduated from this to *L. mexicana mexicana* in a line of dog sarcoma cells (Mattock & Peters 1973). The main disadvantage of tissue culture models, apart from the technical problems involved, is the limited period during which useful observations can be made on the action of drugs to which they are exposed, i.e. in most cases some four days. Experience has shown that with most drugs showing some activity against either *T. cruzi* or *Leishmania* amastigotes in tissue culture the effect is only becoming maximal after this period; older cultures tend to become too overgrown for accurate observation and *T. cruzi* begins to transform into the trypomastigote stage (Fig. 1).

The few observations we have made on the action of drugs against *T. cruzi* are in line with those of earlier workers. Like da Silva & Kirchner (1962) we found primaquine to be ineffective against amastigotes, as were diamidines, trivalent and pentavalent antimonials. Amphotericin B proved to be slightly more toxic to the amastigotes than to the host cells. The nitrofurfurylidene compound, nifurtimox (Bayer 2502, Lampit), totally inhibited growth in parasites exposed to a concentration of 1–10 µg/ml for 72 h. Toxicity to host cells was observed after exposure to 20 µg/ml for the same time. Growth was also totally inhibited by 10 to 20 µg/ml after 48 h or 50 µg/ml concentration for 24 h. The therapeutic index of nifurtimox in this system, as indeed has been shown in man, is very narrow. Marsden *et al.* (1972) report that nifurtimox is only curative in mice at high, subtoxic dose levels that are continued for a long time, in spite of the fact that this drug rapidly clears most circulating trypomastigotes. Brener (1966) found that two other nitrofurantoin compounds, NF 902 and Furadantin sodium, at 7 µg/ml produced marked morphological changes in the amastigotes within 24 to 48 hours. Against circulating trypomastigotes nitrofurazone was very active *in vivo* (in mice) (Brener 1971), but again it is not curative against the amastigotes *in vivo*.

Nitrofurazone has, in contrast, been curative in some human infections with *T. rhodesiense* and *T. gambiense*, presumably because only trypomastigotes were present. Could the 'capriciousness' of its action (Hawking 1963) be related to the presence in later stages of infection with these African trypanosomes of amastigote tissue forms, as proposed by Soltys & Woo (1970) and Ormerod & Venkatesan (1971)?

Primaquine too exerts some action against circulating trypomastigotes in mice (Brener 1971) but, as mentioned above, has no action against the amastigotes in tissue culture, nor apparently *in vivo*.

It appears then that we can refer to 'resistance to therapy' in *T. cruzi* infection, but can we also refer to 'drug resistance'? Although there have been several references to drug-resistant strains of *T. cruzi*, these have been strains in which resistance has been induced by exposing epimastigotes in liquid culture to, for example, primaquine and to nitrofurazone (Amrein 1965). 'Resistance to therapy' develops because of the failure of any drugs we know at present to offer a sufficient degree of selective toxicity against the amastigote tissue forms, and to understand why this is so it is necessary to take a close look at the parasite–host relationship.

Leishmania

Before we consider the parasite–host relationship, however, let us consider the response to drugs of *L. mexicana mexicana* (Bray's L 11 strain) in the dog Sticker sarcoma cell line (SAMSO Série 503, kindly provided by Professor Lamy of the Pasteur Institute, Paris). The preliminary data that we have

TABLE 1

Preliminary data showing drug concentrations that prevent development of *L. mexicana mexicana* (Bray L 11 strain) in dog Sticker sarcoma cells (SAMSO série 503) in tissue culture at 33 °C, and concentrations toxic to host cells (original data provided by Miss N. Mattock)

Drug	Concentration and duration of exposure		Effect on intracellular parasites[a]	Effect on host cells	Notes
	µg/ml	(h)			
Pentamidine	50	(48)	—	Toxic	[b]
isethionate	20	(72)	+ +	Nil	20 (96) non-toxic to host
	10	(96)	+ +	Nil	cells, no action on extra-
	1	(96)	0	Nil	cellular amastigotes
Primaquine	20	(48)	—	Toxic	10 (96) non-toxic to host
phosphate	10	(72)	+ +	Nil	cells
	5	(72)	+ +	Nil	
	1	(96)	0	Nil	
Lithium Sb^{III}	10	(72)	—	Toxic	[b]
thiomalate	5	(96)	+	Nil	0.01-1.0 (96) slight effect
(Anthiomaline)	1	(96)	0	Nil	on extracellular amasti-gotes
Sodium Sb^{III}	100	(48)	—	Toxic	[b]
gluconate	50	(96)	0	Nil	50 (96) slight effect on
(Triostam)					extracellular amastigotes
Sodium Sb^{V}	10	(72)	—	Toxic	
gluconate	5	(96)	0	Nil	
(Pentostam)					
Nifurtimox	500	(48)	—	Toxic	100 (96) non-toxic to host
(Bayer 2502,	100	(24)	+ +	Nil	cells
Lampit)	50	(96)	+ +	Nil	
	25	(96)	0	Nil	
Cycloguanil	1.0	(72)	—	Toxic	
hydrochloride	1.0	(48)	+ +	Nil	
	0.5	(96)	0	Nil	
Amphotericin B	50	(48)	—	Toxic	5 (96) non-toxic to host
	10	(72)	—	Toxic	cells
	10	(48)	+ +	Nil	
	5	(48)	+ +	Nil	
	1	(72)	+ +	Nil	
	0.5	(96)	+ +	Nil	
	0.1	(72)	0	Nil	

[a] Cultures were observed for up to 96 h after first exposure to drug. At this time intracellular amastigote numbers are considerably reduced by active drugs, but all parasites may not yet have been eliminated.

— = effect on amastigotes cannot be distinguished because of toxic change in host cells;
+ = some reduction of parasite numbers compared with untreated controls;
+ + = few or no parasites present;
0 = parasite numbers approximately the same as in controls.

[b] The effect on extracellular parasites is assessed by observing the numbers taken up by host cells exposed to drug before the addition of a standard inoculum of amastigotes. This technique has not yet been applied to all the drugs shown above.

obtained so far in this system are summarized in Table 1. Neither the pentavalent antimonial, sodium stibogluconate (one of the best drugs in clinical use against cutaneous infections), nor two trivalent derivatives, lithium antimony thiomalate and sodium antimonyl gluconate, completely inhibit growth of the amastigotes even after exposure for 96 h to drug concentrations that are non-toxic to the host cells. Beveridge (1963) noted that pentavalent antimonials also have little effect on promastigotes in culture medium, and suggested that they have first to be metabolized by the organism to the trivalent form before they are active *in vivo*.

There is a considerable variation in the response to sodium stibogluconate in different *in vivo* models. Moreover, as mentioned above, Ercoli (1966) demonstrated clearly that resistance can arise to this type of compound (in his case the related pentavalent Glucantime) during the course of therapy in the absence of an effective immune response mediated by host cells. Clinically the trivalent antimonial, stibophen, has proved of value and we intend to examine this in our tissue culture system.

Pentamidine isethionate, a very effective drug for the treatment of visceral infection with *L. donovani*, has proved to be only marginally active against the amastigotes of *L. mexicana*, with a therapeutic index of about 2. Another clinically useful compound, cycloguanil, is marginally active at a dose level that is just tolerated by the host cells. However it is the slowly released repository formulation of the embonate that is employed clinically. This is known to produce persistent but extremely low blood levels (well below 1 μg/ml) over several months. Neal (1972) has been able to demonstrate only slight, if any, activity with the embonate in hamsters infected with a variety of *Leishmania* isolates, including one from a man whose lesion responded rapidly to this compound.

Nifurtimox has an inhibitory action on *L. mexicana* amastigotes but the therapeutic index appears to be similar to that in the *T. cruzi* model. Only one compound that we have tested so far has shown itself to be both inhibitory at a very low concentration, and selectively toxic. Amphotericin B has a therapeutic index of about 10 in tissue culture. In Brazil it has been used successfully for the treatment of kala azar in children who no longer respond to pentamidine, and against mucocutaneous lesions. Side effects are common with therapeutic doses, and it should therefore be used only as a second-line drug in resistant cases (Prata 1963; Sampaio *et al.* 1971).

So far we have only been able to study the response of a single parasite strain in a particular host cell to a small number of drugs. Quite clearly the programme must be extended to cover a wide spectrum of *Leishmania* species, and, within each species, isolates from many different sources. These sources will, we hope, include individual patients at different times during the course of therapy, different patients with similar lesions, patients with the same type of lesion but exhibiting different responses to the same drug, and so on. We find ourselves confronted from the start with the problem of deciding exactly what constitutes a leishmanial species (or subspecies). In order to help resolve this question we have been obliged to institute, in collaboration with our colleagues in the field, an investigation into the biochemical characteristics of *Leishmania* isolates that may, we hope, eventually provide a biochemical classification of this genus. Our preliminary data (Chance *et al.* 1973) indicate some interesting distinctions as well as affinities, but further elaboration of this topic is beyond the scope of the present paper.

Unlike *T. cruzi*, several *Leishmania* species have displayed clinically a clear-cut resistance to pentavalent antimonials, to pentamidine and to cycloguanil. Sen Gupta (1968) has underlined that post-kala azar dermal leishmanoid does not respond to antimonials, and responds only poorly to diamidines. This condition is an interesting example of a 'dissociated immunity' in which the viscera no longer support the organisms, whereas the skin does. An interesting feature of such cases is that *L. donovani*, on transfer to the hamster, display a normal response to antimonials (Beveridge & Neal 1967). A remarkable and paradoxical situation was described by Ercoli (1970), who stated that *L. enriettii* may be found in the viscera of the guinea pig after the dermal lesions have been cured with antimonials. This would appear to imply that the viscerally located amastigotes are resistant to the drugs.

While diamidines have generally proved of most value against visceral leishmaniasis, both experimentally and in man, Neal (1964) found that pentamidine was only active at toxic doses against *L. tropica major* infection in mice. Clinically, in addition to the case of post-kala azar dermal leishmanoid described above, Manson-Bahr (1959) and Wijers (1971) found that East African kala azar responds poorly to diamidines, and a similar situation appears to exist in the Sudan and Somaliland.

Although cycloguanil embonate has given good results in the treatment of cutaneous and mucocutaneous leishmaniasis in Panama, Costa Rica and the Lebanon, treatment failure is not uncommon (Walton *et al.* 1968) and Walton (1970) has shown that these patients may not respond to subsequent doses of this compound. They may be cured, however, by stibophen. Neal (1972) found little correlation between the *in vivo* response to cycloguanil embonate in man and that in the hamster.

The most serious situation as regards drug resistance is seen in patients with diffuse cutaneous leishmaniasis in whom there appears to be a complete failure of cell-mediated immunity. Convit *et al.* (1959) in Venezuela, followed by

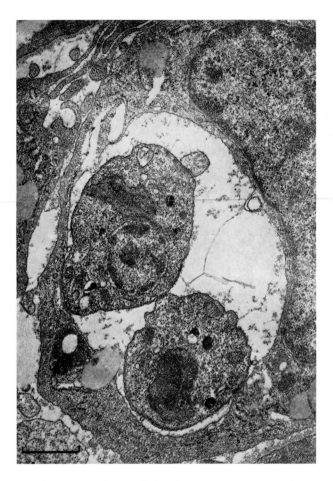

Fɪɢ. 2. Electron micrograph showing two *T. cruzi* in mouse heart muscle. One trypomastigote (with adherent flagellum) and one amastigote lie within a vacuole in a host cell of undetermined origin. Bar = 1 μm. (Original electron micrograph by P. J. Gardener.)

Balzer *et al.* (1960) in Ethiopia, drew attention to the failure of both pentavalent antimonials and diamidines in these patients. Although at first the Venezuelan cases were attributed to an organism described as *L. pifanoi*, it now seems most likely that this form of cutaneous leishmaniasis may arise in any anergic individual as a result of infection with any of the dermatropic *Leishmania* that cause the common form of skin ulceration in any given locality. Thus the Ethiopian cases are caused by the local variety of *L. tropica*, those in Venezuela by a local strain, probably of *L. mexicana pifanoi*, and those in the Amazon delta by *L. mexicana amazonensis*. All these organisms therefore appear to have

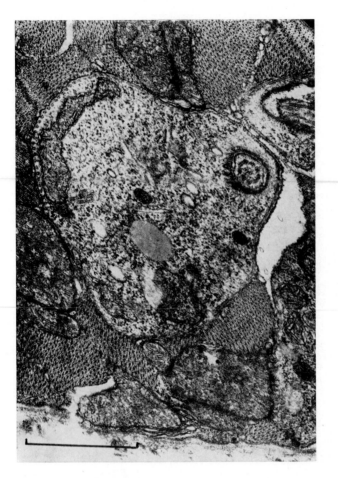

FIG. 3. Electron micrograph of a *T. cruzi* amastigote in mouse heart muscle to show the intimate anatomical relationship that commonly develops between the parasite and the host
tissues. Bar = 1 μm. (Original electron micrograph by P. J. Gardener.)

the ability, in the absence of a satisfactory host response, rapidly to develop
resistance to antileishmanial drugs.

Does our limited experience in tissue culture models and the above clinical
evidence indicate that in leishmaniasis, as in *T. cruzi* infection, chemotherapy
does little to affect the intracellular amastigote stages and only attacks the
parasites extracellularly in association with host immunity? Certainly this is
true of *T. cruzi*, where we have shown that the circulating trypomastigotes are
susceptible to drugs. In leishmanial infection are the parasites only susceptible
during the brief periods when they are being released from one dying host cell

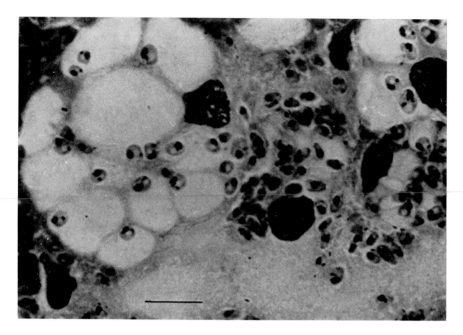

FIG. 4a. Amastigotes of *L. mexicana amazonensis* (strain PH8) in a smear made from a granuloma on the foot of a hamster. Note the marked vacuolation of the cytoplasm of several of the host macrophages.

and waiting to be taken up by another? To consider this question too we must take a close look at the host–parasite relationships.

THE IMPORTANCE OF THE HOST–PARASITE RELATIONSHIP

Morphological relationships

With the exception of the tissue stages of the African trypanosomes to which reference was made above, the parasites may be considered as dwelling in tissue spaces and in the peripheral circulation, where they are freely exposed to circulating and diffused chemical agents, antibodies, phagocytes, etc. Of the organisms discussed in this paper, the African trypanosomes are not only the most susceptible to chemotherapy but also the most capable of developing drug resistance. Their very accessibility ensures this.

The situation is similar in the trypomastigote stages of *T. cruzi* (Fig. 2), as already discussed, although in this case we really do not know whether repeated

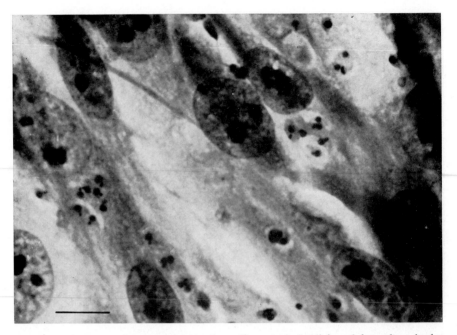

FIG. 4b. Amastigotes of *L. mexicana mexicana* (Bray strain L 11) in a 6-day culture in dog
Sticker sarcoma cells (SAMSO série 503) kept at 33 °C. An early stage of host cell vacuolation
can be seen around several parasites. Bar = 10 μm. (Original micrographs by Miss N.
Mattock; Giemsa stain.)

exposure of trypomastigotes to drugs leads to drug resistance *in vivo*, since
parasitic relapses are due to the production of fresh waves of trypomastigotes
from the amastigote tissue forms. The latter are most commonly in very
intimate anatomical contact with their host cells. This is seen particularly well
in electron micrographs (Figs. 3, 4).

   Leishmania amastigotes are believed to reside in phagocytic cells of the skin
and viscera, the site depending on the species and strain. The amastigote stage
is probably the only one that occurs in the vertebrate host, at least in mammals.
The contact with the host cells, while showing certain differences from that of
T. cruzi, is equally intimate, and it is easy to envisage the difficulties inherent in
the passage of a drug or antibody from the serum to the interior of the parasite.
Moreover, these amastigotes dwell in precisely those host cells that should be
concerned in their destruction. They must therefore have a finely evolved
mechanism which enables them to survive unharmed, and indeed to thrive and
multiply in the host cells (Fig. 5). One can readily understand how difficult
it is to find selectively toxic compounds with which to attack the amastigotes
of either *T. cruzi* or *Leishmania*.

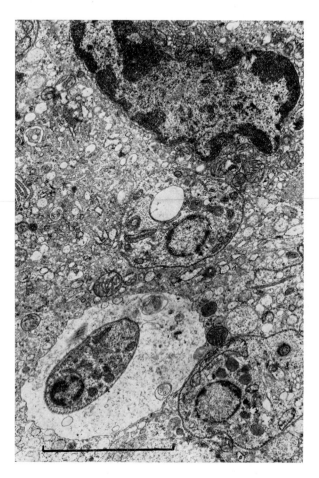

FIG. 5. Electron micrograph showing a macrophage from a granuloma on a hamster nose containing three amastigotes of *L. chagasi* (strain M884). Two of the parasites lie in intimate contact with the cytoplasm of the host cell, while the third is situated within a membrane-lined vacuole. Bar = 5 μm. (Original electron micrograph by P. J. Gardener.)

Host immunity

The paradoxical nature of the host responses in *T. cruzi* infection, and in visceral, cutaneous and diffuse forms of leishmaniasis, have been touched on above and are considered in more detail in reviews by Köberle (1968) and Bray (1972), respectively. What is not known in these infections is the role, if any, played by antigenic variation in the relapse pattern seen in both Chagas' disease and leishmaniasis. Antigenic variation is of major importance in the African trypanosomiases, and is possibly of importance also in the development of drug resistance by these organisms.

Finally we are left with two other unknown factors concerning the host–parasite relationship. The first of these is the possible role of interferon in the response to intracellular infection by these parasites. The second is the possible immunosuppressive effect that the infections themselves may have on the host. Here are yet two more questions to ponder in our consideration of the phenomenon of drug action and drug failure in Chagas' disease and the leishmaniases.

SUMMARY

Drug resistance is a common phenomenon in the African trypanosomiases, rare in infection with *T. cruzi* and relatively uncommon in the leishmaniases. Preliminary studies of drug responses of the intracellular amastigote stages of *T. cruzi* and *Leishmania* species emphasize that few drugs exert a selective toxicity against them. It is suggested that compounds used *in vivo* against these infections act essentially on free extracellular parasites, whether the circulating trypomastigotes of *T. cruzi* or the static amastigotes of *Leishmania*. To a large degree therefore, it is argued, the problem in these conditions is rather one of 'resistance to therapy' than of 'drug resistance', except in certain types of leishmaniasis, namely post-kala azar dermal leishmanoid and diffuse cutaneous leishmaniasis, where true drug resistance occurs. The intimate contact between parasite and host is considered to create a serious obstacle to the development of compounds with selective toxicity against these organisms.

ACKNOWLEDGEMENTS

The studies discussed here are being carried out by the author and his colleagues, in particular Miss N. Mattock, Dr M. L. Chance, Mr P. J. Gardener, Dr R. E. Howells and Dr D. H. Molyneux, with generous support from the Wellcome Trust and from the Division of Parasitic Diseases, World Health Organization, Geneva. The author wishes to acknowledge also the collaboration of Drs R. Lainson and J. J. Shaw in Belém, Professor R. S. Bray and Dr R. W. Ashford in Addis Ababa, and Dr A. Herrer in Panama.

References

AMREIN, Y. U. (1965) Genetic transfer in trypanosomes: 1. Syngamy in *Trypanosoma cruzi*. *Exp. Parasitol.* **17**, 261-263

BALZER, R. J., DESTOMBES, P., SCHALLER, K. F. & SÉRIÉ, CH. (1960) Leishmaniose cutanée pseudolépromateuse en Ethiopie. *Bull. Soc. Pathol. Exot.* **53**, 293-298

BEVERIDGE, E. (1963) in *Experimental Chemotherapy* (Schnitzer, R. J. & Hawking, F., eds.), vol. 1, pp. 257-287, Academic Press, New York

BEVERIDGE, E. & NEAL, R. A. (1967) Chemotherapy of cutaneous and visceral leishmaniasis in laboratory animals. *Dermatol. Int.* **6**, 163-164

BRAY, R. S. (1972) Leishmaniasis in the Old World. *Br. Med. Bull.* **28**, 39-43

BRENER, Z. (1965) Comparative studies of different strains of *Trypanosoma cruzi. Ann. Trop. Med. Parasitol.* **59**, 19-26

BRENER, Z. (1966) Chemotherapeutic studies in tissue cultures infected with *Trypanosoma cruzi:* the mode of action of some active compounds. *Ann. Trop. Med. Parasitol.* **60**, 445-451

BRENER, Z. (1968) Quimioterapia da doença de Chagas, in *Medicina Tropical (Libro Homenajo al Professor Dr Felix Pifano)*, (Anselmi, A., ed.), pp. 351-363, Editorial Fournier, Mexico

BRENER, Z. (1971) Study of the action of some active drugs against *Trypanosoma cruzi* blood forms. *Rev. Inst. Med. Trop. São Paulo* **13**, 302-306

BRENER, Z. & CHIARI, E. (1967) Susceptibilidade de diferentes amostras de *Trypanosoma cruzi* a vários agentes quimioterápicos. *Rev. Inst. Med. Trop. São Paulo* **9**, 197-207

CHANCE, M. L., PETERS, W. & GRIFFITHS, H. W. (1973) A comparative study of DNA in the genus *Leishmania. Trans. R. Soc. Trop. Med. Hyg.* **67**, 24-45

CONVIT, J., ALARCON, C. J., MEDINA, R., REYES, O. & VARGAS, F. K. (1959) Leishmaniasis tegumentaria difusa. Nueva entidad clinico-patologica parasitaria. *Arch. Venez. Med. Trop. Parasitol. Med.* **3**, 218-251

ERCOLI, N. (1966) Drug responsiveness in experimental cutaneous leishmaniasis. *Exp. Parasitol.* **19**, 320-326

ERCOLI, N. (1970) Studies on the control of experimental leishmaniasis. *J. Parasitol.* **56**, 93-94

GONZÁLEZ CAPPA, S. M. & KAGAN, I. G. (1969) Agar gel and immunoelectrophoretic analysis of several strains of *Trypanosoma cruzi. Exp. Parasitol.* **25**, 50-57

GRAY, A. R. & ROBERTS, C. J. (1971) The cyclical transmission of strains of *Trypanosoma congolense* and *T. vivax* resistant to normal therapeutic doses of trypanocidal drugs. *Parasitology* **63**, 67-89

HAWKING, F. (1963) in *Experimental Chemotherapy* (Schnitzer, R. J. & Hawking, F., eds.), vol. 1, pp. 129-256, Academic Press, New York

KÖBERLE, F. (1968) Chagas' disease and Chagas' syndromes: the pathology of American trypanosomiases. *Adv. Parasitol,* **6**, 63-116

LAINSON, R. & SHAW, J. J. (1972) Leishmaniasis of the New World: taxonomic problems. *Br. Med. Bull.* **28**, 44-48

MACLENNAN, K. J. R. (1970) in *The African Trypanosomiases* (Mulligan, H. W., ed.), pp. 799-821, Allen & Unwin, London

MANSON-BAHR, P. E. C. (1959) East African kala-azar with special reference to the pathology, prophylaxis and treatment. *Trans. R. Soc. Trop. Med. Hyg.* **53**, 123-136

MARSDEN, P. D., MILES, M. A., PATTERSON, J. W. & PETTITT, L. E. (1972) Preliminary studies on the efficacy of Bayer 2502 (Lampit) for treatment of *Trypanosoma cruzi* (strain 7) infection in CF1 mice. *Trans. R. Soc. Trop. Med. Hyg.* **66**, 508-510

MATTOCK, N. & PETERS, W. (1972) An *in vitro* system for chemotherapy studies on amastigote forms of *T. cruzi* and *Leishmania. Trans. R. Soc. Trop. Med. Hyg.* **66**, 10

MATTOCK, N. & PETERS, W. (1973) Chemotherapy of leishmaniasis: a method for screening potential leishmanicides. *Trans. R. Soc. Trop. Med. Hyg.* **67**, 22

NEAL, R. A. (1964) Chemotherapy of cutaneous leishmaniasis: *Leishmania tropica* infections in mice. *Ann. Trop. Med. Parasitol.* **58**, 420-430

NEAL, R. A. (1972) Effect of dihydrofolate reductase inhibitors on experimental cutaneous leishmaniasis, with especial emphasis on *Leishmania* isolates from Latin America. *Rev. Inst. Med. Trop. São Paulo,* **14**, 341-351

ORMEROD, W. E. & VENKATESAN, S. (1971) The occult visceral phase of mammalian trypanosomes with special reference to the life cycle of *Trypanosoma (Trypanozoon) brucei. Trans. R. Soc. Trop. Med. Hyg.* **65**, 722-736

PRATA, A. (1963) Treatment of kala-azar with amphotericin B. *Trans. R. Soc. Trop. Med. Hyg.* **57**, 266-268

SAMPAIO, S. A. P., CASTRO, R. M., DILLON, N. L. & COSTA MARTINS, J. E. (1971) Treatment of mucocutaneous (American) leishmaniasis with amphotericin B: report of 70 cases. *Int. J. Dermatol.* **10**, 179-181

SEN GUPTA, P. C. (1968) in *Medicina Tropical (Libro Homenajo al Professor Dr Felix Pifano)*, (Anselmi, A., ed.), pp. 73-79, Editorial Fournier, Mexico

SILVA, L. H. P. DA & KIRCHNER, E. (1962) Experimental chemotherapy of *Trypanosoma cruzi* infection in tissue culture. A comparative study on the action of primaquine, carbidium sulphate and the aminonucleoside of stylomycin. *Rev. Inst. Med. Trop. São Paulo* **4**, 16-28

SOLTYS, M. A. & WOO, P. (1970) Further studies on tissue forms of *Trypanosoma brucei* in a vertebrate host. *Trans. R. Soc. Trop. Med. Hyg.* **64**, 692-694

WADDY, B. B. (1970) in *The African Trypanosomiases* (Mulligan, H. W., ed.), pp. 711-725, Allen & Unwin, London

WALTON, B. C. (1970) The indirect fluorescent antibody test for evaluation of effectiveness of chemotherapy in American leishmaniasis. *J. Parasitol.* **56**, 480-481

WALTON, B. C., PERSON, D. A., ELLMAN, M. H. & BERNSTEIN, R. (1968) Treatment of American cutaneous leishmaniasis with cycloguanil pamoate. *Am. J. Trop. Med. Hyg.* **17**, 814-818

WIJERS, D. J. B. (1971) A ten years' study of kala-azar in Tharaka (Meru district, Kenya). Part II: Relapses. *East Afr. Med. J.* **48**, 551-558

WILLIAMSON, J. (1970) in *The African Trypanosomiases* (Mulligan, H. W., ed.), pp. 125-221, Allen & Unwin, London

WILSON, R. E. (1972) The effect of five-membered ring compounds on the epimastigote form of *Trypanosoma cruzi*. M. Sc. thesis, Dept of Microbiology, California State College, Long Beach

Discussion

Martinez-Silva: How do you determine the effectiveness of a drug on parasites?

Peters: We allow the host cells to grow for a day or two, infect them with the organisms and start treatment a day or two later. We take coverslips out and stain them and so on after 24, 48, 72 and 96 h.

Martinez-Silva: We have done similar work on the effects of drugs on *T. cruzi* and, in general, our results are the same as yours. We inoculate the cells and five days later, when we see a heavy infection, we start giving the drug. We change the medium to which the drug is added three times a week. After removing the drug we observe the cells daily for the presence of parasites in the medium. With some drugs, such as amphotericin B, no parasites were observed in the medium for a week; however, if incubation was extended, parasites began to be seen. With other substances such as antitumour drugs (actinomycin D) the same schedule totally suppresses infection, but this favourable effect could not be reproduced *in vivo* in mice. We conclude, maybe incorrectly, that the well balanced host–parasite relationship existing in tissue culture is easy to change with drugs because of the many factors involved. This seemed to be confirmed with a substance, synthesized by a colleague, thioxanthone sulph-oxide, which gave good results *in vitro* but did not affect the course of infection *in vivo* at all.

Peters: We are not using this system as a drug screen but are simply trying to show how certain drugs work that are known to have a clinical action. A new drug tested in this way naturally may not work at all *in vivo*.

Martinez-Silva: It is well known that *T. cruzi* induces interferon but inter-feron has no effect at all on the course of *T. cruzi* infection. We used poly (I, C), a potent interferon-inducer, in mice as well as in tissue culture, and followed the course of infection in these models (Martinez-Silva *et al.* 1970). Results were similar *in vitro* in both treated and control groups; in mice, how-ever, because of the toxicity of poly (I, C), the result was an enhancement of the infection.

Peters: A synthetic RNA inducer of interferon that we tested in the tissue culture system appeared to have the paradoxical effect of giving better growth of organisms with no obvious toxic effects on the host cells.

Bray: How does it do that? There must be cells in the tissue culture that are producing interferon.

At the other end of the scale, I believe that some unpublished work of Dr D. J. Bradley indicates that leishmania in an immune animal no longer synthesize DNA, although the parasites sit there and can be seen after staining —they are not incorporating tritiated thymidine. We have to be careful about just looking at a parasite without some other criteria of viability. In our cytotoxic experiments for two years now we have been concerned about whether we are looking at a dead parasite: our experiment may have suc-ceeded—that is we killed the beast—but may be registered as negative because we have stained an apparently perfectly good parasite. The same thing may apply to *L. enriettii* in the inner organs: is it alive? On occasion, at least, one should inoculate these tissue cultures into an animal and, if parasites are present, see whether they are infective.

Newton: It might be dangerous to assume that a parasite is not synthesizing DNA just because it doesn't incorporate tritiated thymidine.

Bray: I agree, but at least it is an indication that something may be wrong.

Newton: It is an indication that the parasite does not have a functional 'salvage pathway' or that it is impermeable to tritiated thymidine.

Bray: Normally they are taking up tritiated thymidine, and under some conditions they are not taking it up. At least it makes one suspicious about the organism in the latter case.

I didn't entirely agree with you, Professor Peters, about the non-importance of drug resistance in sleeping sickness. Certainly in the days before Mel B

(melarsoprol), resistance to tryparsamide was a nuisance in West Africa with
T. gambiense infection.

In curing diffuse cutaneous leishmaniasis with pentamidine in Ethiopia,
Bryceson (1969, 1970) got what he thought were conversions from delayed
hypersensitivity-negative to delayed hypersensitivity-positive in a few cases,
but we now know that all these patients relapsed. Only three cases of diffuse
cutaneous leishmaniasis were completely cured and have never relapsed.
Every one of them is still negative in delayed hypersensitivity tests and their
lymphocytes are completely inactive in relation to the antigen. So your warning
about diffuse cutaneous leishmaniasis and getting rid of the last parasite is
quite correct. I believe that these patients are, as it were, at the 'leishmanatous'
leishmaniasis end of the spectrum and that the clone of lymphocytes responsible
for dealing with leishmanial antigen has been utterly wiped out in them so
that one won't be able to get it back by 'transfer factor' or any other attempted
reactivation.

Peters: I cannot comment on that, but I do agree that simply because one
sees a parasite does not necessarily mean it is alive. However, we can often
obtain positive skin cultures with plenty of leishmanial organisms from apparently normal healthy rodents. I did not, incidentally, intend to imply that
drug resistance was not important in African sleeping sickness.

Lumsden: Hawking (1962) showed that the organisms in the cases resistant
to melarsoprol were drug-resistant when he transferred them into mice. But it
seemed to me that nitrofurazone had a definite application in a special clinical
situation. That is in the odd 5% of cases that are melarsoprol-resistant and
cannot be cured in any other way, when it is justifiable to take the risks associated with nitrofurazone. Didn't both Apted and Robertson (see Robertson
1962) get successful cures with this drug in these situations?

de Raadt: That is true, but because only infections resistant to Mel B or
Mel W are treated with nitrofurazone, this drug has little chance of being
properly evaluated, simply because of the way the patients are selected. I do
not think that the accessibility of the parasite to the drug plays a role because
there is a genuine phenomenon of drug resistance, for instance against Mel B,
which is still a great problem in Africa. When such resistant strains are inoculated into mice, they show clearly the reduced sensitivity to the drug. This
problem is related to current practice in treating human trypanosomiasis. In
order to avoid adverse side reactions small doses are given at the beginning of
treatment and increased step by step later. This, of course, is an invitation for
resistance to occur.

Njogu: We are now using nitrofurazone for the cases resistant to Mel B.
Dr Baker isolated a strain of *T. brucei* from a fly in Ethiopia recently which

when tested for drug sensitivity was found to be resistant to several of the drugs we tested. What is the mechanism of drug resistance here? If this strain was *T. rhodesiense* and if this trend spread, we would be in real danger. As far as I know the bad usage of drugs in Ethiopia is not widespread.

Baker: How resistant was that strain? The criteria you used seemed to be extremely delicate ones—quite justifiably because you were testing it before possibly giving it to a human volunteer—but I didn't think it was significantly resistant clinically.

Njogu: We were using Walker & Watts' (1970) criteria for drug resistance, which are rather different from others. The strain was considered to be resistant if the minimum curative dose of the drug was higher than the usual curative dose, irrespective of whether the strain was sensitive to higher doses below the maximum tolerated dose. It was resistant to Suramin (at 1.5 × normal dose), Ethidium (12.5 × normal dose) and Berenil (7 × normal dose) but sensitive to Mel B and Antrycide.

Baker: Walker's drug levels were exceedingly low, probably less than the therapeutic dose, if one can extrapolate from mice to men.

Bray: From Hutchinson's work (1971) in Ethiopia there is no doubt that Mel B was remarkably successful in some human cases, provided that one takes into account that this was a new disease to these people and that they were coming to treatment fairly late and fairly moribund. Hutchinson was very pleased with the drug in these circumstances. Suramin didn't get much of a test because this was an extremely vicious strain where central nervous system symptoms were turning up on occasions while the primary chancre was still there. Nearly all the patients he treated were CNS cases, so Mel B was the main drug in use.

Baker: But what can be the mechanism for clinical resistance in Ethiopia, where there is no history of prior, possibly inadequate, treatment?

Goodwin: Perhaps, like the mepacrine-resistant Wewak strain of malaria, it just happens to be there.

Newton: I think Dr Njogu's point was whether we knew anything about the mechanism of resistance developing as a result of exposing organisms to low or normal concentrations of drugs. The answer seems to be that we know very little indeed.

Baker: Surely there can be a spectrum of resistance in any organism, and Dr Njogu's strain may simply be a little more resistant to drugs than other strains.

Njogu: I agree. The point is that it is resistant to several types of drugs, and if this resistance is very great, it would be dangerous if an epidemic occurred.

de Raadt: There is no doubt that resistance against the maximum tolerated dose occurs and that such strains retain their resistance after cyclical transmission (van Hoeve & Grainge 1966).

Baker: Does this resistance develop spontaneously without previous exposure to the drug?

Peters: There are other parallels. One well-known example occurs in malaria in rodents, which has certainly never been treated with any drugs. In the low-lying areas of tropical West Africa, *Plasmodium berghei yoelii* has an inherent resistance, if you want to call it that, to chloroquine, mepacrine and various other drugs. The Katanga highlands form of *P. berghei berghei*, which is what we call sensitive, just shows a different baseline level of response. It is simply made that way. In terms of acquired resistance there is a certain amount of information, for example, from the work of Frank Hawking (1937), who reported a reduced uptake of arsenicals by resistant trypanosomes.

Goodwin: It is not so surprising that they should be different; it would be more surprising if they were all the same.

Newton: I think the use of the term 'resistance' in this discussion has become rather confusing. Perhaps we should use 'lack of sensitivity' or 'insensitivity' to describe innate resistance to a drug and keep 'resistance' for the situation which develops after exposure to a drug.

Zeledón: Camolar (cycloguanil) was used for the first time against leishmaniasis in Costa Rica by Peña-Chavarría *et al.* (1965), who were interested in finding a drug which would be effective when given in one or two shots only. With Camolar in an oil suspension they obtained good results with a single shot. Glucantime was introduced into Costa Rica fairly recently and people are already being infected with strains apparently resistant to it. The injections are very painful and since the patients live far away from our medical centres, after two or three injections they don't return to finish the treatment. That is why Dr Peña-Chevarría was looking for a repository effect. You mentioned that we need new lines, Professor Peters, and this form of therapy for leishmaniasis is worth remembering.

Peters: I think the problem with Glucantime is patient resistance. I would not like to accept that the parasites are themselves resistant to Glucantime. A repository drug is obviously very important in the treatment of any condition where one cannot reach the patients, or when they run home because they have to work their farms and so on.

Zeledón: I saw a patient who within the last few years has had three complete courses of treatment with Glucantime. He has relapses every few months.

Goodwin: There is a well-known case of a man with kala azar who was treated with course after course of diamidines and pentavalent antimonials of all kinds. Eventually he had his spleen out and the case was written up (Morton & Cooke 1948) as having been cured. However, he later relapsed and died of the disease. At various times I transmitted his parasites to hamsters and on every occasion they were shown to be sensitive to antimony. It was not drug resistance but drug failure—an unusual way in which the patient dealt with the drug.

I am quite sure that one can find, in different parts of the world, strains of parasites which are more resistant to antimony, for some reason, than they are elsewhere. I am not in the least surprised that Professor Peters didn't find any activity from pentavalent antimonials of the type joined through oxygen to the carbon. These drugs, under whatever name, are simply solutions of antimony pentoxide in a highly hydroxylated organic medium and making them is cookery, not chemistry. One can make such a drug to contain any amount of antimony, and to have any degree of toxicity; one has to choose a method of making it which provides a reasonable product, with reasonable activity and reasonably low toxicity. When one puts it into a patient about 80 or 90 % of the antimony it contains is excreted by the kidneys in the first few hours, so one is relying on what is left in the animal, soaked into the tissue cells, which later reduce it to trivalent antimony (Goodwin & Page 1943). This is the killer, hopefully, of the parasite but unfortunately sometimes of the patient. This is very difficult to test in tissue culture, and my heart goes out to those doing it.

The use of cycloguanil or pyrimethamine in leishmaniasis constitutes an almost unbelievable situation. Professor Trager said earlier (p. 283) that folate was needed and that the parasite can't manage on PABA. Neither Ralph Neal nor I have ever found these substances to have any activity on this parasite in the laboratory. Perhaps we have stumbled on something that acts on the parasite so that the host's defence mechanisms get at it more effectively.

Bray: Berberine sulphate acts something like this in leishmaniasis. Parasites couldn't care less about it and yet it does appear occasionally to cure oriental sore.

Newton: Antrycide may act in a similar way. It appears not to be trypanocidal *in vivo* or *in vitro*; it reduces the rate of growth to a level at which host defence mechanisms compete with and overcome the parasite. Sen *et al.* (1955) have shown that in immunosuppressed or splenectomized animals Antrycide will not clear an infection.

Njogu: A. C. Zahalsky (unpublished results) in our laboratory put a very heavy dose of Antrycide into rats infected with *T. brucei*. The trypanosomes seemed to have been stopped dead as they were dividing.

Bray: In order to prove that the hyrax parasite was the same as a human parasite I infected myself with it and then, once that came up, I decided I wanted to cure myself. When I looked at the array of chemotherapeutics available I had the lesion cut out by a surgeon.

Baker: This doesn't necessarily prove it was the same parasite; it may prove that you are a hyrax!

Peters: Whatever drugs we give, we are simply providing one small bit of assistance to the host. It is really the host's immune processes, if he has any, that are going to get rid of the infection. That is the only lesson we can learn from all this.

Trager: You also raised a good point about the possible activity of lysosomes against intracellular parasites, Professor Peters. Clearly these parasites, from their point of view, have solved their problem, because they even get into a cell like a macrophage which is the digester *par excellence*. The main function of macrophages is to produce lysosomes and the primary lysosomal vacuoles just don't empty their contents into the place where the parasite is, even if it is in a vacuole in a membrane-bounded structure. Of course, in some circumstances it seems not even to be in that. If *L. donovani* is in a membrane-bounded vacuole, the acid phosphatase is not being secreted into that vacuole. Dr C. de Duve has suggested experiments with drugs that might stimulate lysosome formation and activity. It might be interesting to see whether such drugs would have some effect, at least in tissue culture, on the intracellular parasites.

Newton: Also parasites are only resistant to lysosomal digestion so long as they are viable.

Bray: It has been assumed in the past that resistance to macrophage digestion is some function of the parasite wall, particularly in the mycobacteria with their peculiar waxy wall, and that surfactants might alter the wall so that the macrophage can start getting at the parasite. That has not been followed up very far.

Goble: We did some work on surfactants, but that is a long story (Goble *et al.* 1960).

Baker: Akiyama & Haight (1971), working with *L. donovani* in tissue cultures found that parasites in a vacuole were subsequently killed.

Martinez-Silva: In that work the formation of vacuoles was followed by lysis of the promastigote, while the parasites escaping vacuolization evolved into amastigote-like forms. In our studies of *T. cruzi* in tissue-cultured fibroblasts the host–parasite relationship seems to be so smooth that the cells continue to metabolize and divide like non-infected ones. Division of infected cells can proceed and lead to formation of colonies. In some cases we have observed division of cells with 23 parasites, which were distributed between both daughter cells.

Vickerman: We are studying the uptake of strains of *L. mexicana* by mouse peritoneal macrophages in culture. These certainly have a lysosome response. Acid phosphatase is present in the vacuole surrounding the parasite, but we are not sure that this is an infective strain. We would like to be able to do it again with an infective strain.

Baker: Were those parasites going to survive or be killed?

Trager: Jones & Hirsch (1972) at the Rockefeller made available to macrophages live toxoplasmas and toxoplasmas which had been killed with glutaraldehyde. The macrophages had their lysosomes previously labelled by exposure to Thorotrast. In the electron microscope Jones and Hirsch could see the primary lysosomal vacuoles labelled with Thorotrast granules, which show up as black dots. The live toxoplasmas were in membrane-bounded vacuoles. However, in no instance was there any fusion of the Thorotrast-containing vesicles with these vacuoles containing live toxoplasmas. On the contrary, the membranes become surrounded by mitochondria and endoplasmic reticulum. But in the vacuoles which had taken up the glutaraldehyde-killed toxoplasmas, there was very active fusion of the Thorotrast-containing vesicles with the vacuoles.

Bray: It would be extremely interesting to add the products of lymphocyte activation to the same system, whether it be *Toxoplasma* or *Leishmania*, and see whether one gets something the same as in leprosy and in listeriosis (Godal *et al.* 1971; Mackaness 1969), where these products convert the macrophage into what Mackaness calls the 'angry macrophage', which should then start pouring its enzymes in. Mackaness says that you can make a macrophage so angry you daren't put your finger in the culture!

References

AKIYAMA, H. J. & HAIGHT, R. D. (1971) Interaction of *Leishmania donovani* and hamster peritoneal macrophages. A phase-contrast microscopical study. *Am. J. Trop. Med. Hyg.* **20**, 539-545

BRYCESON, A. D. M. (1969) Diffuse cutaneous leishmaniasis in Ethiopia. I: Clinical and histological features of the disease. *Trans. R. Soc. Trop. Med. Hyg.* **63**, 708-737

BRYCESON, A. D. M. (1970) Diffuse cutaneous leishmaniasis in Ethiopia. II: Treatment. *Trans. R. Soc. Trop. Med. Hyg.* **64**, 369-379

GOBLE, F. C., BOYD, J. L. & FULTON, J. D. (1960) Effects of certain surface-active poly-oxyethylene ethers in experimental protozoal infections. *J. Protozool.* **7** (4), 384-390

GODAL, T., REES, R. J. W. & LAMVIK, J. O. (1971) Lymphocyte mediated modification of blood derived macrophage function *in vitro;* including inhibition of growth of intracellular mycobacteria. *Clin. Exp. Immunol.* **8**, 625-637

GOODWIN, L. G. & PAGE, J. E. (1943) A study of the excretion of organic antimonials using a polarographic procedure. *Biochem. J.* **37**, 198-209

HAWKING, F. (1937) Studies on chemotherapeutic action. I: The absorption of arsenical compounds and tartar emetic by normal and resistant trypanosomes and its relation to drug-resistance. *J. Pharmacol. Exp. Ther.* **59**, 123-156

HAWKING, F. (1962) Estimation of the correlation of melarsoprol (Mel B) and Mel W in biological fluids by bioassay with trypanosomes *in vitro. Trans. R. Soc. Trop. Med. Hyg.* **56**, 354-363

HUTCHINSON, M. P. (1971) Human trypanosomiasis in South-West Ethiopia. *Ethiop. Med. J.* **9**, 3-69

JONES, T. & HIRSCH, J. (1972) Interaction of *Toxoplasma gondii* with mammalian cells. II: The absence of lysosomal fusion with phagocytic vacuoles containing living parasites. *J. Exp. Med.* **136**, 1173-1194

MACKANESS, G. B. (1969) The influence of immunologically committed lymphoid cells on macrophage activity *in vivo. J. Exp. Med.* **129**, 973-992

MARTINEZ-SILVA, R., LOPEZ, V. A. & CHIRIBOGA, J. (1970) Effects of Poly I-C on the course of infection with *Trypanosoma cruzi. Proc. Soc. Exp. Biol. Med.* **134**, 885-888

MORTON, T. C. & COOKE, J. N. C. (1948) Splenectomy in kala-azar. *Lancet* **2**, 920

PEÑA-CHAVARRÍA, A., KOTCHER, E. & LIZANO, C. (1965) Preliminary evaluation of cycloguanil (Pamoate) in dermal leishmaniasis. *J. Am. Med. Ass.* **194**, 1142-1144

ROBERTSON, D. H. H. (1962) Chemotherapy of African trypanosomiasis. *Practitioner* **188**, 80-83

SEN, H. G., DUTTA, B. N. & RAY, H. N. (1955) Effect of splenectomy on antrycide therapy of *Trypanosoma evansi* infections in rats. *Nature (Lond.)* **175**, 778-779

VAN HOEVE, K. & GRAINGE, E. B. (1966) Observations on Mel B sensitivity after cyclical transmission. *East Afr. Trypanosomiasis Res. Organ. Rep. 1965*, pp. 63-64

WALKER, P. J. & WATTS, J. M. A. (1970) Drug sensitivity of two strains of *T. brucei* from Gambela, Ethiopia. *East Afr. Trypanosomiasis Res. Organ. Rep. 1970*, p. 58.

General Discussion

Goble: I started looking for drugs for *T. cruzi* about 28 years ago and after 14 years I began working on the possibility of a vaccine. Antigens common to the different strains of *T. cruzi* exist and there is cross-resistance to *in vivo* challenge between strains (Goble 1970). There is no way of predicting the pathogenicity for man of strains which show little virulence in the lower animals. The behaviour of such strains in higher primates is not well enough known to allow any guesses as to the possible danger of attenuated strains for man. At present, therefore, a living vaccine is unthinkable.

Physical methods of preparing killed vaccine have generally resulted in more active preparations than those employing chemical inactivation (Goble *et al.* 1964). Disruption of organisms by freezing-thawing, by ultrasonication and by shaking with ballotini are probably less controllable than disruption by pressure at low temperature under inert atmosphere. Preparations made by the last method, using pressures less than 10 000 p.s.i. (6.9×10^6 N/m^2), have been shown to immunize mice (Yanovsky *et al.* 1969) and to yield sera with more typical complement fixation curves than preparations made with pressures of 20 000 p.s.i. (13.8×10^6 N/m^2) or more (González Cappa & Kagan 1969). The above type of antigen has been tested in man. It produces minor local reactions and antibody production is detectable by complement fixation, indirect immunofluorescence and direct agglutination. The antibody levels were achieved with 0.001 of the dose (mg/kg) used in mouse experiments in which protection was affected (Parodi *et al.* 1971). I have no knowledge of any test of the efficacy of such preparations in the vaccine prophylaxis of Chagas' disease in man. Maybe someone else can add something to this.

Martinez-Silva: We infected a group of mice by the intraperitoneal route with purified ribosomes of *T. cruzi*. Four weeks later we challenged them, together with a control group, but the results did not show a statistically significant difference in protection. We are still working on this aspect in order to find an effective immunogenic agent against *T. cruzi*.

Newton: Why ribosomes?

Martinez-Silva: Ribosomes were shown to be effective against mycobacterial infections by Youmans & Youmans (1969). Ribosomes from *Salmonella, Pseudomonas aeruginosa* and gram-positive cocci have been reported to have protective effects. The mechanism by which ribosomes confer resistance against a challenge of the homologous microorganism is not well known. Dr Pulido's description of the properties of the antigen responsible for complement fixation (pp. 280-283) make me think that a nucleoprotein may be present in the ribosomes or in a subunit of the ribosomes.

Newton: I didn't know of this work, but I find it very surprising.

Bray: It is true of leishmania as well. Ribosomes are said to be highly immunogenic. But their immunogenicity falls off very fast with storage, particularly at low temperature.

Newton: Is there any degree of specificity?

Bray: I don't think this is known; it has only been done with *Leishmania tropica major*.

Bowman: Where the ribosome is the antigen and antibody is produced, how does the antibody then get at hapten groups of the ribosomes in the body of the parasite?

Bray: We are not necessarily talking about antibodies, but about it being immunogenic and productive of cell-mediated immunity.

As well as vaccines, there has also been a search for adjuvants that can be used in man. Obviously polypeptides may be useful, but there is the possibility of a new adjuvant. Lymphocyte activation products are the products after lymphocytes have been activated either with something like phytohaemagglutinin, concanavalin A or pokewood, or by specific antigen if they are from immune animals. When these substances are inoculated into the animals they have a number of effects, one of which seems to be to change the architecture of draining lymph nodes in such a way that they begin to look as if they have already been immunized. It seems just possible that this action might turn out to be an adjuvant action. So lymphocyte activation products may have an adjuvant action and be used for immunization in conjunction with antigen.

Zeledón: We are thinking here about a cell-mediated immunogenic mechanism, as shown in experimental *T. cruzi* infection by Roberson & Hanson (1971) in the United States. If we use parts of the parasite to produce humoral antibodies we might precipitate an immune deviation phenomenon, and this might be the wrong way to approach it.

Bray: There may already be such a mechanism in the infection. The blood-circulating forms may turn the immune system away from the tissue forms; equally the tissue forms might start parasitizing lymph nodes and spleen and start to suppress the humoral response. If a parasite does both these things, obviously the two immune systems can start to interact, perhaps not favourably to the patient.

de Raadt: Protection against African trypanosomiasis depends, of course, on the elucidation of the mechanism of antigenic variation. Even if the basic antigenic type for a certain area is well known, I feel that the trypanosome would be clever enough to overcome the vaccination. But if it could be proved, by means of immunofluorescence of the chancre or post-mortem material, that the common antigens play an important role in the development of immune pathological lesions, then maybe it would be worth vaccinating people not against infection but against the harmful effects of the infection by immunizing them against the common antigen.

Baker: Do you think that the chancre response to *T. rhodesiense* might be a delayed hypersensitivity reaction?

de Raadt: No. It is likely to be due to an Arthus phenomenon rather than cell-mediated immunity, because the secondary phase of the chancre, its characteristic phase, comes at the same time as the first humoral antibodies appear in the circulation. This is when, for the first time, parasites reach detectable levels in the circulation as well. This is mere assumption because histopathologically one cannot easily differentiate cell-mediated immunity from the Arthus phenomenon.

Njogu: I made homogenates from trypanosomes, separated them into soluble and particulate fractions and coupled these chemically to rabbit gammaglobulins to increase their size. I then immunized goats, with or without Freund's complete adjuvant, infected the goats with homologous strains, and tested these in mice for over two months. The only thing I proved was that the soluble fraction was the only one that gave any protection. During the period of testing the mice became positive and then the trypanosomes disappeared but I never managed to get complete disappearance of trypanosomes from the goats.

We did a survey of *T. brucei*, *T. vivax* and *T. congolense* in different geographical areas to find if there were any common antigens so that we could use a cocktail for immunization. Some strains were common to different areas, but most of the strains from different geographical areas were very different antigenically, so the possibility of having a cocktail vaccine has been ruled out.

de Raadt: I think we are talking about two different things. The term 'common antigen' is often confused with 'basic antigen'. Common antigens in the sense of cytoplasmic and nuclear antigens are the antigens which do not elicit protective antibodies. You have been looking for a combination of surface antigens which would overlap the various basic variants present in a certain geographical area.

Njogu: We were cross-reacting strains from different geographical areas to see which ones cross-reacted antigenically with one another. We hoped we would get homology between cross-reacting strains from different areas. If we found that these were common over a wide area then we would have a cocktail for immunizing cattle. In fact, although a few were cross-reacting, most of them were not.

Maekelt: It is of tremendous practical importance to have a drug effective against *T. cruzi in vitro* which can be used in blood banks in concentrations which are not toxic for the recipient. We have had to throw away more than 21 000 blood samples from antibody carriers (donors) in the last 12 years.

Newton: Isn't crystal violet satisfactory?

Maekelt: Venezuelan people don't like blue blood!

Lumsden: Irradiated vaccines seem to hold some possibilities. In African trypanosomiasis sterile immunity doesn't seem to be associated with the common antigens but with the variant antigens. The irradiated organisms still presumably go on producing antigens and shedding antigens when they are used as a vaccine.

Goble: According to Dr Gómez Núñez some work has been done at IVIC, Caracas, on irradiated *T. cruzi*, and Chiari *et al.* (1968) and I have done similar studies. *T. cruzi* can take a terrific amount of radiation and still remain alive. My work was inconclusive. Chiari found that culture organisms were not immunogenic after they were irradiated with 120 000 rads, and blood forms were not immunogenic after 30 000 rads.

Lumsden: Dr E. Sadun (personal communication) irradiated African salivarian organisms with something like 20 000 rads and they appeared to be unable to reproduce, but immunogenic.

Goble: This work is still quite inconclusive. It may be that this is a matter of the dose of irradiation, which at some level selects out an organism that is immunogenic but not invasive.

de Raadt: The main point is whether the irradiated trypanosomes would continue making a range of different variants. That has not been proved yet.

Lumsden: No, but they do have the possibility of continuing to produce some exoantigen.

Martinez-Silva: With *T. cruzi* the D_{37}, i.e. the radiation dose required to reduce the original population to 37%, is about 4000 rads (Martinez-Silva *et al.* 1969). However, parasites must be subjected to high radiation doses before 100% of them are inactivated. Inactivation of growth and infectivity by radiation is accompanied by loss of immunogenicity. For immunity to be induced, at least with the usual numbers, of 1×10^6 to 1×10^7 parasites, the organisms must be able to multiply in the host.

Bray: Has anyone tried to irradiate parasitized tissue cultures and use the tissue cells as a vaccine?

Martinez-Silva: We did and had exactly the same results—that is, no immunity was induced.

Köberle: I have had 20 years' experience of autopsy and experimental work on Chagas' disease. In the acute phase we see a more or less intensive parasitism (sometimes a tremendous one) but in the chronic phase of the disease pseudocysts are extremely rare. Sometimes we see an enormous destruction of ganglion cells soon after infection, during the acute phase or shortly after it, in man and in experimentally infected animals. Therefore we believe that the destiny of the Chagas' patient is determined in the acute phase.

Some years ago everybody in Brazil was speaking about the importance of *endogenous* reinfection during acute outbreaks of chronic Chagas' disease. Nobody had verified the presence or possibility of these acute outbreaks. Another hypothesis was that *exogenous* reinfection occurs when the patients live in highly infected areas. Rodrigues da Silva (1966) showed in Bahia through a meticulous investigation that 'repeated reinfections are not essential for the appearance of morbid manifestations in Chagas' disease'.

We must admit that there is no definite proof of either hypothesis. So we suggest a compromise between the two concepts. That is, that the most important damage occurs in the acute phase, but additional damage may take place in the chronic phase of the disease. Now you can select your attitude! You may leave the patient untreated but protected against a new acute infection, or you may cure the chronic disease and let the patient return to his infected home without any protection. The probability is very high that he will get a new acute phase which is much worse than his old chronic one. It is obvious that in these circumstances treatment is only indicated if the disease can be eradicated in certain areas, thus preventing the acute reinfection of cured patients. This is the main problem. The situation is tragic. Chagas' disease is therefore not simply a matter for curative medicine but a tremendous challenge for preventive medicine.

*   *   *

Newton: After a symposium as broad as this one, the task of making the concluding remarks poses a considerable problem. Clearly, I cannot attempt to sum up all the discussions of the last three days. At the outset, I said that I believed the main aim of the symposium should be to attempt to define the most important lines for future research on trypanosomiasis and leishmaniasis. As a result of our discussions I think most of us have learned a great deal about many aspects of these diseases, but it is perhaps more important that we shall leave the meeting with a much more acute awareness of the main areas of ignorance.

Our discussions have emphasized the need for much more basic information about the different strains and species of parasites, particularly those responsible for cutaneous leishmaniasis and Chagas' disease in different areas of South America. We still know relatively little about the factors affecting infectivity for both insect vectors and mammalian hosts; in leishmaniasis it was pointed out that we don't even know exactly how the parasites are delivered into the skin of the mammalian host. We are still uncertain whether toxins are produced by trypanosomes and leishmania and we can only speculate about the way these protozoa cause damage to host tissues. Antigenic variation in African trypanosomes will, I suspect, provide a problem for immunologists, biochemists and geneticists for many years to come; we don't even know whether such variation occurs in *T. cruzi*. *Leishmania* and *T. cruzi* must enter cells to replicate in the mammalian host; how they get in, how they select particular cells and what stimulates them to leave the bloodstream are all key questions to which we have no answers. We are still unable to grow certain developmental stages of these parasites, we don't know whether they undergo sexual division at some stage in their life cycles, and there are huge gaps in our knowledge of their metabolism. When we turn to chemotherapy, we cannot define precisely the mechanism of action of any trypanocide and we have no clear knowledge of the mechanisms by which parasites become resistant.

All of these deficiencies in our knowledge have, I think, been brought into sharp focus by our discussions and I hope the published proceedings of the symposium will attract more workers from various disciplines to tackle these and the many other problems which remain to be resolved before we gain control of the various forms of trypanosomiasis and leishmaniasis.

References

CHIARI, E., MANSUR NETO, E. & BRENER, Z. (1968) Some effects of gamma-radiation on *Trypanosoma cruzi*, culture and blood forms. *Rev. Inst. Med. Trop. São Paulo* **10** (3), 131-137

GOBLE, F. C. (1970) South American trypanosomes, in *Immunity to Parasitic Animals* (Jackson, G. J., Herman, R. & Singer, I., eds.), vol. 2, 597-689, Appleton-Century-Crofts, New York

GOBLE, F. C., BOYD, J. L., GRIMM-WEHNER, M. & KONRATH, M. (1964) Vaccination against experimental Chagas' disease with homogenates of culture forms of *Trypanosoma cruzi*. *J. Parasitol.* **50** (3), Section 2, p. 19, abstr. 8

GONZÁLEZ CAPPA, S. M. & KAGAN, I. C. (1969) Agar gel and immunoelectrophoretic analysis of several strains of *Trypanosoma cruzi*. *Exp. Parasitol.* **25**, 50-57

MARTINEZ-SILVA, R., LOPEZ, V. A., COLON, J. I. & CHIRIBOGA, J. (1969) *Trypanosoma cruzi:* effects of gamma radiation on growth and infectivity. *Exp. Parasitol.* **25**, 162-170

PARODI, A. S., YANOVSKY, J. F., SZARFMAN, A., SCHMUNIS, G. A. & TRAVERSA, O. C. (1971) Humoral antibodies in human volunteer injected with experimental immunizing antigen against Chagas' disease. *Medicina (B. Aires)* **31**, 369-371

ROBERSON, E. L. & HANSON, W. L. (1971) Effect of antithymocyte serum on the course of trypomastigotes and amastigotes and on mortality of CF₁ mice during acute Chagas' disease. *Am. Soc. Parasitol. (Progr. and Abstrs.) 46th Ann. Meet.* pp. 42-43

RODRIGUES DA SILVA, G. (1966) *Doença de Chagas de Familias de Duas Areas Restritas da Cidade do Salvador, Bahia*, Fund. Gonçalo Moniz, Bahia

YANOVSKY, J. F., TRAVERSA, O. C. & TARATUTO, A. L. (1969) *Trypanosoma cruzi:* Experimental immunization of mice. *Exp. Parasitol.* **26**, 73-85

YOUMANS, A. S. & YOUMANS, G. P. (1969): Factors affecting immunogenic activity of mycobacterial ribosomal and ribonucleic acid preparations. *J. Bact.* **99**, 42-50

Index of contributors

*Entries in **bold** type refer to papers, other entries to contributions to discussions*

Indexes compiled by William Hill

Subject index